AF323150

PROSTATE CANCER
Cell and Molecular Mechanisms in Diagnosis and Treatment

CANCER SURVEYS

Advances and Prospects in Clinical, Epidemiological and Laboratory Oncology

---

SERIES EDITOR: L M Franks, MD

Published for the

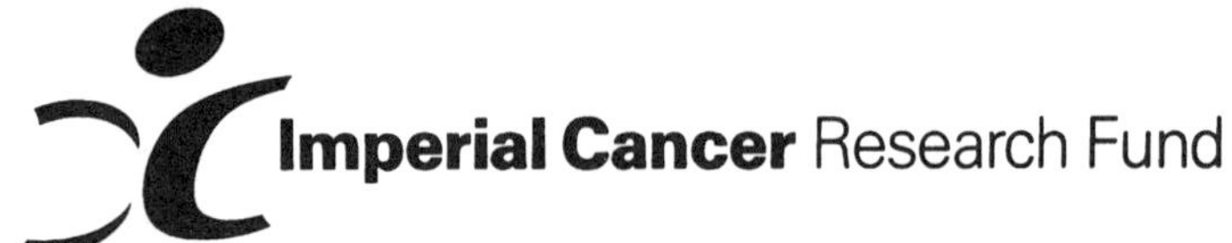

PROSTATE CANCER
Cell and Molecular Mechanisms in Diagnosis and Treatment

Guest Editor
J T Isaacs

COLD SPRING HARBOR LABORATORY PRESS 1991

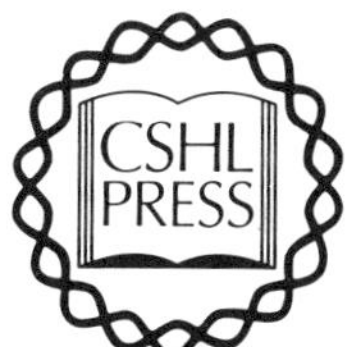

CANCER SURVEYS
*Prostate Cancer: Cell and Molecular Mechanisms
in Diagnosis and Treatment*
Volume 11

Cover and book design by Leon Bolognese & Associates, Inc.

All Cold Spring Harbor Laboratory Press publications may be ordered directly from Cold Spring Harbor
Laboratory Press, 10 Skyline Drive, Plainview, New York 11803-9729. Phone: Continental US & Canada
1–800–843–4388; all other locations (516) 349–1930. FAX: (516) 349–1946.

Contents

PROSTATE CANCER
Cell and Molecular Mechanisms in Diagnosis and Treatment

Introduction: Survey of Outstanding Problems in the Management of Prostatic Cancer

JOHN T ISAACS

Prostatic cancer varies widely in its clinical aggressiveness. In some patients, prostatic cancer metastasizes rapidly, killing the patient within 1 year of initial clinical presentation; other patients may live for many years with localized disease without apparent metastases. If prostatic cancer is truly localized, then radical prostatectomy can be used to cure the patient. Aggressive prostatic screening of men as they age should allow more prostatic cancers to be diagnosed at a curable phase in their natural history. As logical as such an approach is, there are major problems with aggressive screening for prostatic cancer. Necropsy studies indicate that 10% of men 50–60 years old and 50% of those 70–80 years old have histological cancers in their prostates. These histologically localized prostatic cancers are heterogeneous, with only a small subset having undergone all the required malignant changes required to produce a clinically aggressive tumour. The majority of these histologically localized prostate tumours never become fully malignant, despite host longevity. The majority of histologically localized prostatic cancers will remain subclinical and will never require treatment. At present, it is not possible to predict which histologically localized cancers will progress to clinical cancer and which will not. Thus, the ability to predict which tumours will require therapy becomes a critical issue as greater emphasis is placed upon screening for earlier detection of prostatic cancer.

This issue is critical, since if a patient with histologically localized prostatic cancer is left untreated until definitive clinical evidence of metastatic disease outside of the prostate, the opportunity to cure that patient with presently available therapy is lost. However, it is impractical, unwarranted and unnecessary to treat definitively (eg with surgical resection) all men with histologically localized prostatic cancer, since in the majority of these men the disease will never become clinically significant. There is an urgent need for diagnostic methods to identify which histologically localized prostatic cancers have, and which have not, progressed to a stage that will produce clinical disease requiring therapeutic intervention.

To develop such diagnostic methods, the molecular and cellular changes

Cancer Surveys Volume 11: *Prostate Cancer*
© 1991 Imperial Cancer Research Fund. 0-87969-368-1/91. $3.00 + .00

associated with prostatic carcinogenesis and progression to a metastatic state must be resolved. Although the factors involved in prostatic carcinogenesis are not totally known, there is substantial experimental and clinical evidence that the development of a fully malignant cancer cell from a normal cell requires multiple steps. Each event involves genetic alterations in two general classes of cellular genes: tumour suppressor genes and oncogenes. In the first section of this monograph, the current understanding of the role of various genetic changes in prostatic carcinogenesis is summarized by leading experts in the field. These experts not only review what is already known but also describe new experimental approaches seeking to answer more fully many of the unknown fundamentals of prostatic carcinogenesis and progression. In the second section, cellular factors are discussed. These discussions focus on the role of stromal-epithelial cell interactions and the role of various growth factors in prostatic cancer growth and progression. These chapters clarify the present state of knowledge in this rapidly expanding area of the tumour biology of prostatic cancer.

The new approaches described should soon yield diagnostic methods for accurate substaging of histologically localized prostatic cancer into those needing and those not needing therapy. When this happens, aggressive approaches to prostatic cancer screening will be not only logical but practical. Unfortunately, even with such aggressive screening for prostatic cancer, it is likely that substantial numbers of men will be diagnosed at a time when the disease is not confined to the prostate. At present, approximately 60% of new cases of prostatic cancer detected each year are no longer confined to the organ by the time of diagnosis. Thus, at the present time, the majority of prostatic cancer patients are not candidates for curative local surgery. Patients with non-confined disease eventually require systemic androgen ablation therapy. The annual death rate from prostatic cancer has not fallen at all over the 50 years since androgen ablation became standard therapy for metastatic disease. Nearly all men with metastatic prostatic cancer treated with androgen ablation do respond, demonstrating that at least a portion of their cancer cells are androgen responsive. Unfortunately, however, almost all of these patients eventually relapse to a state unresponsive to further anti-androgen therapy. The major reason for the failure of androgen ablation therapy to cure the disease is that the cancer in each patient with metastatic disease is heterogeneously composed of clones of both androgen dependent and independent prostatic cancer cells before therapy is initiated.

To increase the cure rate for metastatic prostatic cancer, a combined approach will be required in which some type of therapy, targeted at the androgen independent cancer cells, is combined with hormonal therapy against androgen dependent cancer cells to combat simultaneously all of the heterogeneous tumour cell populations present within an individual patient. At present, there is no effective therapy for androgen independent prostatic cancer cells. In the final section of this monograph, an overview of the limitations of androgen ablation therapy is presented along with a series of chapters describing new approaches to the therapeutic management of androgen independent prostatic cancer cells. These new approaches offer a real hope for better therapies even for metastatic prostatic cancer.

Familial Risk Factors for Prostate Cancer

B S CARTER[1] • G D STEINBERG[2] • T H BEATY[1] • B CHILDS[3]
P C WALSH[2]

[1]*Department of Epidemiology, Genetic Epidemiology Division, School of Hygiene and Public Health;* [2]*James Buchanan Brady Urological Institute, Johns Hopkins Hospital;* [3]*Department of Pediatrics, Johns Hopkins Hospital, Johns Hopkins Medical Institutions, Baltimore, Maryland 21205*

INTRODUCTION: CANCER GENETICS

Molecular approaches to the understanding of human neoplastic disease have revealed that multiple genetic alterations are an essential component of the tumorigenic process (Weinberg, 1989; Fearon *et al*, 1990). These genetic alterations involve two classes of genes: tumour suppressor genes and oncogenes. Tumour suppressor genes may be considered genes whose products normally regulate growth and differentiation in a negative fashion and thus indirectly suppress neoplastic development. Oncogenes, on the other hand, are genes that, when activated, contribute in a positive manner to transformation to the neoplastic phenotype. The mutational inactivation of tumour suppressor genes coupled with the mutational activation of oncogenes leads to the development of cancer. Furthermore, genetic alterations involved in the transformation of normal cells to the malignant state can both be inherited in the germline and occur somatically in tissue where the cancer arises (Knudson, 1985). Identification of the genetic targets of neoplastic transformation has been approached through the analysis of somatic genetic alterations in the DNA of sporadic tumours, as well as through the genetic study of families with an inherited predisposition for the development of cancer. The interplay between these two approaches has led to the characterization of several gene mutations that are involved in the development of both inherited and sporadic forms of cancer. For example, the *p53* tumour suppressor gene, which has been shown to be somatically mutated in a variety of human tumours (Nigro *et al*, 1989), is also a target of the inherited mutational event causing Li Fraumeni cancer family syndrome (Nelson *et al*, 1990). Also, the retinoblastoma gene *(RB)* is altered in the hereditary and sporadic forms of retinoblastoma and is also a target of somatic alterations in a variety of other human tumour types (Lee *et al*, 1988, 1990), including prostate cancer (Bookstein *et al*, 1990).

Prostate cancer is the most common cancer diagnosed and the second leading cause of cancer mortality in men in the USA (Silverberg and Lubera, 1989). Although prostate cancer is not widely recognized as a familial cancer, there is substantial evidence that it does indeed cluster in families. The fact that a positive family history is a risk factor for prostate cancer suggests that genetic factors may be involved in the development of the disease. The genetic epidemiological approach offers a systematic method for investigating potential genetic factors that may be involved in prostatic carcinogenesis. The identification of genes involved in an inherited form of prostate cancer would be useful for diagnosis and treatment of groups of men at high risk of disease, as well as serving as a model for prostatic carcinogenesis in general.

GENETIC EPIDEMIOLOGICAL INVESTIGATION OF PROSTATE CANCER

The genetic epidemiological method for investigation of the familial aspects of cancer follows a logic that aims to answer the following questions. Is the disease familial? Is familial susceptibility inherited? Are the inherited risk factors genetic? (King, 1982). We and others are pursuing this logic in studying the familial aspects of prostate cancer. Several tools, including the case-control study, complex segregation analysis and genetic linkage analysis, are available to answer these questions. If susceptibility genes for prostate cancer can be identified, a more general understanding of their mode of inheritance, modification by environmental risk factors and total impact on public health can be obtained. As this understanding develops, a group of men who may benefit from early screening and treatment for prostate cancer may be identified.

Is Prostate Cancer Familial?

Several studies have noted the familial aggregation of prostate cancer. Early evidence for this clustering was found by Woolf (1960) in the Utah Mormon population in the USA. He studied the fathers and brothers of 228 cases of prostate cancer and age matched control relatives. Examination of death certificates revealed that 15 of 355 case relatives compared with 5 of 355 control relatives died of prostate cancer, thus demonstrating an approximately threefold increased risk of prostate cancer to the relatives of cases (0.02<p<0.05). In another early study, Morganti *et al* (1956) found 11 cases of prostate cancer among the relatives of 183 prostate cancer cases but only 1 case among control relatives. Meikle *et al* (1985), in a study of 150 cases of early prostate cancer (all cases diagnosed before age 62), found a relative risk of four in the brothers of probands compared with the brothers-in-law of the probands who were selected as the control group. Several other studies with smaller numbers of cases have also noted an increased occurrence of a positive family history of prostate cancer as compared with control groups (Schuman *et al,* 1971; Krain, 1974).

Two large studies are of particular note in answering the question of whether or not prostate cancer clusters in families. Cannon *et al* (1982) published a study on the genetic epidemiology of prostate cancer in the Utah Mormon population. The study made use of the Utah Mormon Genealogical Database (Skolnick *et al,* 1979) in conjunction with the Utah Cancer Registry to study the familial aggregation of 2821 cases of prostate cancer occurring in Utah during the years 1958–1981. The analysis technique employed involved quantifying the degree of relatedness through calculation of the Malecot coefficient of kinship (Malecot, 1948) for each possible pair of cases on the basis of information about common ancestors available through the genealogical database. A summary statistic, the mean coefficient of kinship, was used to describe the degree of familiality of various cancer sites in the population. For each cancer site, mean kinship was compared between the population of affected individuals and suitable age matched controls. Of all the cancer sites studied, prostate cancer had the fourth highest mean kinship after lip, skin melanoma and ovarian cancer. Prostate cancer had a higher familiality than both colon and breast carcinoma—two solid tumours that are well recognized as having a familial component.

A more recent study by our group (Steinberg *et al,* 1990) employed the case control approach to clarify the impact of a positive family history of prostate cancer on a man's risk of this disease. Extensive cancer pedigrees were obtained by telephone interview from 691 men with prostate cancer and 640 spouse controls. Fifteen percent of the cases but only 8% of the controls had a father or brother affected with prostate cancer (p<0.001). As seen in Table 1, men with a first degree relative (father or brother) affected were at twice the risk of developing prostate cancer compared with men with no relatives affected. The risk was attenuated but still significant if a man had only a second degree relative affected (grandfather or uncle). The greatest elevation in risk, however, was seen for those with both a first degree and a second degree relative affected with disease. When considering the relatives of the cases alone in a conditional logistic regression analysis (Table 2), it was noted that there was a trend of increasing risk with increasing number of affected family members such that men with two or three first degree relatives affected had a 5- and 11-fold increased risk for the development of prostate cancer.

Taken together, the aforementioned studies provide strong evidence that prostate cancer does indeed cluster in families. As seen in the Steinberg *et al* (1990) study, the nature of this clustering is such that the closer genetically a man is to an affected relative and the greater number of relatives affected in a man's family, the greater his risk of prostate cancer.

TABLE 1. Standard logistic regression analysis: relative risks of developing prostate cancer for men with affected relatives, adjusted for age of the proband[a]

Affected relatives	Relative risk (95% confidence interval)
First degree	2.0 (1.2–3.3)
Second degree	1.7 (1.0–2.9)
First and second degrees	8.8 (2.8–28.1)

[a]Steinberg *et al*, 1990

Is Familial Clustering of Prostate Cancer Due to Inherited Factors?

The aforementioned studies have provided evidence that prostate cancer aggregates in families. These studies, however, do not allow the aetiological nature of prostate cancer clustering to be determined. For example, such clustering may be due to genetic risk factors for disease or it may be due to common exposure of relatives to environmental carcinogens. There are features of such clustering, however, that may suggest a genetic component. The genetic contribution to disease of complex origin such as cancer is often most salient in the families of cases of early onset (Childs and Scriver, 1986). Therefore, one feature of an inherited form of prostate cancer may be increased clustering of disease in families of cases with early onset. In addition, it is possible to assess whether or not the pattern of inheritance seen in families is consistent with Mendelian inheritance at a single locus by employing complex segregation analysis or pedigree analysis (Elston, 1980).

Some insight into the nature of prostate cancer clustering is provided by the study of Cannon *et al* (1982) described previously. The impact of age on the familiality of disease was characterized by calculating the relative odds for the development of prostate cancer for brothers of men with varying ages at onset of prostate cancer. As seen in Table 3, Cannon *et al* found that the young brothers (<65 years old) of younger cases (<65 years old) were at higher risk of prostate cancer than were the older relatives of older patients.

We have also investigated the effect of age at onset on the familiality of prostate cancer as an extension of our previous study of 691 prostate cancer

---

TABLE 2. Conditional logistic regression analysis: age adjusted relative risk of prostate cancer according to number of first degree relatives affected with disease[a]

Number of first degree affected relatives (besides proband)	Relative risk (95% confidence interval)
One	2.2 (1.4–3.5)
Two	4.9 (2.0–12.3)
Three	10.9 (2.7–43.1)

[a]Steinberg *et al*, 1990

TABLE 3. Relative odds of developing prostate cancer in brothers of prostate cancer cases by age[a]

Age of probands	Age of brothers		
	<65	65–79	80+
<65	5.97[b]	2.77[b]	2.29
65–79	2.77[b]	2.04[a]	2.52[b]
80+	2.29	2.52[a]	1.14

[a]Cannon et al. 1982
[b]p<0.001
[c]p<0.01

families (Carter BS, Beaty TH, Steinberg GS, Childs B and Walsh PC, unpublished). Our aim has been to assess whether or not there is an increased clustering of prostate cancer in families of men with early onset of prostate cancer that may be suggestive of a genetic form of the disease. Accordingly, Cox proportional hazards analysis was performed to assess whether there was increased clustering of prostate cancer in families of cases with early onset. The proportional hazards analysis revealed that two factors, age at onset of disease and whether multiple family members were affected, were the most important determinants of risk of prostate cancer in these families. The combination of effects of early onset in the proband and having multiple relatives affected was such that the brother or father of a proband diagnosed at age 40 with an additional first degree relative affected was at 10–11-fold higher risk of prostate cancer than a brother or father of a proband diagnosed at age 70 with no additional relatives affected.

In addition, a complex segregation analysis of the 691 prostate cancer families was done to test the hypothesis of a Mendelian form of prostate cancer. This analysis revealed that prostate cancer clustering can be explained by Mendelian inheritance of a rare autosomal gene producing prostate cancer at an early age. Other models postulating random environmental transmission of disease were rejected because they fitted the data less well than the Mendelian model. According to the estimates of gene frequency obtained from the segregation analysis, only a relatively small overall percentage (10–12% of prostate cancer occurring by age 85) of prostate cancer was inherited in Mendelian fashion. This percentage is similar to the proportion of breast and colon cancer thought to be inherited in Mendelian fashion (Lynch and Lynch, 1980; Newman *et al*, 1988).

Are the Inherited Risk Factors for Prostate Cancer Genetic?

The aforementioned work which suggests that prostate cancer not only is familial but also has a distinct Mendelian subtype provides a framework for genetic linkage studies to map genes influencing prostate cancer risk. These further studies are required to confirm segregation analyses, which provide evidence for Mendelian inheritance, and to map the genes involved in the inherited predisposition. To date, genetic linkage studies of prostate cancer have not been reported. As an aetiologically heterogeneous disease that occurs late in life, several difficulties for performing genetic linkage studies in prostate cancer families should be considered.

Disease heterogeneity at multiple levels may pose difficulty in mapping susceptibility genes for prostate cancer. As the most common cancer in US men, with the most rapid age related rise in incidence of any solid tumour (Cook *et al*, 1969), multiple cases will occur in some families by chance alone or as a result of exposure to common environmental risk factors. The genetic analyses described in this chapter reveal the family structures and persons most suitable for genetic linkage analyses. Families with multiple affected members and early onset of disease are most likely to have a Mendelian form of prostate cancer suitable for linkage analysis.

Locus heterogeneity may also be important in prostate cancer in that more than one form of inherited prostate cancer may exist. Our previous segregation analysis did not show whether predisposition to prostate cancer was determined by a single susceptibility locus operating in all families or two or more different loci operating in different families. Studies of extended pedigrees with sufficient power to test for linkage heterogeneity will be important to assess heterogeneity at this level.

Studies of genetic alterations in primary human prostate cancers provide clues about candidate genomic regions for linkage analyses. Allelic loss at chromosomes 16q, 10q and 8p is common in prostate tumours (Bergerheim, 1990; Carter *et al*, 1990). Studies of allelic loss in other tumour systems such as colon cancer have revealed associations between the genomic regions identified by somatic loss of heterozygosity in tumour DNA and those identified by linkage analysis as harbouring genes that cause inherited forms of the disease. For example, most sporadic colon cancers exhibit allelic loss at the *DCC* gene locus on chromosome 18q21 (Fearon *et al*, 1990). The hereditary non-polyposis colon cancer syndrome (Lynch type I) also maps to this region, raising the possibility that the same locus is altered in both inherited and sporadic forms of colon cancer (Lynch *et al*, 1985; Geitvik *et al*, 1987). Thus, regions identified by loss of heterozygosity in prostate cancer may serve as useful starting points for mapping the genes involved in Mendelian forms of the disease.

MODEL OF INHERITED PROSTATE CANCER IN THE SETTING OF MULTISTEP CARCINOGENESIS

The genetics of prostate cancer are probably similar to those of colon, breast and other cancers, where a subset of the disease occurs in persons who inherit in the germline one or more of the causal genetic alterations required for neoplastic transformation. In other individuals, sporadic cases of disease may occur as these genes are altered at the tissue level through random or environmentally induced errors in cellular processes. The existence of these subsets of individuals in whom prostate cancer develops is consistent with theories of multistep carcinogenesis.

According to this model, the development of the full neoplastic phenotype in both hereditary and non-hereditary forms of prostate cancer depends on multiple genetic alterations. Current understanding of the molecular events that characterize these genetic alterations suggests that there may be considerable differences in the types of genes affected and the relative impact of various genetic alterations on the development of cancer. Oncogenes and perhaps more frequently tumour suppressor genes are thought to be the two major classes of genes involved in this process. Studies of colorectal cancer have suggested that it is the accumulation rather than the order of genetic changes that is important in the development of cancer (Fearon et al, 1990). In addition, there are probably very few loci that must absolutely be altered to develop a given cancer type. Some genetic alterations may push a cell further towards the development of the neoplastic phenotype or influence the subsequent rate of accumulation of additional genetic alterations differently from others through effects on cell proliferation and growth. In persons with early onset hereditary prostate cancer, presumably one of the key steps necessary for tumour development is inherited such that the majority of people with this inherited defect will accumulate the additional genetic alterations required for the development of prostate cancer. This will be reflected as early onset and high penetrance of disease in these susceptible individuals. In addition, exposure to environmental carcinogens superimposed on a susceptible genotype may also influence the age at onset and penetrance of cancer in susceptible individuals. In the sense that one inherits only an initial step in the development of cancer, Knudson has pointed out that the term "hereditary cancer" may be a misnomer. That which is inherited is actually a susceptibility or predisposition to cancer development (Knudson, 1985).

This model of germline inheritance of prostate cancer has several implications regarding the nature of the specific genetic defect likely to be involved. Because the genetic defect is transmitted in the germline, it must be compatible with development that is sufficiently normal to allow reproduction. To confer specificity to the prostate gland, a gene with tissue specific expression such as occurs with the Wilms' tumour gene, *WT1*, may be involved. Another possibility is analogous to the situation with the *RB* and *p53* genes which, although expressed ubiquitously, give rise only to specific tumour types when inherited as mutant alleles as, for example, in hereditary retinoblastoma or the Li Fraumeni syndrome. Likewise, inherited mutations in other ubiquitously expressed genes may confer a specific prostate cancer susceptibility.

Because of the relationship between inherited and non-inherited forms of cancer, molecular genetic characterization of the subset of prostate cancer inherited in Mendelian fashion should provide significant insights into the genetic mechanisms that occur in prostate tumorigenesis in general.

CLINICAL IMPLICATIONS OF FAMILIAL PROSTATE CANCER

Although the genetic loci involved in inherited prostate cancer have not yet been identified, a considerable amount of information about familial aspects of this disease is already available to the clinician. The data presented regarding the familial aspects of prostate cancer have important clinical implications. Epidemiological studies to date have revealed no other risk factor as consistently and strongly associated with the development of prostate cancer as that of a positive family history of disease. Men with a positive family history of disease constitute an easily identifiable high risk group who could benefit from appropriate screening. We have previously suggested that men with a positive family history of disease after age 40 should undergo yearly digital rectal examination (Steinberg *et al*, 1990). Other emerging techniques such as serial serum prostatic specific antigen determination, transrectal ultrasound or magnetic resonance imaging of the prostate may serve as screening tools for this high risk population.

SUMMARY

This chapter describes the application of the genetic epidemiological approach to the study of human prostate cancer. We review the evidence for the familial clustering of prostate cancer and the Mendelian nature of this aggregation. The nature of this clustering is such that the closer genetically a man is to an affected relative and the greater number of relatives affected in a man's family, the greater his risk of prostate cancer. A complex segregation analysis of the 691 prostate cancer families showed that prostate cancer clustering can be explained by Mendelian inheritance of a rare autosomal gene producing prostate cancer at an early age. A model of inherited prostate cancer in the setting of multistep carcinogenesis is presented. The implications of these data for clinicians who diagnose and treat prostate cancer are also discussed.

References

Bergerheim U (1990) Doctoral dissertation, pp 95–105, Ludwig Institute for Cancer Research, Karolinska Institute, Stockholm, Sweden

Bookstein R, Rio P, Madreperla SA *et al* (1990) Promoter deletion and loss of retinoblastoma gene expression in human prostate carcinoma. *Proceedings of the National Academy of Sciences of the USA* **87** 7762–7766

Cannon L, Bishop DT, Skolnick M, Hunt S, Lyon JL and Smart CR (1982) Genetic epidemiology of prostate cancer in the Utah Mormon genealogy. *Cancer Surveys* **1** 47–69

Carter BS, Ewing CM and Ward WS *et al* (1990) Allelic loss of chromosomes 16q and 10q in human prostate cancer. *Proceedings of the National Academy of Sciences of the USA* **87** 8751–8755

Childs B and Scriver CR (1986) Age at onset and causes of disease. *Perspectives in Biology and Medicine* **29** 437–460

Cook PJ, Doll R and Fellingham SA (1969) A mathematical model for the age distribution of cancer in man. *International Journal of Cancer* **4** 93–112

Elston RC (1980) Segregation analysis, In: Harris H and Hirschhorn K (eds). *Advances in Human Genetics,* vol 11, pp 63–120, Plenum Press, New York

Fearon ER and Vogelstein B (1990) A genetic model for colorectal tumorigenesis. *Cell* **61** 759–767

Fearon ER, Cho KR and Nigro JM *et al* (1990) Identification of a chromosome 18q gene that is altered in colorectal cancers. *Science* **247** 49–56

Geitvik GA, Hoyheim B, Gedde-Dahl T *et al* (1987) The Kidd (JK) blood group locus assigned to chromosome 18 by close linkage to a DNA-RFLP. *Human Genetics* **77** 205–209

King MC (1982) Genetic and epidemiological analysis of cancer in families: breast cancer as an example. *Cancer Surveys* **1** 33–46

Knudson AG (1985) Hereditary cancer, oncogenes and anti-oncogenes. *Cancer Research* **45** 1437–1443

Krain LS (1974) Some epidemiologic variables in prostatic carcinoma in California. *Preventive Medicine* **3** 154–159

Lee WH, Bookstein R and Lee EY-HP (1988) Studies on the human retinoblastoma susceptibility gene. *Journal of Cellular Biochemistry* **38** 213–227

Lee WH, Bookstein R and Lee EY-HP (1990) Molecular biology of the human retinoblastoma gene, In: Klein G (ed). *Tumor Suppressor Genes,* pp 169–200, Dekker, New York

Lynch PM and Lynch HT (1980) Preface, In: Lynch PM, Lynch HT (eds). *Colon Cancer Genetics,* pp IX–XI, Van Nostrand Reinhold, New York

Lynch HT, Schuelke GS, Kimberling WJ *et al* (1985). *Cancer* **56** 939–951

Malecot G (1948) *Les mathematiques de l'heridite,* Masson et Cie, Paris

Meikle AW, Smith JA and West DW (1985) Familial factors affecting prostatic cancer risk and plasma sex steroid levels. *Prostate* **6** 121–128

Morganti G, Gianferrari L, Cresseri A, Arrigoni G and Lovati G (1956) Recherches clinico-statistiques et genetiques sur les neoplasies de la prostate. *Acta Gènètica Statistica* **6** 304–305

Nelson CG, Kim DH, Kassel J *et al* (1990) Germline p53 mutations in a familial syndrome of breast cancer, sarcomas, and other neoplasms. *Science* **250** 1233–1248

Newman B, Austin MA, Lee M and King MC (1988) Inheritance of human breast cancer: evidence for autosomal dominant transmission in high risk families. *Proceedings of the National Academy of Sciences of the USA* **85** 3044–3048

Nigro JM, Baker SJ, Preisinger AC *et al* (1989) Mutations in the p53 gene occur in diverse human tumor types. *Nature* **342** 705–708

Schuman LM, Mandel J, Blackard C, Bauer H, Scarlett J and McHugh R (1971) Epidemiologic study of prostate cancer: preliminary report. *Cancer Treatment Reports* **61** 181–186

Silverberg E and Lubera JA (1989) Cancer statistics. *CA-A Cancer Journal for Clinicians* **38** 14–15

Skolnick M, Bean LL, Dintelman SM and Mineau G (1979) A computerized family history data base system. *Sociology and Social Research* **63** 506–523

Steinberg GS, Carter BS, Beaty TH, Childs B and Walsh PC (1990) Family history and the risk of prostate cancer. *Prostate* **17** 337–347

Weinberg RA (1989) Oncogenes, anti-oncogenes, and the molecular basis of multistep carcinogenesis. *Cancer Research* **45** 1437–1443

Woolf CM (1960) An investigation of the familial aspects of carcinoma of the prostate. *Cancer* **13** 739–744

The authors are responsible for the accuracy of the references.

Genetic Changes Associated with Prostate Cancer in Humans

W B ISAACS • B S CARTER

Department of Urology, Johns Hopkins University School of Medicine, Baltimore, Maryland 21205

INTRODUCTION: GENETIC CHANGES IN COMMON SOLID TUMOURS

The past several years have seen a dramatic increase in our knowledge of the genetic changes occurring in human cancer cells. This progress is largely due to the development of molecular techniques, such as the polymerase chain reaction, and the availability of localized, polymorphic DNA probes, which have revolutionized the basic approaches to identifying and understanding genetic changes that occur in cancer. Extensive investigations of common human tumours (eg breast, colorectal, lung and bladder) using such techniques have led to the realization that genetic alterations, including point mutations, deletions, translocations and amplifications, are a common feature of primary human cancers (Hansen and Cavenee, 1987; Cavenee *et al*, 1990; Peehl, this issue).

Oncogenes and Tumour Suppressor Genes

The emerging picture of carcinogenesis is one in which a collaboration exists between oncogene activation and anti-oncogene (tumor suppressor gene) inactivation, resulting in the expression of the malignant phenotype. The *ras*, *myc* and *erb*B-2 genes are oncogenes, activated through genetic alteration in a variety of human tumours. Although significant progress has been made in understanding the role of these and other oncogenes in human cancers (reviewed in Cooper, 1990), the advances made in the area of tumour suppressor genes have been particularly striking. Indeed, it is now apparent that loss of gene activity is just as important in the tumorigenic process as is gene activation. The

Cancer Surveys Volume 11: *Prostate Cancer*
© 1991 Imperial Cancer Research Fund. 0-87969-368-1/91. $3.00 + .00

first tumour type in which inactivation of a tumour suppressor gene was demonstrated is retinoblastoma. From studies from a number of laboratories, it has become evident that Knudson's "two-hit" hypothesis is correct, in that the two different alleles of the retinoblastoma (*RB*) gene must be inactivated before tumour development (Godbout *et al*, 1983; Knudson, 1985). Frequently, one allele is inactivated by deletion and the other by mutation. Introduction of a cloned intact copy of the *RB* gene into retinoblastoma cells with concomitant restitution of normal growth control has been reported, demonstrating the capacity of this gene to suppress the tumorigenic phenotype (Huang *et al*, 1988).

The most commonly used technique to search for tumour suppressor genes has been determination of the frequency of allelic loss at various chromosomal loci. "Allelotyping" is the term coined by Vogelstein and coworkers to describe the process whereby each chromosomal arm is analysed with polymorphic DNA probes to determine whether loss of alleles has occurred in the affected cells (Vogelstein *et al*, 1989). This process possesses a number of advantages over conventional karyotype analysis in that metaphase chromosomes are not required, and losses of much smaller chromosome regions are discernible. Allelic deletions leading to reductions to homozygosity at specific loci have been detected in a wide variety of human tumours, including Wilms' tumour, osteosarcoma, bladder cancer, renal cell carcinoma, breast cancer, small cell lung cancer, cervical cancer and colorectal cancer (Koufos *et al*, 1984; Hansen *et al*, 1985; Yokota *et al*, 1987, 1989; Zbar *et al*, 1987; Callahan and Cambell, 1989; Vogelstein *et al*, 1989; Tsai *et al*, 1990). A number of these cancer types are associated with allelic loss at multiple sites. In colorectal cancers, deletions at both 17p and 18q are observed in over 70% of tumours analysed. Mapping of the deletions on 17p to the region between 17p13.3 and 17p12 has led to the identification of the *p53* gene as a tumour suppressor gene, which is inactivated in colorectal cancer (Baker *et al*, 1989). Baker *et al* (1990a) have recently demonstrated the ability of wild type *p53* to suppress the growth of colorectal carcinoma cells containing only mutant forms of this protein. Thus, the paradigm established by the study of retinoblastoma may hold for a wide variety of human cancers, with the number of tumour suppressor genes quite possibly being rather large—some being tumour specific and others being inactivated in a number of different tumour types.

To date, at least five candidate tumour suppressor genes have been cloned. These include the Wilms' tumour gene (*WT1*) on chromosome 11p (coding for a zinc finger protein) (Call *et al*, 1990), the neurofibromatosis gene (*NF1*) on chromosome 17q (Cawthon *et al*, 1990), the *DCC* gene on chromosome 18q (a putative cell adhesion molecule) (Fearon *et al*, 1990), the *p53* gene on chromosome 17p (Baker *et al*, 1989) and the *RB* gene on chromosome 13q (Friend *et al*, 1986). Clues that led to the identification of these genes included consistent cytogenetic abnormalities, cell-cell and monochromosome-cell hybrids, homozygous deletions and deletion mapping employing loss of heterozygosity. In addition, multiple studies have suggested the locations of putative suppressor genes on chromosomes 3p and 9q involved in renal, cervical and lung cancers (3p) and bladder cancer (9q) (Yokota *et al*, 1987, 1989; Zbar *et al*, 1987; Tsai *et al*, 1990). As mentioned above, two of these genes (*RB* and *p53*) have been shown to be capable of suppressing the tumorigenic phenotype when reintroduced into tumour cells. A recent study by Bookstein *et al* (1990a) has shown that the *RB* gene product is altered in the prostate cancer cell line DU-145 and that suppression of tumorigenicity is observed upon introduction of the cloned intact *RB* gene into these cells. Two other prostate cancer cell lines examined in the same study had apparently normal *RB* gene products. A subsequent study by this group documented a deletion in the promoter of the *RB* gene, leading to the lack of expression of this gene in a metastatic prostatic cancer specimen (Bookstein *et al*, 1990b).

The critical role of alterations in the *p53* gene in the pathogenesis of a wide variety of human neoplasms is becoming increasingly more apparent. Previously thought to be an oncogene, it has only been within the past year that the "dominant negative" nature of *p53* has been explained. When mutated in critical regions, the p53 protein can act as an oncogene, cooperating with *ras* to transform primary rodent fibroblasts (Parada *et al*, 1984; Hinds *et al*, 1989). Presumably, this phenomenon is caused by the dimerization of mutant and wild type p53 proteins, which inactivates the latter (Gannon *et al*, 1990). In wild type form, the p53 protein is a key cell cycle regulatory factor, acting as a brake of uncontrolled proliferation in a way not yet clearly defined. What has become abundantly clear, however, is that the *p53* gene is either deleted or mutated or both (one copy mutated, one copy deleted) in most common human tumours. Reports describing allelic loss of chromosome 17p in the majority of human colon, breast, small cell lung and bladder cancers have appeared within the past several years (Yokota *et al*, 1887; Callahan and Campbell, 1989; Vogelstein *et al*, 1989; Tsai *et al*, 1990). In each of these tumour types, mutations in the remaining *p53* allele have been detected. Additionally, some tumours have been analysed that retain two *p53* alleles, with either one or both demonstrating mutations (Nigro *et al*, 1990). This latter finding raises the interesting possibility that an intermediate step in transformation may exist consisting of heterozygosity of *p53* alleles, one mutated and the other wild type. The frequency of such a condition in colorectal tumours has recently been demonstrated by Baker *et al* (1990b) to be 17%, leading the authors to suggest that point mutations are the rate limiting step in *p53* gene inactivation, rapidly followed by allelic loss. No studies of the status of the *p53* gene in human prostate cancer have been reported.

What is the significance of chromosomal deletions in general and, specifically, of the identification of tumour suppressor genes? At present, the mechanisms by which such deletions occur are not clear. Presumably, a deletion leading to the inactivation of growth control genes results in a positive selection and clonal expansion of the affected cell. That frequent chromosomal deletions are a hallmark of primary human cancers is indicative, at the very least, of the development of substantial genetic instability in cancer cells, resulting in rather massive alterations in the genome, as well as the frequent point mutations that have been observed in certain oncogenes (eg *ras*). The ability of such deletions to unmask inactivated tumour suppressor genes has opened new avenues to identify and elucidate the pathways that normally regulate cellular proliferation and differentiation.

Genetic Markers of Tumour Progression

Perhaps the most exciting aspect of the demonstration of specific allelic loss in human cancers, at least from a clinical point of view, is the ability of various aspects of these deletions to be both correlative with and predictive of tumour progression. Vogelstein *et al* (1989), using markers for every non-acrocentric autosomal arm to probe a large number of colorectal tumours, found that patients with more than the median number of allelic deletions had a worse prognosis than other patients, demonstrating that frequency of allelic loss in a given tumour was a better predictor of disease progression than pathological grade. James *et al* (1988), studying a number of loci in glial tumours, found loss of chromosome 10 sequences only in the most malignant histological stage of glioma, demonstrating that malignancy stage specific somatic losses of heterozygosity can provide a genotypic, rather than phenotypic, analysis of tumour progression.

The ability to assess tumour aggressiveness on the basis of molecular markers has particular relevance to prostate cancer. It has been estimated on the basis of necropsy studies that nearly one-third of men over the age of 50 (some 11 million US men) have lesions within the prostate that are histologically identifiable as prostate cancer (Carter and Coffey, 1989). The vast majority of these lesions never give rise to symptoms, presumably because the molecular events necessary for tumour progression have not occurred. The presence of these lesions of unknown malignant potential presents the urologist with a dilemma, since there is no reliable way to predict which lesions will remain latent and which will progress. Obviously, the development of molecular markers that could predict tumour aggressiveness would be helpful in determining the appropriate therapeutic regimen for men diagnosed with this disease. Indeed, the number of men in this situation could dramatically increase in the near future as proposed, intensive screening programmes aimed at early detection of prostate cancer are initiated.

GENETIC CHANGES IN PROSTATE CANCER

In contrast to the situation in other common solid tumours, there have been few reports of genetic alterations in human prostate cancer. At present, little is known regarding either the activation of oncogenes or the inactivation of tumour suppressor genes in this disease. Certainly, this will rapidly change.

ras Gene Mutations in Prostate Cancer

The possible role of mutated *ras* genes in prostate cancer has been suggested by a number a previous studies. Thompson *et al* (1989) demonstrated that *ras* and *myc* oncogenes can cooperate to transform the cells of reconstituted mouse prostate gland. Treiger and Isaacs (1988) showed that transfection of the v-Ha-*ras* gene into Dunning rat prostatic cancer cells resulted in their conversion from a low to a high metastatic phenotype. In an analysis of DNA from human prostate cancer tissue, Peehl *et al* (1987) showed that one of eight cancer specimens contained an activated Ki-*ras* gene as detected by a 3T3 transfection assay.

To address further the question of the role of *ras* gene involvement in either the initiation or progression of human prostatic cancer, we have examined prostatic cancer cell DNA for the presence of *ras* gene mutations using differential oligodeoxynucleotide hybridization of DNA amplified using the polymerase chain reaction (PCR) (Carter *et al*, 1990a). Included in this study were 24 primary prostate tumours (23 acinar tumours and 1 ductal tumour) and 5 prostate cell lines, examined at codons 12, 13 and 61 of the Ki-*ras*, Ha-*ras*, and N-*ras* genes. Only two mutations were detected: an A to G transition causing a glutamate to arginine substitution at codon 61 of the Ha-*ras* gene in a primary prostatic duct adenocarcinoma and a G to T transversion causing a glycine to valine substitution at codon 12 of the Ha-*ras* gene in a prostate cell line (TSU-Pr1) derived from a lymph node metastasis. The presence of these mutations has been confirmed by direct sequencing of the PCR amplified products. We have recently extended this study to include analysis of paraffin embedded samples, including 12 metastatic prostate cancer lesions, 10 primary ductal adenocarcinomas and 16 samples of benign prostatic hyperplasia (BPH). Of these samples, only one, a metastatic deposit, had a *ras* gene mutation. These results demonstrate that activation of *ras* oncogenes is not a common event in either the initiation or progression of prostatic neoplasia.

Loss of Heterozygosity in Prostate Cancer

We have turned our attention to the role of tumour suppressor gene inactivation in prostate cancer. Cytogenetic analyses of prostate cancer have not revealed consistent chromosomal deletions (recently reviewed in Brothman *et al*, 1990). One study by Atkin and Baker (1985), however, showed that four of four patients with late stage prostate carcinomas exhibited chromosome 10q deletions and three of four exhibited chromosome 7q deletions. In addition, deletions of 10q have been observed in several prostate cancer cell lines (Konig *et al*, 1988; Brothman *et al*, 1990).

To pursue these observations at a molecular level, we studied allelic loss in prostate cancer using polymorphic DNA probes (listed in Table 1) for chromosomes 10q and 7q as well as probes for chromosomes containing docu-

TABLE 1. Chromosomal locations of polymorphic DNA probes employed to study loss of heterozygosity and restriction endonucleases revealing polymorphism[a]

Chromosomes	Probe name	Restriction endonuclease
3p	EFD 145.1	*Taq*
7q	G3	*Taq*
9q34	EFD 126.3	*Taq*
10p13-pter	MHZ15	*Taq*
10p13-pter	TBQ7	*Taq*
10q22-q23	1-101	*Taq*
10q22-qter	EFD75	*Taq*
10p24-qter	HUK-8	*Bam*HI
10q26	HOAT1	*Msp*
11p15	EJ988	*Taq*
13q	MHZ47	*Taq*
13q14	68RS20	*Rsa*I
16p12-p13.3	16/32	*Taq*
16q22-q24	79-2-23	*Taq*
16q22	HP2α	*Bam*HI
17p13	144D6	*Msp*
18q21	15-65	*Msp*

[a]From Carter *et al*, 1990b

mented and putative tumour suppressor genes (3p, 9q, 11p, 13q, 17p, 18q), as mentioned above. We examined 28 primary prostate cancer specimens, most of which were localized, stage B lesions, measuring <2 cm in diameter. The results of these analyses are summarized in Tables 2 and 3 (Carter *et al*, 1990b). We found that the majority (61%) of the tumours in the study exhibited allelic loss on at least one of the chromosomes examined. The regions most frequently deleted are found on the long arms of chromosomes 10 and 16. Analysis of the latter was originally included in the study as a control chromosome, not known to harbour any tumour suppressor genes or to exhibit frequent allelic deletions in human tumours (see below). Thus, whereas allelic loss on chromosome 10q was predicted from previous karyotype analyses, allelic loss on chromosome 16q is a novel finding. For neither 10q nor 16q, however, have any candidate tumour suppressor genes been identified (see below).

Preliminary deletion mapping of three prostatic tumours deleted on 10q that were informative for multiple markers on this arm suggests that the gene of interest lies in the region 10q24-qter (Carter *et al*, 1990b). Other than restriction to the long arm, no subchromosomal localization could be assigned for the deletions on chromosome 16.

In addition to our study, Bergerheim *et al* (in press) have examined ten primary tumour specimens, as well as eight metastatic lesions, for allelic loss on every non-acrocentric autosomal chromosomal arm. Chromosomes 10 and 16, along with chromosome 8, most frequently exhibited allelic loss in this

TABLE 2. Allelic loss in 28 human prostate tumours[a]

Tumour	Chromosomes arms on which allelic markers were lost	Chromosome arms on which allelic markers were retained
4		3p,9q,10p,13q,16p,16q,17p
5	13q	3p,10p,10q,11p,16p,16q,17p,18q
10	10q,16q	9q,10p,11p,13q,16p
11		3p,7q,10p,10q,13q,16p,16q,18q
13	16q,18q	3p,10q,13q,16p,17p
14	10q	13q,17p
18		3p,7q,9q,10p,10q,11p,13q,16p,17p
20	10q	7q,11p
23	17p	7q,9q,10p,10q,11p,16q,18q
24	3p	10p,17p,16q,18q
25	18q	7q,10p,10q,17p
26		3p,7q,10p,11p,17p,18q
29[b]		7q,10q,13q,16q,17p 10p,16p
30		3p,7q,9q,10p,10q,11p,18q
35	10q	7q,9q,10p,11p,13q,16p,16q,17p,18q
38		7q,10p,10q,16q,17p,18q
42	16q	3p,7q,10p,10q,11p,18q
46		3p,7q,9q,10p,10q,11p,16q,18q
71	10q	7q,17p
73	7q	10q,17p
78		9q,10p,10q,13q,16q,17p
79		9q,10p,10q,17p
80		9q,10q,13q,16q
81		7q,9q,10p,10q,16q,17p
74[c]	10q	7q
75[c]	17p	7q
76[c]	9q,16q	7q,10q,13q
77[c]	9q,13q	10q

[a]From Carter *et al*, 1990b
[b]Prostatic ductal carcinoma
[c]Patients failing androgen ablation therapy

study. Taken together, these results provide evidence for the specificity of allelic loss on chromosomes 10 and 16 in prostate cancer.

Two additional tumour types, breast and hepatocellular carcinoma, have recently been identified in which allelic loss on chromosome 16q is a frequent event (Sato *et al*, 1990; Tsuda *et al*, 1990). It is not clear at the present time whether the affected gene on chromosome 16q is the same in each of these tumour types. The gene for the epithelial cell adhesion molecule, E-cadherin, located on chromosome 16q22.1 (Natt *et al*, 1989), has been proposed as an important modulator of the invasive potential of a variety of cultured human carcinoma cells (Frixen *et al*, in press). The status of this interesting candidate "invasion suppressor" gene in prostate cancer is an area of current investigation (Bussemakers *et al*, 1991).

In addition to detection of allelic loss on chromosomes 10q and 16q, approximately one-fifth of the prostatic tumours analysed in our study were

TABLE 3. Summary of allelic loss by chromosomes[a]

	Chromosome										
	3p	**7q**	**9q**	**10p**	**10q**	**11p**	**13q**	**16p**	**16q**	**17p**	**18q**
Deleted	1	2	2	0	7	0	3	0	5	3	2
Informative	10	19	13	18	24	11	13	8	16	18	12
Percent	10	10	15	0	29	0	23	0	31	17	17

[a]From Carter *et al*, 1990b

deleted at chromosomes 17p, 18q and 13q. These regions harbour the tumour suppressor genes *p53*, *DCC* and *RB*, respectively. Thus, the possibility exists that inactivation of these genes plays a part in at least a subset of prostatic neoplasms. The importance of *RB* gene inactivation in prostate cancer has been suggested by the studies of Bookstein *et al* (1990a,b). With regard to the *p53* gene, preliminary experiments performed in this laboratory suggest that at least two prostate cancer cell lines (TSU and PC-3) contain mutations in the coding sequence of the *p53* gene and that the growth of these lines can be suppressed by the introduction of a wild type copy of this gene. Obviously, a closer examination of the roles of these genes in prostatic cancer is warranted, particularly with respect to progression of this disease.

In relation to tumour progression, we observed that whereas just over half of the clinically localized tumours demonstrated allelic loss, four of four metastatic tumours, even when analysed at a limited number of chromosomal loci, showed allelic loss. Although the number of metastatic tumours analysed is too low to be conclusive, these results suggest that increased frequency of allelic loss may be correlated with tumour aggressiveness. In the case of colon cancer, a strong correlation between allelic loss and tumour progression has been demonstrated (Kern *et al*, 1989; Vogelstein *et al*, 1989). Obviously, analysis of greater numbers of prostatic tumours is required to clarify this question in this tumour type.

SUMMARY

We have detected allelic loss in a majority of prostate cancers analysed. These losses have been detected on several chromosomes known to harbour tumour suppressor genes important in the development of other tumour types. Elevated rates of loss of heterozygosity on chromosome 16q and 10q suggest that tumour suppressor genes important in the pathogenesis of prostate cancer may be present on these chromosomes. Conversely, determination of the frequency of *ras* gene mutations in prostate cancer tissue suggests that these genetic alterations play a minor part in both the initiation and progression of this disease in humans.

Acknowledgements

This work was supported by the Edwin Beer Program of the New York Academy of Medicine and National Institutes of Health grants CA-09314 and DK-19300.

References

Atkin NB and Baker MC (1985) Chromosome study of five cancers of the prostate. *Human Genetics* **70** 359–364

Baker SJ, Fearon ER, Nigro JM *et al* (1989) Chromosome 17 deletions and p53 gene mutations in colorectal carcinomas. *Science* **244** 217–221

Baker SJ, Markowitz S, Fearon ER, Willson JKV and Vogelstein B (1990a) Suppression of human colorectal carcinoma cell growth by wild-type p53. *Science* **249** 912–915

Baker SJ, Preisinger A, Jessup JM *et al* (1990b) p53 gene mutations occur in combination with 17p allelic deletions as late events in colorectal tumorigenesis. *Cancer Research* **50** 7717–7722

Bergerheim USR, Kunimi K, Collins VP and Ekman P Deletion mapping of chromosomes 8 10 and 16 in human prostatic carcinoma. *Genes, Chromosomes and Cancer* (in press)

Bookstein R, Shew J, Chen P, Scully P and Lee W-H (1990a) Suppression of tumorigenicity of human prostate carcinoma cells by replacing a mutated Rb gene. *Science* **247** 712–715

Bookstein R, Rio P, Madreperla S *et al* (1990b) Promoter deletion and loss of retinoblastoma gene expression in human prostate carcinoma. *Proceedings of the National Academy of Sciences of the USA* **87** 7762–7766

Brothman A, Peehl D, Patel A and McNeal J (1990) Frequency and pattern of karyotypic abnormalities in human prostate cancer. *Cancer Research* **50** 3795–3803

Bussemakers MJG, Isaacs WB, Carter BS, van de Ven WJM, DeBruyne FMJ and Schalken JA (1991) E-cadherin is a candidate tumor suppressor gene implicated in prostate cancer. *Journal of Urology* **145** 294A

Call KM, Glaser T, Ito CY *et al* (1990) Isolation and characterization of a zinc finger polypeptide gene at the human chromosome 11 Wilms' locus. *Cell* **60** 509–520

Callahan R and Campbell G (1989) Mutations in human breast cancer: an overview. *Journal of the National Cancer Institute* **81** 1780–1786

Carter HB and Coffey DS (1990) The prostate: an increasing medical problem. *The Prostate* **16** 39–48

Carter BS, Epstein JI and Isaacs WB (1990a) Ras gene mutations in human prostate cancer. *Cancer Research* **50** 6830–6832

Carter BS, Ewing CM, Ward SW *et al* (1990b) Allelic loss of chromosomes 16q and 10q in human prostate cancer. *Proceedings of the National Academy of Sciences of the USA* **87** 8751–8755

Cavenee WK, Ponder B and Solomon E (eds) (1990) Genetics and cancer. *Cancer Surveys* **9**, 3 and 4, Oxford University Press, Oxford

Cawthon RM, Weiss R, Xu G *et al* (1990) A major segment of the neurofibromatosis type 1 gene: cDNA sequence, genomic structure and point mutations. *Cell* **62** 193–201

Cooper GM (1990) *Oncogenes*, pp 141–159, Jones and Bartlett, Boston

Fearon ER, Cho KR, Nigro JM *et al* (1990) Identification of a chromosome 18q gene that is altered in colorectal cancers. *Science* **247** 49–56

Friend SH, Bernards R, Rogelj S *et al* (1986) A human DNA segment with properties of the gene that predisposes to retinoblastoma and osteosarcoma. *Nature* **323** 643–646

Frixen UH, Behrens J, Sachs M *et al* E-cadherin-mediated cell-cell adhesion prevents invasiveness of human carcinoma cells. *Journal of Cell Biology* (in press)

Gannon JV, Greaves R, Iggo R and Lane DP (1990) Activating mutations in p53 produce a common conformational effect. *EMBO Journal* **9** 1595–1602

Godbout R, Dryja TP, Squire J, Gallie BL and Phillips RA (1983) Somatic inactivation of genes on chromosome 13 is a common event in retinoblastoma. *Nature* **304** 451–453

Hansen MF and Cavenee WK (1987) Genetics of cancer predisposition. *Cancer Research* **47** 5518–5527

Hansen MF, Koufos A, Gallie BL *et al* (1985) Osteosarcoma amd retinoblastoma: a shared chromosoal mechanism revealing recessive prediposition. *Proceedings of the National Academy of Science USA* **82** 6216–6220

Hinds P, Finlay CA and Levine AJ (1989) Mutation is required to activate the p53 gene for cooperation with the ras oncogene and transformation. *Journal of Virology* **63** 739–746

Huang HJ, Yee J-K, Shew J-Y *et al* (1988) Suppression of the neoplastic phenotype by replacement of the Rb gene in human cancer cells. *Science* **242** 1563–1566

James DJ, Carlbom E, Dumanski JP *et al* (1988) Clonal genomic alterations in glioma malignancy stages. *Cancer Research* **48** 5546–5551

Kern SE, Fearon ER, Tersmette KWF *et al* (1989) Allelic loss in colorectal carcinoma. *Journal of the American Medical Association* **261** 3099–3103

Knudson AG (1985) Heritary cancer, oncogenes and antioncogenes. *Cancer Research* **45** 1437–1143

Konig JJ, Hagemeijer A, Smit B, Kamst E, Romijn J and Schroder FH (1988) Cytogenetic characterization of an established xenografted prostatic prostatic carcinoma cell line (PC-82). *Cancer Genetics and Cytogenetics* **34** 91–99

Koufos A, Hansen MF, Lampkin BC *et al* (1984) Loss of alleles at loci on chromosome 11 during genesis of Wilms' tumor. *Nature* **309** 170–172

Natt E, Magenis RE, Zimmer J, Mansouri A and Scherer G (1989) Regional assignment of the human loci for uvomorulin and chymotrypsinogen B with the help of two overlapping deletions on the long arm of chromosome 16. *Cytogenetics and Cell Genetics* **50** 145–148

Nigro JM, Baker SJ, Preisinger AC *et al* (1990) Mutations of the p53 gene occur in diverse human tumour types. *Nature* **342** 705–708

Parada LF, Land H, Weinberg RA, Wolf D and Rotter W (1984) Cooperation between gene encoding p53 tumour antigen and ras in cellular transformation. *Nature* **312** 649–651

Peehl DM, Wehner N and Stamey TA (1987) Activated Ki-ras oncogene in human prostatic adenocarcinoma. *The Prostate* **10** 281–289

Sato T, Tanigami A, Yamakawa K *et al* (1990) Allelotype of breast cancer: cumulative allele losses promote tumor progression in primary breast cancer. *Cancer Research* **50** 7184–7189

Thompson TC, Southgate J, Kitchener G and Land H (1989) Multistage carcinogenesis induced by ras and myc oncogenes in a reconstituted organ. *Cell* **56** 917–930

Treiger BF and Isaacs JT (1988) Expression of a transfected v-Ha-ras oncogene in a Dunning rat prostate adenocarcinoma and the development of high metastatic ability. *Journal of Urology* **140** 1580–1586

Tsai Y, Nichols P, Hiti A, Williams Z, Skinner D and Jones P (1990) Allelic losses of chromosomes 9 11 and 17 in human bladder cancer. *Cancer Research* **50** 44–47

Tsuda H, Zhang W, Shimasato Y *et al* (1990) Allele loss on chromosome 16q associated with progression of human hepatocellular carcinoma. *Proceedings of the National Academy of Sciences of the USA* **87** 6791–6794

Vogelstein B, Fearon ER, Kern SE *et al* (1989) Allelotype of colorectal carcinomas. *Science* **244** 207–211

Yokota J, Wada M, Shimosato Y, Terada M and Sugimura T (1987) Loss of heterozygosity on chromosome 3 13 and 17 in small-cell carcinoma and on chromosome 3 in adenocarcinoma of the lung. *Proceedings of the National Academy of Sciences of the USA* **84** 9252–9256

Yokota J, Tsukada Y, Nakajima T *et al* (1989) Loss of heterozygosity on the short arm of chromosome 3 in carcinoma of the uterine cervix. *Cancer Research* **49** 3598–3601

Zbar B, Braugh H, Talmudge C and Linehan M (1987) Loss of alleles of loci on the short arm of chromosome 3 in renal cell carcinoma. *Nature* **327** 721–724

The authors are responsible for the accuracy of the references.

Searching for Suppressor Genes in Prostate Cancer

DONNA M PEEHL

*Department of Urology, Stanford University School of Medicine,
Stanford, California 94305*

Introduction
Somatic cell hybrids
Novel suppressor genes
Chromosomal aberrations
In vitro transformation
Summary

INTRODUCTION

It is generally accepted that the development of invasive, metastatic cancer is a multistep process, beginning with an initiation event and followed by numerous stages of progression. The molecular mechanisms underlying neoplastic evolution are believed to be primarily of two types: activation of dominant oncogenes by mutation or amplification or rearrangement, and loss of suppressor gene activity by mutation or deletion (Weinberg, 1989; Stanbridge and Nowell, 1990).

Colorectal cancer provides one of the most well characterized examples of how different molecular events, including oncogene activation and suppressor gene loss, are involved in the development of neoplasia (Fearon *et al*, 1990). Comparatively little is known about the molecular changes occurring at the onset and throughout the progression of prostate cancer. Activation of known oncogenes does not seem to be common in prostate cancer, although mutation of the *ras* gene may be a late event (Peehl *et al*, 1987; Carter *et al*, 1990). Reports of suppressor gene inactivation in prostate cancer are rudimentary, with loss of retinoblastoma gene expression noted in several samples of advanced prostatic carcinomas (Bookstein *et al*, 1990).

This review will focus on approaches that can be used to identify and characterize suppressor genes whose loss may be involved in the development of prostate cancer. The study of somatic cell hybrids between normal and cancer cells is one such approach that led to the original conception of the existence of suppressor genes. Karyotypic analysis of tumour samples or cultured cells has been another frequently used technique to look for gross loss of genetic material which is visible at the level of light microscopy. A more sensitive and specific method now available to detect minute genetic changes involves the

Cancer Surveys Volume 11: *Prostate Cancer*
© 1991 Imperial Cancer Research Fund. 0-87969-368-1/91. $3.00 + .00

use of polymorphic DNA probes specific for different regions spanning all of the chromosomal arms. Another molecular means of detecting loss of gene activity is subtraction hybridization, which permits the cloning of genes expressed in normal but not in malignant cells. Finally, in vitro transformation models involving the introduction of oncogenes and mutagenesis can be developed to induce genetic changes that may be representative of actual changes that occur in vivo during tumour progression.

Regardless of the approach, the search for specific molecular events occurring at each stage of tumour development seems particularly appropriate for prostate cancer. Several characteristics of prostate cancer that must eventually be explained by molecular events include: (a) the preponderance of cancer arising in the peripheral, but not the central, zone of the prostate (McNeal *et al*, 1988); (b) the multifocal origin of prostate cancer (McNeal and Bostwick, 1986); (c) the relationship of intraepithelial neoplasia (dysplasia) to invasive cancer (McNeal, 1988) and (d) the correlations between volume, differentiation and malignant potential (McNeal *et al*, 1986).

SOMATIC CELL HYBRIDS

Characterization of somatic cell hybrids created by fusing normal with malignant cells led to the recognition that the normal phenotype was dominant and that loss of genetic material was required for the re-expression of the malignant phenotype (Harris, 1988). The fact that the prerequisite genetic loss was specific and not random led to the concept of suppressor genes—genes whose products regulate key functions in normal cells and which are lost or inactivated in malignant cells (Sager, 1989).

Although suppressor gene products have yet to be identified from the study of somatic cell hybrids, certain chromosomes with suppressor functions have been implicated from these investigations. Chromosome 11 was identified as the specific chromosome lost when suppressed (non-tumorigenic) hybrids derived from fusion of normal human fibroblasts to HeLa (cervical carcinoma) cells gave rise to tumorigenic segregants (Srivatsan *et al*, 1986). Suppressor activity on chromosome 11 was verified by directly introducing chromosome 11 into HeLa cells, which blocked their tumorigenic potential (Oshimura *et al*, 1990).

In fact, the introduction of chromosome 11 can partially or wholly suppress other, but not all, types of tumour cells besides HeLa (Oshimura *et al*, 1990). This finding indicates that either a common suppressor gene has been lost among diverse tumours or that several different suppressor genes are present on chromosome 11. Evidence in support of the former postulate is that certain hybrids derived from the fusion of cancer cells with other cancer cells are tumorigenic without additional chromosome loss, implying the loss of a common suppressor gene between the two types of cancer cells (Weissman and Stanbridge, 1983). On the other hand, the suppressor gene lost in Wilms' tumour is on chromosome 11 (Koufos *et al*, 1984), yet somatic cell hybrids of Wilms' × HeLa cells were non-tumorigenic, suggesting that different suppressor genes on chromosome 11 were lost in each tumour type.

In addition, it would appear that different types of cells may use different suppressor genes to suppress the malignant potential of HeLa cells. Chromosomes 1 and 4 were lost when tumorigenic segregants arose from HT1080 × HeLa hybrids (Pasquale *et al*, 1988), in contrast to the loss of chromosome 11 from fibroblast × HeLa hybrids. This perhaps relates to the mechanism of suppression, which will be discussed more fully below.

Taking the approach of somatic cell hybridization to search for suppressor genes in the prostate, we created hybrids between normal prostatic epithelial and HeLa cells (Peehl *et al*, 1990). Because cancer arises much more frequently in the peripheral zone than in the central zone of the prostate, we thought it of interest to compare the characteristics of hybrids made from cells of the two different zones.

As expected from previous studies of normal × malignant somatic cell hybrids, the prostate × HeLa hybrids were non-tumorigenic whether the parental prostatic cells were derived from the central or the peripheral zone. No phenotypic differences distinguished hybrids from the central versus peripheral zones. Work is in progress to isolate tumorigenic segregants, which should arise as chromosomes are lost during serial passage of the prostate × HeLa hybrids. Identification of the loss of specific chromosomes may point towards suppressor genes lost in prostate adenocarcinoma. Whether different suppressor genes are involved in central versus peripheral zone tumours is a question that may also be answered through the study of somatic cell hybrids.

Another important aspect of studying somatic cell hybrids has relevance with regard to prognostic indicators and perhaps to therapy. It appears that differentiation is a key element in suppression of the malignant phenotype in somatic cell hybrids (Peehl and Stanbridge, 1982; Harris and Bramwell, 1987). In vitro, non-tumorigenic hybrid cells appear to be transformed and undifferentiated (Stanbridge and Wilkinson, 1978), but in vivo, the differentiated phenotype of the normal parent is often expressed by suppressed hybrid cells. Examples are fibroblast × HeLa suppressed hybrids, which express a fibroblastic phenotype when injected into nude mice, and non-tumorigenic keratinocyte × HeLa hybrids, which resemble keratinocytes in vivo (Stanbridge *et al*, 1982). These differentiated phenotypes are lost upon reversion to tumorigenicity after loss of chromosomes by the hybrids.

The expression of the differentiated phenotype of the normal parent by somatic cell hybrids in vivo has led to a novel approach for obtaining monoclonal antibodies that react with differentiation specific antigens (Stanbridge *et al*, 1986). Isolation of antibodies that react with differentiation antigens of prostate cells would be significant for prostate cancer, since histological differentiation is currently the best prognostic indicator for prostate cancer (Gleason, 1977). Traditional approaches towards identification of differentiation antigens and corresponding antibodies have not been overwhelmingly successful for the prostate, and somatic cell hybrids could theoretically prove useful for this purpose. Unfortunately, we found that prostate × HeLa hybrids did not express a secretory epithelial phenotype in vivo (Peehl *et al*, 1990). Rather, suppression was associated with a squamous epithelial appearance.

The expression of a squamous phenotype by prostate × HeLa hybrids may relate to the fact that even normal prostate cells, when injected subcutaneously into nude mice, become squamous. Development of a squamous epithelium is a characteristic response of the prostatic epithelium to certain abnormal conditions, such as high levels of estrogen (Mostofi and Price, 1979), but the mechanisms governing the expression of the discrete differentiation pathways of secretory versus squamous development are unknown. Perhaps the appropriate conditions for the expression of the secretory phenotype are not being provided in the nude mouse. One wonders whether the induction of a squamous phenotype in prostate derived cells after injection into nude mice may explain the poor take of prostate cancer cells or tissues in nude mice (Reid *et al*, 1980); perhaps growth is prevented by inappropriate squamous differentiation.

In any case, until this difficulty is overcome, prostate × HeLa hybrids will not be useful for studying the role of prostate specific differentiation in the suppression of prostate cancer or for identifying new differentiation specific antigens. Prostate cells fused with malignant cells other than HeLa may provide a more appropriate model for the suppression of prostate cancer, and efforts are in progress to prepare prostate cancer cell lines with mutations suitable for the biochemical selection necessary for creating somatic cell hybrids. Such hybrids between normal and malignant prostate cells might also yield more relevant information about specific suppressor genes lost in prostate cancer cells, and whether the same suppressor genes are commonly lost among different prostate cancers. Our preliminary results from fusing a strain of prostate cancer cells to HeLa cells indicated that the resulting hybrids were suppressed, suggesting that prostate cancer has different genetic defects from HeLa cells (Terris MK, Peehl DM and Stamey TA, unpublished results).

NOVEL SUPPRESSOR GENES

The family of suppressor genes will undoubtedly turn out to be as large as the family of oncogenes. Already several diverse categories of suppressor genes have been noted, including those involved in DNA repair (Parshad *et al*, 1990) and inhibition of angiogenesis (Rastinejad *et al*, 1989). In fact, the ability of chromosome 11 to suppress many diverse tumour types may lie in the presence of several different suppressor genes on this chromosome, such as one encoding host regulatory mechanisms against human papillomavirus (Schwab, 1989) in addition to the well known Wilms' tumour locus (Van Heyningen *et al*, 1985).

One approach to identifying novel suppressor genes is to make "subtraction libraries" from normal and tumorigenic cells. Messenger RNA from populations of normal and cancer cells is cross-hybridized, and unreacted material is separated and cloned. The application of this method to human mammary epithelial cells resulted in the recognition of a number of genes that were expressed in normal cells but whose expression was reduced or lost in transformed and tumorigenic counterparts (Trask *et al*, 1990). Fibronectin and keratin 5 were two of those genes, but a third was a previously unrecognized gene referred to as "*NB-1*" (Yaswen et al, 1990). Recently, this gene was demonstrated to be a member of the calmodulin family. Normal human prostatic epithelial cells are among the few cell types that express *NB-1* in vitro, and *NB-1* gene expression appears to be decreased in prostate cancer derived cell populations (Yaswen *et al*, 1990). The role of *NB-1* in prostate cells is being scrutinized. Since calcium is recognized as a key regulator of cellular differentiation and calmodulin is a primary mediator of cellular response to calcium flux, the possibility that a calmodulin like gene is a suppressor gene in the prostate has very interesting ramifications regarding the role of differentiation in the development of prostate cancer.

CHROMOSOMAL ABERRATIONS

Recognition of consistent chromosomal deletions in hereditary cancers via karyotypic analysis was the starting point for the eventual molecular cloning of the suppressor genes lost in retinoblastoma and Wilms' tumour. Similarly, karyotypic analysis led to the identification of the specific oncogene that was activated by translocation in chronic mylogenous leukemia (Ben-Neriah *et al*, 1986). It is therefore evident that karyotypic analysis can yield important clues about the genetic changes involved in cancer. Yet, until recently, karyotypic analysis was not a feasible approach for the characterization of prostate cancer.

Because prostate cancers, even those of high malignant grade, are slow growing, it has been virtually impossible to karyotype them directly. From the few studies accomplished in this manner, a deleted chromosome 10 was implicated in prostate cancer (Atkin and Baker, 1985; Lundgren *et al*, 1988). Improved culture techniques have now permitted karyotypic analysis of cells cultured directly from primary prostatic tumours, resulting in the largest studies to date of prostate cancer cell strains (Brothman *et al*, 1989, 1990 and in press). Clonal aberrations were noted in approximately one-third of the 50 cell strains that were examined, but no consistent changes were noted. However, double minute chromsomes were seen in a number of cases, as has been described in some other studies of prostate cancer cells (reviewed in Brothman *et al*, 1990). It may be that a previously uncharacterized oncogene is commonly amplified in prostate cancer; such a possibility bears further investigation.

IN VITRO TRANSFORMATION

Transformation of normal cells by viral infection or DNA transfection of oncogenes is a common experimental method for inducing one of the possible events in tumorigenic progression. The transforming abilities of SV40 are well established, and therefore SV40, although not implicated in any naturally occurring human tumour, is often introduced into cells to initiate early stages of tumour development.

The introduction of SV40 into neonatal prostatic epithelial cells led to the isolation of cells with an extended lifespan and some transformed properties, such as anchorage independent growth and reduced growth factor requirements (Kaighn *et al*, 1980). The use of DNA transfection to introduce SV40 transforming genes into prostate cells circumvented the problems associated with viral replication and maintenance, and immortal cell lines were established with this method (Kaighn *et al*, 1989).

Cells immortalized with SV40 transforming genes theoretically provide a base for introducing further oncogenic events, including loss of suppressor genes, to create tumours. However, attempts to do so in SV40 transformed prostate cells either by the introduction of additional oncogenes or by chemical mutagenesis have been unsuccessful (Kaighn *et al*, 1980; Peehl DM and Stamey TA, unpublished results). Why this should be is unclear. Certainly, the recognition of transformation events in vitro in epithelial cells is often difficult, but even in vivo selection for tumorigenic variants was unsuccessful. Possibly the apparent lack of successful transformation to tumorigenicity is related to the inadequacy of nude mice tumorigenic assays for prostate cells (for discussion, see Somatic Cell Hybrids, above).

Failure to create a model for investigating the aetiology and progression of prostatic cancer by in vitro transformation is in contrast to encouraging results in another urological system. Normal human urothelial cells were first transformed to immortality with SV40 genes and then made tumorigenic by the addition of the *ras* oncogene or by chemical mutagenesis (Meisner *et al*, 1988; Reznikoff *et al*, 1988). The chromosomal losses that accompanied transformation to tumorigenicity were similar to those found in naturally occurring transitional cell carcinomas, validating the power of this approach for identifying specific genetic changes involved in malignant transformation. An interesting observation in this model was that although *ras* transformation yielded transitional cell carcinomas, chemical transformation resulted in squamous carcinomas of varying degrees of differentiation. Further studies may provide information regarding the regulation of differentiation in malignant progression.

Although instability of the karyotype is characteristic of virally transformed cells, neither SV40 transformed prostatic cells nor urothelial cells spontaneously transformed to malignancy. Specific changes induced by the introduction of other oncogenes or by mutagenesis were required to convert urothelial cells to tumorigenicity. Prostatic epithelial cells could not be transformed in vitro with *ras* or *myc* or adenovirus E1A and E1B, or combinations of these oncogenes. Yet, in a reconstituted mouse organ model, introduction of *ras* plus *myc* did lead to cancer (Thompson *et al*, 1989). However, the resultant tumours were clonal, again suggesting that specific additional events (perhaps involving suppressor gene inactivation) were required, which apparently did not occur in the in vitro transformation model.

In vitro transformation by human papillomavirus (HPV) may be a more realistic approach than using SV40 to alter prostatic epithelial cells. Papillomavirus has been implicated as an aetiological agent in cervical cancer (Arends *et al*, 1990), and use of the sensitive polymerase chain reaction has permitted the detection of HPV in prostate cancers (McNicol and Dodd, 1990). HPV has been used to transform a variety of epithelial cells in culture, including cervical cells, which are a natural target (DiPaolo *et al*, 1990), and breast cells, which are not (Band *et al*, 1990). Generally, human epithelial cells are immortalized but not made tumorigenic by the introduction of HPV DNA. Chromosomal changes occur in HPV transformed cells but, as for SV40 transformed cells, additional specific changes such as the introduction of the *ras* oncogene are required to induce the tumorigenic phenotype (DiPaolo *et al*, 1990). It may be possible to transform adult prostatic epithelial cells with HPV, since improved techniques for culture as well as for DNA transfection are now available (Brash *et al*, 1987; Peehl *et al*, 1988).

SUMMARY

Prostate cancer poses many challenges for clinicians. Methods for early detection are not satisfactory, and in fact more efficient detection will lead to even further dilemmas. We know from necropsy studies that the occurrence of prostate cancer is much higher than the clinical incidence (Yatani *et al*, 1982). Obviously, only some of the prostate cancers detected early would progress to a health threatening state if left untreated—the question is, which ones? This is a question that must be addressed, because prostate cancer has the highest occurrence rate of any cancer among males in the US, and current approaches to eradicating early stage prostate cancers involve expensive surgical or irradiation techniques. Even for primary prostatic tumours of more advanced stages, current prognostic indicators are not ideal.

What is the potential of specific suppressor genes lost in prostate cancer for identifying useful prognostic indicators? Even though numerous molecular events, including loss as well as gain of gene activity, have been delineated for colon cancer, no single genetic change has proven prognostic. Rather, increasing malignant potential of colon cancer seems to be correlated with an accumulation of several genetic events. On the other hand, a specific chromosomal abnormality, a deletion of chromosome 17p, does appear to be a prognostic indicator for distinguishing high grade from low grade transitional cell carcinoma (Olumi *et al*, 1990). Whether loss of chromosome 17p will prove to be a better prognostic marker than other parameters, however, is still unknown. At present, no consistent genetic changes have been associated with any stage of prostate cancer, so we are a long way from determining whether such changes will prove their hypothetical usefulness as new and improved prognostic indicators.

The other clinical realm in which the identification of loss of suppressor genes in prostate cancer might prove a resource is therapy. Suppressor gene products obviously provide key regulatory functions, perhaps linked to differentiation, in normal cells. Restoration of these regulatory functions in cancer cells, either by directly supplying the lost regulatory element or by circumventing the missing element by other means, is a novel therapeutic approach that might offer hope even in metastatic disease. Realization of this dream will require much more knowledge of the precise nature of the suppressor gene products lost in cancer, and a detailed understanding of the hierarchy of regulation of growth and differentiation in normal cells. Although studies to obtain such information are still limited for prostate cancer, work in other areas of cancer biology might point the way towards successful clinical application of molecular parameters such as loss of suppressor genes.

References

Arends MJ, Wyllie AH and Bird CC (1990) Papillomaviruses and human cancer. *Human Pathology* **21** 686–698

Atkin NB and Baker MC (1985) Chromosome study of five cancers of the prostate. *Human Genetics* **70** 359–364

Band V, Zajchowski D, Kulesa V and Sager R (1990) Human papilloma virus DNAs immortalize normal human mammary epithelial cells and reduce their growth factor requirements. *Proceedings of the National Academy of Sciences of the USA* **87** 463–467

Ben-Neriah Y, Daley GQ, Mes-Masson A-M, Witte ON and Baltimore D (1986) The chronic myelogenous leukemia-specific p210 protein is the product of the *bcr/abl* hybrid gene. *Science* **233** 212–214

Bookstein R, Rio P, Madreperla SA *et al* (1990) Promoter deletion and loss of retinoblastoma gene expression in human prostate carcinoma. *Proceedings of the National Academy of Sciences of the USA* **87** 7762–7766

Brash DE, Reddel RR, Quanrud M, Yang K, Farrell MP and Harris CC (1987) Strontium phosphate transfection of human cells in primary culture: stable expression of the simian virus 40 large-T-antigen gene in primary human bronchial epithelial cells. *Molecular and Cellular Biology* **7** 2031–2034

Brothman AR, Lesho LJ, Somers KD, Schellhammer PF, Ladaga LE and Merchant DJ (1989) Cytogenetic analysis of four primary prostatic cultures. *Cancer Genetics and Cytogenetics* **37** 241–248

Brothman AR, Peehl DM, Patel AM and McNeal JE (1990) Frequency and pattern of karyotypic abnormalities in human prostate cancer. *Cancer Research* **50** 3795–3803

Brothman AR, Peehl DM, Patel AM *et al* Cytogenetic evaluation of 20 primary prostatic tumors. *Cancer Genetics and Cytogenetics* (in press)

Carter BS, Epstein JI and Isaacs, WB (1990) ras gene mutations in human prostate cancer. *Cancer Research* **50** 6830–6832

DiPaolo JA, Popescu NC and Woodworth CD (1990) Transformation of human cervical epithelial cells. *Proceedings of the American Association of Cancer Research* **31** 129

Fearon ER, Cho KR, Nigro JM *et al* (1990) Identification of a chromosome 18q gene that is altered in colorectal cancers. *Science* **247** 49–56

Gleason DF (1977) Histologic grading and clinical staging of prostate carcinoma, In: M Tannenbaum (ed). *Urologic Pathology: The Prostate,* pp 171–197, Lea and Febiger, Philadelphia

Harris H (1988) The analysis of malignancy by cell fusion: the position in 1988. *Cancer Research* **48** 3302–3306

Harris H and Bramwell ME (1987) The suppression of malignancy by terminal differentiation: evidence from hybrids between tumour cells and keratinocytes. *Journal of Cell Science* **87** 383–388

Kaighn ME, Narayan KS, Ohnuki Y, Jones LW and Lechner JF (1980) Differential properties among clones of simian virus 40-transformed human epithelial cells. *Carcinogenesis* **1** 635–645

Kaighn ME, Reddel RR, Lechner JF *et al* (1989) Transformation of human neonatal prostate epithelial cells by strontium phosphate transfection with a plasmid containing SV40 early region genes. *Cancer Research* **49** 3050–3056

Koufos A, Hansen MF, Lampkin BC *et al* (1984) Loss of alleles at loci on human chromosome 11 during genesis of Wilms' tumour. *Nature* **309** 170–172

Lundgren R, Kristofferson U, Heim S, Mandahl N and Mitelman F (1988) Multiple structural chromosome rearrangements, including del (7q) and del (10q), in an adenocarcinoma of the prostate. *Cancer Genetics and Cytogenetics* **35** 103–108

McNeal JE (1988) Significance of duct-acinar dysplasia in prostatic carcinogenesis. *Prostate* **13** 91–102

McNeal JE and Bostwick DG (1986) Intraductal dysplasia: a premalignant lesion of the prostate. *Human Pathology* **17** 64–71

McNeal JE, Kindrachuk RA, Freiha FS, Bostwick DG, Redwine EA and Stamey TA (1986) Patterns of progression in prostate cancer. *Lancet* **i** 60–63

McNeal JE, Redwine EA, Freiha FS and Stamey TA (1988) Zonal distribution of prostatic carcinoma: correlation with histologic pattern and direction of spread. *American Journal of Surgical Pathology* **12** 897–906

McNicol PJ and Dodd JG (1990) Detection of human papillomavirus DNA in prostate gland tissue by using the polymerase chain reaction amplification assay. *Journal of Clinical Microbiology* **28** 409–412

Meisner LF, Wu S, Christian BJ and Reznikoff CA (1988) Cytogenetic instability with balanced chromosome changes in an SV40 transformed human uroepithelial cell line. *Cancer Research* **48** 3215–3220

Mostofi FK and Price EB (1979) Tumors of the prostate, In: Firminger HI (ed). *Tumors of the Male Genital System, Atlas of Tumor Pathology,* Second Series, Fascicle 8, pp 117-252, Armed Forces Institute of Pathology, Washington, DC

Olumi AF, Tsai YC, Nichols PW *et al* (1990) Allelic loss of chromosome 17p distinguishes high grade from low grade transitional cell carcinomas of the bladder. *Cancer Research* **50** 7081–7083

Oshimura M, Kugoh H, Koi M *et al* (1990) Transfer of a normal human chromosome 11 suppresses tumorigenicity of some but not all tumor cell lines. *Journal of Cellular Biochemistry* **42** 135–142

Parshad R, Sanford KK, Stanbridge EJ, Satoh H, Barrett JC and Oshimura M (1990) Genes on human chromosome 11 associated with DNA repair and tumor suppression. *Proceedings of the American Association of Cancer Research* **31** 18

Pasquale SR, Jones GR, Doersen C-J and Weissman BE (1988) Tumorigenicity and oncogene expression in pediatric cancers. *Cancer Research* **48** 2715–2719

Peehl DM and Stanbridge EJ (1982) The role of differentiation in the suppression of tumorigenicity in human cell hybrids. *International Journal of Cancer* **30** 113–120

Peehl DM, Wehner N and Stamey TA (1987) Activated Ki-ras oncogene in human prostatic adenocarcinoma. *Prostate* **10** 281–289

Peehl DM, Wong ST and Stamey TA (1988) Clonal growth characteristics of adult human prostatic epithelial cells. *In Vitro* **24** 530–536

Peehl DM, Wong ST, McNeal JE and Stamey TA (1990) Analysis of somatic cell hybrids derived from normal human prostatic epithelial cells fused with HeLa cells. *Prostate* **17** 123–136

Rastinejad F, Polverini PJ and Bouck NP (1989) Regulation of the activity of a new inhibitor of angiogenesis by a cancer suppressor gene. *Cell* **56** 345–355

Reid LCM, Minato N and Rojkind M (1980) Human prostatic cells in culture and in conditioned animals, In: Spring-Mills E and Hafez ESE (eds). *Male Accessory Sex Glands,* Vol 4, pp 617–640, Elsevier/North Holland Biomedical Press, New York

Reznikoff CA, Loretz LJ, Christian BJ, Wu S-Q and Meisner LF (1988) Neoplastic transformation of SV40-immortalized human urinary tract epithelial cells by in vitro exposure to methylcholanthrene. *Carcinogenesis* **9** 1427–1436

Sager R (1989) Tumor suppressor genes: the puzzle and the promise. *Science* **246** 1406–1412

Schwab M (1989) Genetic principles of tumor suppression. *Biochimica et Biophysica Acta* **989** 49–64

Srivatsan ES, Benedict WF and Stanbridge EJ (1986) Implication of chromosome 11 in the suppression of neoplastic expression in human cell hybrids. *Cancer Research* **46** 6174–6179

Stanbridge EJ and Wilkinson J (1978) Analysis of malignancy in human cells: malignant and transformed phenotypes are under separate genetic control. *Proceedings of the National Academy of Sciences of the USA* **75** 1466–1469

Stanbridge EJ and Nowell PC (1990) Origins of human cancer revisited. *Cell* **63** 867–874

Stanbridge EJ, Der CJ, Doersen C-J *et al* (1982) Human cell hybrids: analysis of transformation and tumorigenicity. *Science* **215** 252–259

Stanbridge EJ, Araujo D, Ross P, Butler G, McCullough J and Wilkinson J (1986) A novel approach for obtaining and identifying monoclonal antibodies that react with differentiation-specific antigens using human hybrid cells. *Cancer Research* **46** 4759–4764

Thompson TC, Southgate J, Kitchener G and Land H (1989) Multistage carcinogenesis induced by ras and myc oncogenes in a reconstituted organ. *Cell* **56** 917–930

Trask DT, Band V, Zajchowski DA, Yaswen P, Suh T and Sager R (1990) Keratins as markers that distinguish normal and tumor-derived mammary epithelial cells. *Proceedings of the National Academy of Sciences of the USA* **87** 2319–2323

Van Heyningen V, Boyd PA, Seawright A *et al* (1985) Molecular analysis of chromosome 11 deletions in aniridia-Wilms' tumor syndrome. *Proceedings of the National Academy of Sciences of the USA* **82** 8592–8596

Weinberg RA (1989) Oncogenes, antioncogenes, and the molecular bases of multistep carcinogenesis. *Cancer Research* **49** 3713–3721

Weissman BE and Stanbridge EJ (1983) Complementation of the tumorigenic phenotype in human cell hybrids. *Journal of the National Cancer Institute* **70** 667–672

Yaswen P, Small A, Peehl DM, Trask DK, Sager R and Stampfer MR (1990) Downregulation of a calmodulin-related gene during transformation of human mammary epithelial cells. *Proceedings of the National Academy of Sciences of the USA* **87** 7360–7364

Yatani R, Chigusa I, Akazaki I, Stemmermann GN, Welsh RA and Correa P (1982) Geographic pathology of latent prostatic carcinoma. *International Journal of Cancer* **29** 611–616

The author is responsible for the accuracy of the references.

Genetic Factors and Metastatic Potential of Prostatic Cancer

TOMOHIKO ICHIKAWA[1] • **YAYOI ICHIKAWA**[1] • **JOHN T ISAACS**[1,2]

[1]*Johns Hopkins Oncology Center, Baltimore, Maryland 21205;*
[2]*James Buchanan Brady Urological Institute, Department of Urology,*
Baltimore, Maryland 21205

INTRODUCTION

Models of Metastasis

Studies of experimental and human cancers have demonstrated that transformation of a normal cell to a fully malignant cancer cell requires a series of genetic changes (Nowell, 1976; Nicolson, 1987; Vogelstein *et al*, 1988). This transformation involves gain in function of certain genes coupled with losses or inactivations of other genes (Klein, 1987; Fearon *et al*, 1990). These studies have led to the realization that carcinogenesis is a process of competition between genes that determine the induction versus the suppression of malignancy.

An unresolved question, however, is whether the acquisition of metastatic potential by already tumorigenic cancer cells also involves both positive and negative genetic changes. In this chapter, the mechanism of acquisition of metastatic potential in prostatic cancer was studied utilizing the Dunning rat prostatic cancer system. The original Dunning R-3327 tumour is a spontaneous rat prostatic adenocarcinoma (Dunning, 1963). This is an androgen responsive, slow growing, well differentiated and non-metastatic cancer. From the original tumour, a large variety of additional sublines have spontaneously developed during serial passage (Isaacs, 1987). Within the Dunning system, there is a wide range of tumour phenotypes with regard to androgen sensitivity, growth rate, histological and biochemical differentiation and metastatic potential. Cytogenetic study of 16 Dunning sublines demonstrates that a gain of chromosome 4 is associated with acquisition of increased malignant behaviour, as reflected by an increased tumour growth rate, loss of androgen sensitivity and development of poorly differentiated histology (Isaacs and Hukku, 1988). Gaining an extra copy of chromosome 4 does not, however, necessarily induce the acquisition of high metastatic potential. Previous studies also demonstrate that acquisition of high metastatic potential within the Dunning system is associated with increased cellular motility (Mohler *et al*, 1988; Partin *et al*, 1988).

Ha-*ras* Oncogene and Metastasis

Expression of the mutated Ha-*ras* oncogene or overexpression of the normal *ras* proto-oncogene stimulates proliferation and induces transformation in a number of cell lines (Barbacid, 1987). Viola *et al* (1986) have demonstrated that the level of expression of the Ha-*ras* proto-oncogene in human prostatic cancer seems to correlate with histological grade of the cancer. Sumiya *et al* (1990) have shown immunohistochemically the correlation between expression of *ras* p21 and progression of the stage and grade in human prostatic cancer and the negative expression of *ras* p21 in normal prostate or benign prostatic hyperplasia. Previous studies have demonstrated that initially non-tumorigenic NIH3T3 cells can acquire both a tumorigenic phenotype and a high metastatic potential in nude mice following transfection with the mutated Ha-*ras* oncogene (Bernstein and Weinberg 1985; Greig *et al*, 1985; Thorgeirsson *et al*, 1985; Bradley *et al*, 1986; Egan *et al*, 1987; Hill *et al*, 1988). The acquisition of metastatic potential following Ha-*ras* oncogene transfection is not, however, universal and is dependent on the type of the recipient cell (Muschel *et al*, 1985).

It has been demonstrated that when non-metastatic rat mammary cancer cells are transfected with the mutated v-Ha-*ras* oncogene, an occasional resultant transfectant develops high metastatic potential. There is, however, no simple dose-response relationship between the level of the mutated v-Ha-*ras* expression in these transfectants and the development of metastases (Kyprianou and Isaacs, 1990). These results imply that the acquisition of high metastatic potential by rat mammary cancer cells is not a single step reaction regulated by Ha-*ras* p21 expression but rather a complex process requiring additional changes. Such a possibility is consistent with the fact that metastasis is a multistep process (Poste and Fidler, 1980). Cytogenetic analysis on the same rat mammary cancer system has demonstrated that the frequency of chromosomal changes in the mutated v-Ha-*ras* transfection is significantly higher than that in control transfectants (Ichikawa *et al*, 1990). These studies also suggest that if appropriate chromosomal changes occur, these v-Ha-*ras* RMC1 transfectants acquire high metastatic potential. This suggests that genetic instability induced in the transfectants expressing the mutated v-Ha-*ras* transfected gene is one mechanism for the development of high metastatic potential in the rat mammary cancer system.

Treiger and Isaacs (1988) have demonstrated that expression of the mutated v-Ha-*ras* oncogene can convert a tumorigenic non-metastatic Dunning rat prostatic cell line (ie AT2.1) to a highly metastatic state. Additional studies on the AT2.1 system have demonstated the correlation between increased metastatic potential of mutated v-Ha-*ras* transfectants and decreased expression of fibronectin (Schalken *et al*, 1988) and an increase in cellular motility (Partin *et al*, 1988). Such progressive phenotype changes induced following v-Ha-*ras* transfection suggest that genotypic alterations may be involved.

GENETIC ANALYSIS OF THE METASTATIC PHENOTYPE

Cytogenetic Analysis of v-Ha-*ras* Transfected Prostatic Cancer Cells

To study this possibility further, the relationship between the development of metastatic potential, mutated v-Ha-*ras* expression and genetic instability of the AT2.1 transfected cells has been analysed biochemically, cytogenetically and biologically. Neither the parental AT2.1 nor any of the four control AT2.1 transfectants had spontaneous metastatic potential. In contrast, six of nine v-Ha-*ras* transfectants developed spontaneous metastatic potential; however, there was a wide range of metastatic potentials among these latter transfectants (Ichikawa *et al*, 1991a). Western blotting analysis demonstrated that there was no simple dose-response relationship between the level of the mutated v-Ha-*ras* protein expression and spontaneous metastatic potential by the v-Ha-*ras* AT2.1 transfectants (Ichikawa *et al*, 1991a).

Parental AT2.1 cells had a modal chromosomal number of 71, with seven structurally rearranged chromosomes and three to five small markers (Ichikawa *et al*, 1991a). Only one of four control AT2.1 transfectants had additional numerical changes and additional structural abnormality that were not observed in the parental AT2.1 (Ichikawa *et al*, 1991a). In contrast, all of nine v-Ha-*ras* AT2.1 transfectants had additional numerical and/or structural changes (Ichikawa *et al*, 1991a). Frequency of additional numerical and/or structural chromosomal changes was significantly higher in v-Ha-*ras* AT2.1 transfectants than in the control AT2.1 transfectants (p<0.05). Loss of normal chromosome 10 was observed in all of the v-Ha-*ras* AT2.1 transfectants, whereas a similar loss was observed in only one of the four control AT2.1 transfectants (p<0.05) (Ichikawa *et al*, 1991a).

These results demonstrate that v-Ha-*ras* p21 expression in both mammary and prostatic cancer cells is not sufficient, but might be necessary, to induce metastatic potential. This progression to a high metastatic potential induced by enhanced Ha-*ras* expression involves an increased genetic instability. These results suggest that if the appropriate random chromosomal changes occur, these v-Ha-*ras* transfectants acquire metastatic potential. Such chromosomal changes could also be important in the decreased expression of fibronectin and the increased cellular motility, both of which correlate significantly with high metastatic potential in the Dunning rat prostatic cancer system (Partin *et al*, 1988; Shalken *et al*, 1988).

Somatic Cell Fusion

On the basis of these earlier studies, it was concluded that gains of certain motility functions are associated with acquisition of metastatic potential by prostatic cancer cells. Gains in functions alone, however, may not be the only process required for acquisition of high metastatic potential by prostatic cancer cells, since previous studies have demonstrated that both spontaneous and v-Ha-*ras* transfection induced acquisition of high metastatic potential of Dunning prostatic cancer cells is correlated with a downregulation of the fibronectin gene (Schalken *et al*, 1988). If the progression from no metastatic to high metastatic potential involves only gains in the expression of oncogenes, then fusing a non-metastatic with a highly metastatic prostatic cancer cell should produce a highly metastatic cell hybrid. In contrast, if loss or inactivation of suppressor gene(s) is also involved, then such hybrids should be non-metastatic, since chromosomes from the non-metastatic parental cell should supply the lost suppressor function. Therefore, such somatic cell fusion studies can be used to determine whether gains in function are alone involved in acquisition of high metastatic potential by prostatic cancer cells or whether losses of function are also required.

To test this possibility, two Dunning rat prostatic cancers, the non-metastatic AT2.1 and the highly metastatic AT3.1 sublines, were fused and the metastatic behaviours of the hybrid cells were analysed. When injected subcutaneously into the leg of rats, AT2.1 cells produced no distant metastases in ten animals injected, whereas AT3.1 cells produced distant metastases in all ten animals injected (Ichikawa *et al*, 1991b). AT2.1 cells were fused with AT3.1 cells, and AT2.1 × AT3.1 hybrid clones were isolated. Hybrid clones that conserved all (eg hybrid 1) or nearly all (eg hybrid 2) of the normal and traceable aberrant chromosomes from their parental AT2.1 and AT3.1 cells were identified. When such hybrids were injected subcutaneously into the leg of rats, primary tumours developed in all animals, but no distant metastases were observed in any animals (Ichikawa *et al*, 1991b).

To test whether the suppression of metastatic potential observed in the AT2.1 × AT3.1 hybrids was a specific effect as opposed to a non-specific effect of cell hybridization itself, highly metastatic AT3.1 cells were fused to each other. When AT3.1 × AT3.1 clones were inoculated into animals, they maintained high metastatic potential (Ichikawa *et al*, 1991b). This demonstrates that cell hybridization itself does not suppress the high metastatic potential of the AT3.1 parental cells.

When the non-metastatic AT2.1 × AT3.1 hybrid 1 cells were injected subcutaneously into the flank of rats and primary tumours were passaged in vivo, distant metastases developed in occasional animals (Ichikawa *et al*, 1991b). Five individual lung metastases and three individual axillary lymph node metastases from animals bearing these second and third in vivo passaged AT2.1 × AT3.1 hybrid 1 tumours were established in culture and analysed cytogenetically. These metastatic revertant cells showed between one and six chromosomal changes (ie <5% changes in total chromosomes). All of these changes were simple chromosomal losses. A loss of normal chromosome 2 was consistently observed in all eight metastatic revertants (Ichikawa *et al*, 1991b). One of eight metastatic revertants had only one change—a loss of chromosome 2. When injected into animals to retest metastatic potential, all eight of these metastatic revertant lines showed high metastatic potential (Ichikawa *et al*, 1991b).

These studies demonstrate that high metastatic potential is suppressed in hybrid cells produced by fusing non-metastatic and highly metastatic rat prostatic cancer cells when the hybrid cells retain all chromosomes from their parental cells. This suggests that acquisition of high metastatic potential by rat prostatic cancer cells involves loss of metastasis suppressor gene function. These studies also suggest that for rat prostatic cancer such a metastasis suppressor gene(s) is located on chromosome 2.

Microcell Mediated Chromosome Transfer

A more direct approach to identify a chromosome(s) carrying metastasis suppressor gene(s) is the introduction of specific chromosomes into the highly metastatic cancer cells. Direct demonstrations of the suppression of tumorigenicity or the induction of cellular senescence by means of microcell mediated chromosome transfer have been reported (Saxon *et al*, 1986; Weissman *et al*, 1987; Koi *et al*, 1989; Oshimura *et al*, 1990; Sugawara *et al*, 1990; Yamada *et al*, 1990). In these studies, a normal human chromosome 11 suppresses the tumorigenicity of various kinds of tumour cell lines. We are currently introducing specific human chromosomes, including chromosome 11, into highly metastatic Dunning prostate cancer cells in collaboration with Dr JC Barrett and Dr M Oshimura. Introduction of a normal human chromosome 11 into the highly metastatic Dunning AT3.1 rat prostatic cancer cell line did not suppress its tumorigenicity but suppressed its metastatic ability (Ichikawa T, Ichikawa Y, Isaacs JT, Oshimura M and Barrett JC, unpublished). Further studies on the introduction of human chromosomes into highly metastatic Dunning sublines may permit the identification of the chromosomes carrying metastasis suppressor gene(s).

SUMMARY

When a non-metastatic subline from the Dunning rat prostatic cancer was transfected with the v-Ha-*ras* oncogene, some transfectants acquired metastatic potential. Molecular analysis demonstrated that there was no simple dose-response relationship between v-Ha-*ras* expression and metastatic potential in this prostatic cancer system. Cytogenetic analysis on the same system demonstrated increased genetic instability following v-Ha-*ras* transfection. Progression of prostatic cancer from no metastatic to high metastatic potential may involve the loss of a metastasis suppressor gene. To test this possibility, non-metastatic and highly metastatic Dunning rat prostatic cancer cells were fused. Hybrid clones were isolated that conserved the chromosomes from their parental cells. When these hybrids were injected into animals, none developed distant metastases. When the non-metastatic primary tumours were passaged in vivo, distant metastases developed in occasional animals. Cytogenetic analysis of eight of these metastatic revertants demonstrated a consistent loss of normal chromosome 2. These studies show that metastasis is associated with the loss of a specific chromosome. These studies also suggest that a metastasis suppressor gene for rat prostatic cancer is located on chromosome 2. A more direct approach to identify a chromosome(s) carrying metastasis suppressor gene(s) by using microcell mediated chromosome transfer is currently progressing.

References

Barbacid M (1987) ras genes. *Annual Review of Biochemistry* **56** 779–827

Bernstein SC and Weinberg RA (1985) Expression of the metastatic phenotype in cells transfected with human metastatic tumor DNA. *Proceedings of the National Academy of Sciences of the USA* **82** 1726–1730

Bradley MO, Kraynak AR, Storer RD and Gibbs JR (1986) Experimental metastasis in nude mice of NIH 3T3 cells containing various ras genes. *Proceedings of the National Academy of Sciences of the USA* **83** 5277–5281

Dunning WF (1963) Prostate cancer in the rat. *Monographs of the National Cancer Institute* **12** 351–369

Egan SE, McClarty GA, Jarolim L *et al* (1987) Expression of H-ras correlates with metastatic potential: evidence for direct regulation of the metastatic phenotype in 10T+ and NIH 3T3 cells. *Molecular and Cellular Biology* **7** 830–837

Fearon ER, Cho KR, Nigro JM *et al* (1990) Identification of a chromosome 18q gene that is altered in colorectal cancers. *Science* **247** 49–56

Greig RG, Koestler TP, Trainier DL *et al* (1985) Tumorigenic and metastatic properties of normal and ras-transfected NIH/3T3 cells. *Proceedings of the National Academy of Sciences of the USA* **82** 3698–3701

Hill SA, Wilson S and Chambers AF (1988) Clonal heterogeneity, experimental metastatic ability, and p21 expression in H-ras-transformed NIH 3T3 cells. *Journal of the National Cancer Institute* **80** 484–490

Ichikawa T, Kyprianou N and Isaacs J (1990) Genetic instability and the acquisition of metastatic ability by rat mammary cancer cells following v-H-ras oncogene transfection. *Cancer Research* **50** 6349–6357

Ichikawa T, Schalken JA, Ichikawa Y, Steinberg G and Isaacs JT (1991a) H-ras expression, genetic instability, and acquisition of metastatic ability by rat prostatic cancer cells following v-H-ras oncogene transfection. *The Prostate* **18** 163–172

Ichikawa T, Ichikawa Y and Isaacs JT (1991b) Genetic factors and suppression of metastatic ability of prostatic cancer. *Cancer Research* **51** 3788–3792

Isaacs (1987) Development and characteristics of the available animal model systems for the study of prostatic cancer, In: Coffey DS, Bruchovsky N, Gardner Jr WA, Resnick MI and Karr JP (eds). *Current Concepts and Approaches to the Study of Prostate Cancer*, pp 513–576, Alan R Liss, New York

Isaacs JT and Hukku B (1988) Nonrandom involvement of chromosome 4 in the progression of rat prostatic cancer. *The Prostate* **13** 165–188

Klein G (1987) The approaching era of the tumor suppressor genes. *Science* **238** 1539–1545

Koi M, Morita H, Yamada H, Satoh H, Barrett JC and Oshimura M (1989) Normal human chromosome 11 suppresses tumorigenicity of human cervical tumor cell line SiHa. *Molecular Carcinogenesis* **2** 12–21

Kyprianou N and Isaacs JT (1990) Relationship between metastatic ability and ras oncogene expression in rat mammary cancer cells transfected with v-Hras oncogene. *Cancer Research* **50** 1449–1454

Mohler JL, Partin AW, Isaacs JT and Coffey DS (1988) Metastatic potential prediction by a visual grading system of cell motility: prospective validation in the Dunning R-3327 prostatic adenocarcinoma model. *Cancer Research* **48** 4312–4317

Muschel RJ, Williams JE, Lowy DR and Liotta LA (1985) Harvey ras induction of metastatic potential depends upon oncogene activation and the type of recipient cell. *American Journal of Pathology* **121** 1–8

Nicolson GL (1987) Tumor cell instability, diversification, and progression to the metastatic phenotype: from oncogene to oncofetal expression. *Cancer Research* **50** 1449–1454

Nowell PC (1976) The clonal evolution of tumor cell population. *Science* **194** 23–28

Oshimura M, Kugho H, Kio M *et al* (1990) Transfer of a normal human chromosome 11 suppresses tumorigenicity of some but not all tumor cell lines. *Journal of Cellular Biochemistry* **42** 135–142

Partin AW, Isaacs JT, Treiger B and Coffey DS (1988) Early cell motility changes associated with an increase in metastatic ability in rat prostatic cancer cells transfected with v-Harvey-ras oncogene. *Cancer Research* **48** 6050–6053

Poste G and Fidler IJ (1980) The pathogenesis of cancer metastasis. *Nature* **283** 139–146

Saxon PJ, Srivatsan ES and Stanbridge EJ (1986) Introduction of human chromosome 11 via microcell transfer controls tumorigenic expression of HeLa cells. *EMBO Journal* **15** 3461–4366

Schalken JA, Ebeling SB, Isaacs JT *et al* (1988) Down modulation of fibronectin messenger RNA in metastasizing rat prostatic cancer cells revealed by differential hybridization analysis. *Cancer Research* **48** 2042–2046

Sugawara O, Oshimura M, Koi M, Annab LA and Barrett JC (1990) Induction of cellular senescence in immortalized cells by human chromosome 1. *Science* **247** 707–710

Sumiya H, Masai M, Akimoto S, Yatani R and Shimazaki J (1990) Histochemical examination of expression of ras p21 protein and R 1881-binding protein in human prostatic cancers. *European Journal of Cancer* **26** 786–789

Thorgeirsson UP, Turpeenniemi-Hyjanen T, Williams JE *et al* (1985) NIH/3T3 cells transfected with human tumor DNA containing activated ras oncogenes express the metastatic phenotype in nude mice. *Molecular and Cellular Biology* **5** 259–262

Treiger B and Isaacs J (1988) Expression of a transfected v-H-ras oncogene in a Dunning rat prostate adenocarcinoma and the development of high metastatic ability. *Journal of Urology* **140** 1580–1586

Viola MV, Framowitz F, Oravez MS *et al* (1986) Expression of ras oncogene p21 in prostatic cancer. *New England Journal of Medicine* **314** 133–137

Vogelstein B, Fearon ER, Hamilton SR *et al* (1988) Genetic alterations during colorectal-tumor development. *New England Journal of Medicine* **319** 525–532

Weissman BE, Saxon PJ, Pasquale SR, Jones GR, Geiser AG and Stanbridge EJ (1987) Introduction of a normal human chromosome 11 into a Wilms' tumor cell line controls its tumorigenic expression. *Science* **236** 175–180

Yamada H, Wake N, Fujimoto S, Barrett JC and Oshimura M (1990) Multiple chromosomes carrying tumor suppressor activity for a uterine endometrial carcinoma cell line identified by microcell-mediated chromosome transfer. *Oncogene* **5** 1141–1147

The authors are responsible for the accuracy of the references.

Molecular Methods for Predicting the Metastatic Potential of Prostate Cancer

JACK A SCHALKEN

Urology Research Laboratory, Department of Urology, PO Box 9101, 6500 HB Nijmegen, The Netherlands

INTRODUCTION: THE IMPORTANCE OF EARLY DETECTION OF METASTATIC POTENTIAL IN PROSTATE CANCER

Prostate cancer, the malignancy with the highest incidence rate in the western male population, is characterized by the fact that at clinical presentation, the majority of patients have disease extended beyond the prostate, ie capsular penetration and/or established locoregional or distant metastases. For prostate cancer, the clinical consequences of established metastatic disease are profound, since no curative therapy is available (Scott *et al*, 1980). Systemic palliative methods, based on androgen ablation, are usually successful but of limited duration. The outgrowth of androgen insensitive cells is inevitable and will eventually result in the patient's death (Lepor *et al*, 1984).

Patients with localized tumours can be cured with radical prostatectomy. A considerable proportion of these patients, however, will show clinical progression to metastatic disease. Obviously, identification of those patients at risk is of great importance. It is likely that the number of patients with small localized tumours will steadily increase as a consequence of incidental and/or systematic screening of the male population older than 50 years of age (eg by digital rectal

Cancer Surveys Volume 11: *Prostate Cancer*
© 1991 Imperial Cancer Research Fund. 0-87969-368-1/91. $3.00 + .00

examination [DRE] and serum prostate specific antigen [PSA]). In this group, there are three categories present, which as yet cannot be discriminated: (a) patients with small tumours that do not need any treatment, (b) those that should undergo radical prostatectomy but have a low risk for clinical progression and (c) high risk patients with tumours that are likely to progress to metastatic disease. At present, no accepted method is available to make this distinction, which makes systematic screening programmes at least questionable. Hence, methods to predict metastatic potential of tumour cells are urgently needed. This chapter deals with a molecular approach to this problem.

The approaches described are all based on the question as to whether molecular differences at the DNA, RNA or protein level can be identified that can serve as progression markers for malignant prostatic disease. Furthermore, I will focus on those methods that are potentially instrumental in a clinical setting, ie methods that could be implemented in "molecular uropathology".

MOLECULAR MARKERS FOR PROSTATE CANCER PROGRESSION

Prostate Cancer Metastasis Model Systems

Studies that aim at the identification of molecular markers associated with the metastatic phenotype require the use of well established model systems in which metastatic potential can be evaluated. The Dunning R-3327 rat prostate cancer model systems consists of several sublines all derived from the parental Dunning R-3327 tumour (Dunning, 1963). These sublines represent a spectrum of relevant phenotypic characteristics, including metastatic potential. Furthermore, it appeared to be possible to induce and reverse the metastatic phenotype (Treiger and Isaacs, 1988; Isaacs JT, personal communication; Ichikawa *et al*, this issue). Of the established human prostate cancer derived cell lines, only TSU-Pr1 has metastatic potential (Lizumi *et al*, 1987). Under certain experimental conditions, however, PC-3 can also metastasize (Shervin *et al*, 1989). Of the described prostate cancer xenografts, none has metastatic potential.

Genomic Changes

Tumour progression is usually associated with phenotypic changes, which are determined by the protein expression pattern. Aberrant protein expression patterns, in turn, can find their origin in genomic alterations. Therefore, studies on the involvement of specific genetic changes, such as chromosomal abnormalities, can serve as a lead to identify genes that are implicated in the onset and progression of cancer (Yunis, 1983).

Studies on chromosomal changes associated with the onset and progression of prostate cancer have been greatly hampered by the fact that prostate tumours usually have a low mitotic index, which makes chromosome analysis on so called direct chromosome preparations difficult. Furthermore, prostate cancers are difficult to grow in vitro, even in short term culture. Nonetheless, specific chromosomal changes have been identified in prostate cancer. As summarized by Peehl (1987 and this issue), deletions on chromosomes 1, 2, 5, 17 and Y, trisomy of chromosomes 7, 14, 20 and 22, and structural changes involving chromosomal segments 2p, 7q and 10q are the most common changes reported (Brothman *et al*, 1990). Of these, deletions on 7q and 10q were found in late stage cancers (Atkin and Baker, 1985a,b). These findings, however, are all based on small numbers of patients and should be considered anecdotal rather than indicative of specific changes associated with this disease.

A less complicated technique that overcomes the problems associated with the low mitotic index in prostate tumours is the so-called allelotyping; DNA probes that map to known chromosomal locations and detect restriction fragment length polymorphisms (RFLPs) can be used to identify consistent chromosome deletions. Likewise, allelotyping colorectal carcinomas revealed a frequent deletion of the long arm of chromosome 17, which led to the identification of *p53* as a tumour suppressor gene (Baker *et al*, 1989). Also, a candidate tumour suppressor gene on chromosome 18, *DCC* (deleted in colorectal carcinoma) was identified after an initial lead obtained from RFLP analysis (Fearon *et al*, 1990).

As stated above, the few karyotypes determined from human prostate cancers indicated that deletions in the long arm of chromosomes 10 (10q23-ter) and 7 were found in late stage prostate cancers (Atkin and Baker, 1985a,b). Restriction fragment length polymorphism analyses now provide an adequate technique to test this observation in a large group of patients. Thus, Carter *et al* (1990a) showed that whereas loss of chromosome 10 was indeed frequently observed (in approximately 30% of cases studied), an as yet unreported loss on chromosome 16 occurred even more frequently. It thus appears that of the chromosomes tested, 10q and 16q are candidates to use in studies on the relation between allelic loss and progression of the disease.

Neither chromosomal analyses nor allelotyping enables us to determine subtle changes in the genome, such as point mutations and/or small deletions. These studies require the use of Southern analyses and/or differential hybridization with oligonucleotides. Such approaches are "self limiting", in that they are confined to known genes and/or previously described aberrations. Genes that should be considered "relevant" are oncogenes, tumour suppressor genes and genes that encode growth factors, growth factor receptors, transcription factors, extracellular matrix proteins and cell adhesion molecules. The term "self limiting" therefore seems to be an understatement, since taking all this into account, at least 300 known genes should be studied. Only a few reports are available for point mutations considered important in the aetiology and progression of prostate cancer. The presence of an activated *ras* oncogene in a primary prostate cancer was described by Peehl *et al* (1987), but a study by Carter *et al* (1990b) indicated that the frequency of such mutations is low.

This does not mean, however, that these mutations, when they do occur, may not have an important impact on the biological behaviour of the tumour.

(Monoclonal) Antibodies

Studies of phenotypic changes of cancer cells have been greatly facilitated by the hybridoma technology (Kohler and Milstein, 1975). Antibodies produced by hybridomas detect specific antigens, and when tumour cells or extracts are used as immunogen, appropriate screening procedures can result in the isolation of a reagent that detects tumour specific antigens. The use of monoclonal antibodies as progression markers has an established place in many disciplines, but urological oncology has few examples. Many monoclonal antibodies have been described for bladder and renal cancer (reviewed in Bander, 1987), but none of these has an established usefulness as a progression marker. The situation for prostate cancer is even worse. Several authors have reported on the isolation of prostate cancer monoclonal antibodies (Starling, 1982, 1986; Webb *et al*, 1984; Lindgren, 1985). No reports are available, however, on the use of these antibodies as progression markers. It is therefore evident that the use of monoclonal antibodies in the identification of advanced prostate cancer cells is underexploited.

Of the products of potential "relevant" genes (see above) only *ras* p21 has been studied. Viola *et al* (1986) reported on an inverse relation between *ras* p21 expression and histological tumour grade. Furthermore, p21 *ras* expression was correlated with the frequency of nodal metastases (Fan, 1988). More recently, Sumiya *et al* (1990) also found a higher expression of *ras* p21 in high grade and late stage prostate cancers. In late stage tumours, however, *ras* p21 expression did not correlate with survival.

Another protein with potential relevance for prostate cancer progression is the androgen receptor. In a recent study, however, it was clearly established that expression of the nuclear localized androgen receptor did not correlate with grade, stage and androgen sensitivity of the tumour (Van der Kwast *et al*, 1991). These findings show clearly that androgen receptor content measured by immunocytochemical techniques is not likely to be a useful progression marker.

DNA Probes Detecting Differentially Expressed Genes

Studies at the RNA level by northern blot assays have "constraints" similar to those at the genomic level, ie only previously characterized genes can be studied. However, an overwhelming amount of circumstantial evidence indicates that the above mentioned genes can actually be involved in the onset and progression of cancer. Therefore, the study of these genes and their relation to the aetiology and progression of prostate cancer are of major importance. Buttyan (1987) found increased levels of *myc* transcripts in high grade prostate cancers. In model system studies, several researchers have investigated whether a relation between oncogene expression and prostate cancer progression was evident. So far, no consistent association between the overexpression of proto-oncogenes and the metastatic phenotype was found (Cooke, 1988a,b; Bussemakers *et al*, 1991b).

A direct approach to identify genes that are differentially expressed is based on comparison of steady state mRNA populations, such as differential and subtraction hybridization analyses. These techniques, however, do not enable the identification of genes that are aberrantly expressed (ie different size of transcripts). Unless the level of steady state mRNA has changed, no aberrant expression patterns can be identified. Another constraint of these techniques is that a number of genes can be regulated posttranscriptionally (mRNA stability) or posttranslationally. Such subtle differences cannot be identified with this approach. The advantages of differential/subtraction hybridization analyses are threefold. Firstly, as yet unknown although relevant genes can be isolated. Moreover, genes that are upregulated, as well as those that are downmodulated, can be identified. Hence, both dominant acting genes (eg oncogenes and genes that encode growth factors and growth factor receptors) and recessive genetic elements (eg tumour suppressor genes) can thus be characterized. Secondly, cDNA clones can be routinely characterized by DNA sequence analysis, and the resulting DNA sequences can be compared with nucleic acid/protein data bases. Thirdly, regardless of whether the gene is aetiologically related to the disease or merely a marker for progression, the cDNA can be immediately evaluated for its use in diagnosis by RNA in situ hybridization analysis.

There are different methods for comparing mRNA populations. When comparing mRNA populations, two aspects are of great importance. First is the complexity of the mRNA population, which is usually expressed in nucleotides/cell and can range from $6 \times 10E8$ n/cell for a complex population like the brain to $1 \times 10E8$ n/cell for spleen (Britten *et al*, 1974). Second is that the relative abundance of the mRNA population should be considered. In eukaryotic cells, only few mRNAs are present at high abundancy ($>1\%$); most mRNAs are present at low ($1–0.01\%$) or very low abundancy ($<0.01\%$). Essentially, these two factors determine which approach to use. For transcripts of both high and low abundance ($>0.01\%$), differential screening with cDNA libraries is a valid approach ("differential hybridization analysis"; reviewed in Sargent, 1987). The identification of differentially expressed genes of very low abundance ($<0.01\%$) requires a more sophisticated approach, ie subtraction hybridization analysis.

The "flow scheme" for a differential hybridization assay is depicted in Fig. 1. A cDNA library is constructed from the mRNA population from a metastatic line. The resulting cDNA library represents all transcripts from the metastatic population. The library is plated, and replicate filters are screened differentially. Replica 1 is screened with a DNA probe representing the "metastatic" mRNA population (poly(A)$^+$ mRNA is used as a template for a first strand cDNA reaction; second strand cDNA is then labelled to high spe-

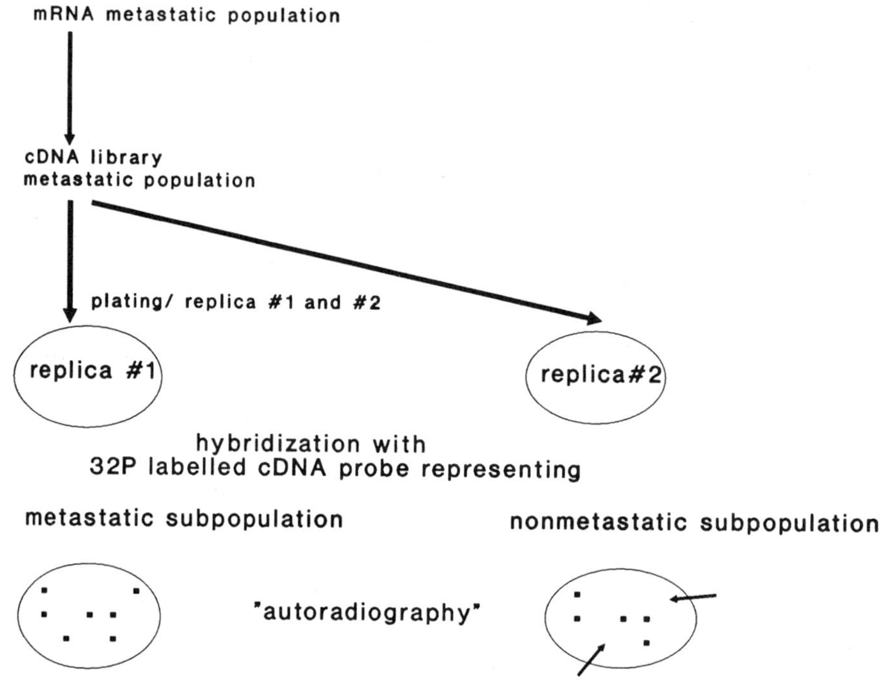

Differences *represent mRNAs overexpressed in the metastatic subline*

Fig. 1. Schematic outline of a differential hybridization assay. The short arrows indicate the position of so-called "differential clones"

cific activity, using the random prime labelling method, according to Feinberg and Vogelstein [1983]). Thus, cDNAs can be detected if the corresponding transcript is present at a relative abundance greater than 0.01% in the template mRNA population that was used to synthesize the probe, ie sensitivity is approximately 0.01%. Likewise, replica 2 is screened with a probe representing the mRNA population of the non-metastatic subline. The differences in the resulting autoradiographs represent cDNA clones that detect transcripts that are overexpressed in the metastatic subline. Usually, transcripts with an expression level below 0.01% are not detectable with this assay.

To improve the sensitivity of the technique, the method of liquid subtraction hybridization analysis is used (Fig. 2). In this approach, first strand cDNA from the metastatic subline is hybridized in solution to excess mRNA from the non-metastatic line (mRNA "driven", subtraction hybridization). When the amount of the transcript of interest in the "driver" mRNA population is constant, then simple first order kinetics can be applied (Young and Anderson, 1985; Travis and Sutcliffe, 1988). Under these conditions, the time needed to obtain an effective enrichment for the mRNAs of interest can be approximately calculated (R_0t value). Subsequently, the single stranded DNA (ssDNA) molecules can be separated from double stranded DNAs (dsDNAs); a cDNA library is then constructed, using the subtracted first strand DNA population.

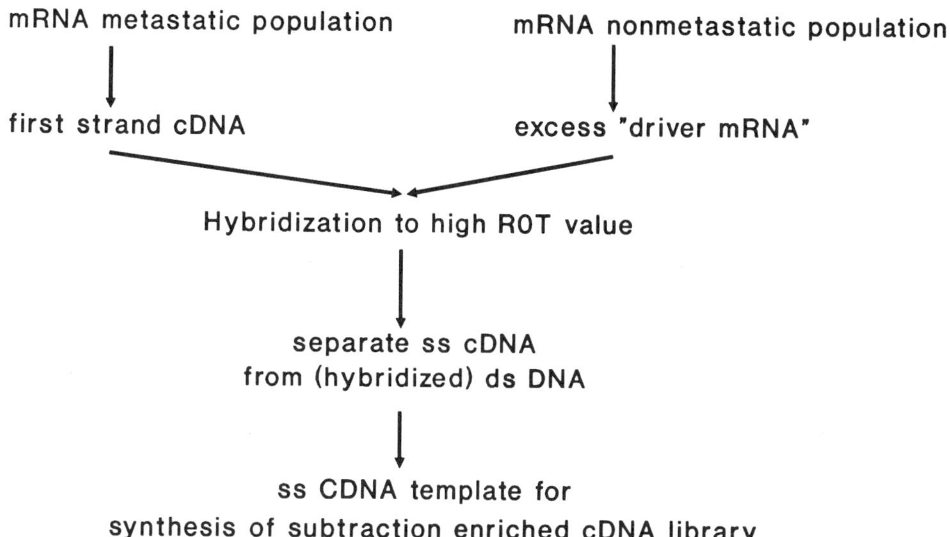

Fig. 2. Schematic outline of the isolation of a subtraction enriched ss-cDNA population for the generation of subtraction enriched cDNA libraries

In this library, an enrichment for cDNAs representing mRNAs overexpressed in the metastatic line, at low abundancy (<0.01%), is effectuated.

Clearly, the reciprocal experiment, ie differential screening of a cDNA library constructed from the non-metastatic subline, or using mRNA from the metastatic line as driver against first strand cDNA from the non-metastatic line, can be used to identify genes downmodulated during metastasis.

The above techniques have been successfully used in the identification of genes induced by growth factors (Lau and Nathans, 1985, 1987; Kartasova *et al*, 1987; Almendral *et al*, 1988). Genes expressed during the induction of differentiation have also been identified in this way (Smits, 1987). Furthermore, comparisons of normal versus malignant tissues using differential hybridization analysis have been successful (Augentlicht and Kobrin, 1982; Yamamoto, 1983; Matrisian *et al*, 1986).

For metastasis, however, few reports are available on the use of this technique to identify genes that are upregulated or downmodulated during this process. Most publications on this topic report only on downregulation of genes during progression. Our group identified fibronectin as being downmodulated in prostatic cancer cells (Schalken *et al*, 1988). Yet another gene, *NM23*, was downregulated in melanoma cells with low metastatic capacity (Steeg *et al*, 1988). *WDNM1* and *WDNM2* are genes downregulated in metastatic mammary adenocarcinoma (Dear *et al*, 1988, 1989). These results indicate that, as in tumorigenesis, suppressor genes might be involved in metastasis ("metastasis suppressor genes"). Recently, we identified two cDNAs by detecting transcripts overexpressed in metastatic rat prostate cancers (Bussemakers *et al*, 1991b). One of these contained long terminal repeat (LTR) like repetitive elements and is most likely not useful for human studies. The other gene appeared to be identical or related to *HMG-I(Y)* (Bussemakers *et al*, 1991a). This codes for a non-histone small nuclear protein presumably implicated in transcription and replication processes. Its overexpression in dedifferentiating cells was reported earlier (Johnson *et al*, 1989). The value as progression marker for prostate cancer needs further investigation.

PERSPECTIVES: NEW TECHNIQUES IN "MOLECULAR UROPATHOLOGY"

The markers described in the previous section may be an aid to the conventional pathological diagnosis of prostate cancer. Some can be used in an immunohistochemical study, an experimental approach used in many laboratories. Others, however, require the use of more state of the art techniques, whose usefulness in a routine setting is not yet established.

Interphase Cytogenetics

Progression markers that can be evaluated for their usefulness in prostate cancer diagnosis are the frequent deletions on chromosomes 10 and 16. Whereas RFLP analysis has few applications in a pathological setting, the so-called interphase cytogenetics does (Hopman *et al*, 1988). In situ hybridization on interphase nuclei, using chromosome specific probes, allows us now to study numerical chromosomal aberrations. Thus, the frequent involvement of chromosomes 9 (loss) and 1 (gain) was studied in a large group of patients with superficial bladder cancer (Hopman *et al*, 1991). Moreover, "chromosome painting", using chromosome specific libraries, may allow the identification of structural chromosomal changes. Unfortunately, chromosome specific probes used for interphase cytogenetics usually recognize the centromeric region of the chromosome but do not detect arm deletions. It is, however, possible to use cosmid clones, thus enabling the analysis of more specific regions for over/underrepresentation in the genome of cancer cells. Owing to the tumour cell heterogeneity in prostate cancers, it is of great importance to define the area of interest. Since it is not yet clear whether reliable in situ interphase cytogenetics (ie on frozen or paraffin sections) will be possible, the nuclei preparations need to be made from pathologically defined sections. The technique, however, is a potentially powerful one for the study of gross genetic aberrations associated with the progression of prostate cancer.

RNA In Situ Hybridization

The progression markers identified by, for instance, differential hybridization analyses are isolated/characterized as cDNA clones. If these represent known genes, antibodies may be available, thus making feasible an immunohistochemical study on the importance for this marker on fresh or stored material. If, however, an unknown gene is thus identified, or if an antibody is not available, RNA in situ hybridization (RISH) can be used to study primary prostate cancers. The use of RISH requires careful tissue handling, since RNA molecules are extremely sensitive to degradation. This aspect of the technique may be an obstacle to its use in (routine) pathology.

Polymerase Chain Reaction

The polymerase chain reaction (PCR) technique is without doubt the most utilized technique in applied molecular biology at the moment. Numerous publications illustrate the potential of this method (for an overview, see Erlich, 1989). It is based on the fact that a small amount of a target sequence can be amplified exponentially using a heat stable DNA polymerase isolated from *Thermus aquaticus* (Erlich, 1989). For a diagnostic approach, one should realize that so far most protocols use nucleic acid preparations obtained from suspensions. If one screens for changes such as deletions or point mutations, an adequate choice of primers is imperative. One major advantage is that the procedure is simple. A disadvantage is that the technique is so sensitive that minor contaminations can interfere with the outcome of the experiment. Moreover, quantification of the amplification is cumbersome.

The recently developed technique, single strand conformation polymorphism PCR, is based on the fact that ssDNA, when run under non-denaturing conditions, will form a secondary conformation that changes in the presence of a point mutation (Orita *et al*, 1989). The various conformations will have a different motility in a non-denaturing gel and can be discriminated accordingly. Similarly, many mutations in the *ras* oncogene were studied (Suzuki *et al*, 1990). If one studies a gene with known hot spots for mutation, this technique will be extremely useful to analyse a large number of patients. The small quantity of RNA necessary for PCR studies further allows the material to be carefully selected (eg by step sectioning). It is therefore likely that PCR based technology will become a routine instrument in molecular uropathological analysis.

SUMMARY

As yet, few molecular markers are available that are likely to be useful in predicting the metastatic potential of prostate cancer cells. The need for such "progression markers" is indicated by the expectation that more localized cancers (ie stage A-2, B-1,2) will be clinically diagnosed in the near future, owing to improvements in diagnostic techniques (eg transrectal ultrasound) and the screening of population groups at risk (males over 50 years old). Few model systems are available for such studies. Animal models are unsuitable for the isolation of monoclonal antibodies that detect epitopes associated with the progression of prostate cancer. Since few cell lines are available, an approach using primary cancer tissue should be undertaken. For the differential hybridization approach described here, the choice of species presents no difficulty, since many DNA sequences are conserved between species. However, no model system fully represents the human situation. Hence, differential hybridization studies using primary prostate cancer tissue need to be considered. Moreover, the group of genes/proteins with potential relevance for cancer progression (eg oncogenes, tumour suppressor genes, genes encoding cell adhesion molecules or growth factors) has not been studied extensively in prostate cancer. Because of the intrinsic heterogeneity of prostate tumours, the use of pathologically defined tissue sections is imperative for a reliable study. This could be achieved either by in situ techniques (whereby tissue morphology is conserved) or by step sectioning. The difficulties associated with the small amount of material obtained from such sections can be overcome by the use of techniques based on the polymerase chain reaction. Taking these considerations into account, a systematic screening of prostate cancer with probes representing the above mentioned genes should be undertaken.

References

Almendral JM, Sommer D, MacDonald-Bravo H, Burckhardt J, Perera J and Bravo R (1988) Complexity of the early genetic response to growth factors in mouse fibroblasts. *Molecular and Cellular Biology* **8** 2140–2148

Atkin NB and Baker MC (1985a) Chromosome study of five cancers of the prostate. *Human Genetics* **70** 359–364

Atkin NB and Baker MC (1985b) Chromosome 10 deletion in carcinoma of the prostate. *New England Journal of Medicine* **312** 315

Augentlicht LH and Kobrin D (1982) Cloning and screening of sequences expressed in a mouse colon tumor. *Cancer Research* **42** 1088–1093

Baker SJ, Fearon ER, Nigro JM *et al* (1989) Chromosome 17 deletions and p53 mutations in colorectal carcinomas. *Science* **244** 217–221

Bander NH (1987) Monoclonal antibodies: state of the art. *Journal of Urology* **137** 603–612

Britten RJ, Graham DE and Neufeld BR (1974) Analysis of repeating sequences by reassociation, In: Grossman L and Moldave K (eds). *Methods in Enzymology* vol 29E pp 363–406, Academic Press, New York

Brothman AR, Peehl DM, Patel AM and McNeal JE (1990) Frequency and pattern of karyotypic abnormalities in human prostate cancer. *Cancer Research* **50** 3795–3803

Bussemakers MJG, Van de Ven WJM, Debruyne FMJ and Schalken JA (1991a) Identification of high mobility group protein I(Y) as a potential marker for prostate cancer by differential hybridization analysis. *Cancer Research* **51** 606–611

Bussemakers MJG, Isaacs JT, Debruyne FMJ, Van de Ven WJM and Schalken JA (1991b) Oncogene expression in prostate cancer. *World Journal of Urology* **9** 58–63

Buttyan R, Sawczuk IS, Benson MC, Siegal JD and Olsson CA (1987) Enhanced expression of the c-*myc* proto-oncogene in high grade human prostate cancers. *Prostate* **11** 327–337

Carter BS, Ewing CM, Ward WS *et al* (1990a) Allelic loss of chromosomes 16q and 10q in human prostate cancer. *Proceedings of the National Academy of Sciences of the USA* **87** 8751–8755

Carter BS, Epstein JI and Isaacs WB (1990b) *ras* gene mutations in human prostate cancer. *Cancer Research* **50** 6830–6832

Cooke DB, Quarmby VE, Mickey DD, Isaacs JT and French FS (1988a) Oncogene expression in prostate cancer: Dunning R-3327 rat dorsal prostatic adenocarcinoma system. *Prostate* **13** 263–272

Cooke DB, Quarmby VE, Petrusz P *et al* (1988b) Expression of *ras* proto-oncogenes in the

Dunning R-3327 rat prostatic adenocarcinoma system. *Prostate* **13** 273–288

Dear TN, Ramshaw IA and Kefford RF (1988) Differential expression of a novel gene WDNM1 in nonmetastatic rat mammary adenocarcinoma cells. *Cancer Research* **48** 5203–5209

Dear TN, McDonald DA and Kefford RF (1989) Transcriptional down regulation of a rat gene WDNM2 in metastatic DMBA-8 cells. *Cancer Research* **49** 5323–5328

Dunning WF (1963) Prostate cancer in the rat. *Monographs of the National Cancer Institute* **12** 351–369

Erlich HA (ed) (1989) *PCR Technology: Principles and Applications for DNA Amplification.* Stockton Press, New York

Fan K (1988) Heterogeneous subpopulations of human prostatic adenocarcinoma cells: potential usefulness of p21 as a predictor for bone metastasis. *Journal of Urology* **139** 318–322

Fearon ER, Cho KR, Nigro JM *et al* (1990) Identification of a chromosome 18q gene that is altered in colorectal carcinomas. *Science* **247** 49–56

Feinberg A and Vogelstein B (1983) A technique for radiolabeling DNA restriction endonuclease fragments to high specific activity. *Analytical Biochemistry* **132** 6–13

Hopman AHN, Ramaekers FCS, Raap AK *et al* (1988) In situ hybridisation as a tool to study numerical chromosomal aberration in solid bladder tumors. *Histochemistry* **89** 307–316

Hopman AHN, Moesker O, Smeets AWGB, Pauwels RPE, Vooijs GP and Ramaekers FCS (1991) Numerical chromosome 1 7 9 and 11 aberrations in bladder cancer detected by *in situ* hybridisation. *Cancer Research* **51** 644–651

Johnson KR, Lehn DA and Reeves R (1989) Alternative processing of mRNAs encoding mamalian high-mobility-group proteins HMG-1 and HMG-Y. *Molecular and Cellular Biology* **9** 2114–2123

Kartasova T, Cornelissen BJC, Belt P and Van de Putte P (1987) Effect of UV 4-NQO and TPA on gene expression in cultured human epidermal keratinocytes. *Nucleic Acids Research* **15** 5945–5962

Kohler G and Milstein G (1975) Continuous cultures of fused cells secreting antibody of predefined specificity. *Nature* **265** 493–495

Lau LF and Nathans D (1985) Identification of a set of genes expressed during G0/G1 transition of cultured mouse cells. *EMBO Journal* **4** 3145–3151

Lau LF and Nathans D (1987) Expression of a set of growth related immediate early genes in Balc/c 3T3 cells: coordinate regulation with c-*fos* or c-*myc*. *Proceedings of the National Academy of Sciences of the USA* **84** 1182–1186

Lepor H, Ross A and Walsh PC (1982) The influence of hormonal therapy on survival of men with advanced prostatic cancer. *Journal of Urology* **128** 335–340

Lindgren J, Pak KY, Ernst C, Rovera G, Steplewski Z and Koprowski H (1985) Shared antigens of human prostate cancer cell lines as defined by monoclonal antibodies. *Hybridoma* **4** 37–45

Lizumi T, Yazaki T, Kanoh S, Kondo I and Koiso K (1987) Establishment of a new prostatic carcinoma cell line (TSU-Pr1). *Journal of Urology* **137** 1304–1306

Matrisian LM, Bowden GT, Kriegg P *et al* (1986) The mRNA coding for the secreted protease transin is expressed more abundantly in malignant than in benign tumors. *Proceedings of the National Academy of Sciences of the USA* **83** 9413–9417

Orita M, Suzuki Y, Sekiya T and Hayashi K (1989) Rapid and sensitive detection of point mutations and DNA polymorphisms using the polymerase chain reaction. *Genomics* **5** 874–879

Peehl DM, Wehner N and Stamey TA (1987) An activated Ki-*ras* oncogene in human prostatic adenocarcinoma. *Prostate* **10** 281–289

Sargent TD (1987) Isolation of differentially expressed genes, In: Berger SL and Kimmel AR (eds). *Methods in Enzymology,* vol 152 pp 423–432, Academic Press, New York

Schalken JA, Ebeling SB, Isaacs JT *et al* (1988) Down modulation of fibronectin mRNA in metastasizing rat prostatic cancer cells revealed by differential hybridization analysis. *Cancer Research* **48** 2042–2048

Scott WW, Menon M and Walsh PC (1980) Hormonal therapy of prostatic cancer. *Cancer* **45**

1929–1936

Shervin DH, Gorny KI and Kukreja SC (1989) Patterns of metastasis by the human prostate cancer cell line PC-3 in athymic nude mice. *Prostate* **15** 187–194

Smits HL, Floyd EE and Jetten AM (1987) Molecular cloning of gene sequences regulated during squamous differentiation of tracheal epithelial cells and controlled by retinoic acid. *Molecular and Cellular Biology* **7** 4017–4023

Starling JJ, Sieg MS, Beckett ML, Schellhammer PF, Ladaga LE, and Wright GL Jr (1982) Monoclonal antibodies to human prostate and bladder tumor-associated antigens. *Cancer Research* **42** 3084–3089

Starling JJ, Sieg SM, Beckett ML *et al* (1986) Human prostate tissue antigens defined by murine monoclonal antibodies. *Cancer Research* **46** 367–374

Steeg PS, Bevilacqua GB, Kopper L *et al* (1988) Evidence for a novel gene associated with low tumor metastatic potential. *Journal of the National Cancer Institute* **80** 200–204

Sumiya H, Masai MN, Akimoto S, Yatani R and Shimazaki J (1990) Histochemical examination of expression of *ras* p21 protein and R1881 binding protein in human prostatic cancers. *European Journal of Cancer* **7** 786–789

Suzuki Y, Orita M, Shiraishi M, Hayashi K and Sekiya T (1990) Detection of ras gene mutations in human lung cancers by single-strand conformation analysis of polymerase chain reaction products. *Oncogene* **5** 1037–1043

Travis GH and Sutcliffe JG (1988) Phenol emulsion enhanced driven subtractive cDNA cloning: Isolation of low abundance monkey cortex specific mRNAs. *Proceedings of the National Academy of Sciences of the USA* **85** 1696–1700

Treiger B and Isaacs JT (1988) Expression of a transfected v-Ha-ra oncogene in a Dunning rat prostatic adenocarcinoma and the development of high metastatic ability. *Journal of Urology* **140** 1580–1583

Van der Kwast TH, Schalken JA, Ruizeveld de Winter JA *et al* (1991) Androgen receptors in endocrine therapy resistant human prostate cancer. *International Journal of Cancer* **48** 189–193

Viola MV, Fromowitz F, Oravez S *et al* (1986) Expression of *ras* oncogene p21 in prostate cancer. *New England Journal of Medicine* **314** 133–137

Webb KS, Paulson DF, Parks SF, Tuck FL, Walther PJ and Ware JL (1984) Characterization of prostate tissue directed monoclonal antibody: alpha-Pro 13 *Cancer Immunology and Immunotherapy* **17** 7–17

Yamamoto M, Maehara Y, Takahashi K and Endo H (1983) Cloning of sequences expressed specifically in tumors of rat. *Proceedings of the National Academy of Sciences USA* **80** 7524–7527

Young BD and Anderson MLM (1985) Quantitative analysis of solution hybridisation, In: Hames BD and Higgins SJ (eds). *Nucleic Acid Hybridization; a practical approach*, pp 47–71, IRL Press, Oxford

Yunis Y (1983) Chromosomal basis of neoplasia. *Science* **221** 335–340

The authors are responsible for the accuracy of the references.

Experimental Oncogene Induced Prostate Cancer

T C THOMPSON[1,2,3] • D KADMON[1,3] • T L TIMME[1,3] • V W MERZ[1,3]
S EGAWA[1,3] • T KREBS[1,3] • P T SCARDINO[1] • S H PARK[1,3]

[1]*Scott Department of Urology,* [2]*Department of Cell Biology, Baylor College of Medicine, Houston, Texas 77030;* [3]*Urology Research Laboratory, Veterans Affairs Medical Center, Houston, Texas 77030*

INTRODUCTION: RELEVANCE AND UTILITY OF THE MOUSE PROSTATE RECONSTITUTION MODEL TO HUMAN PROSTATE CANCER

Important Questions in Prostate Cancer

Prostate cancer represents a serious and increasing medical problem in much of the western world (reviewed in Carter and Coffey, 1990). This malignant disease is particularly worrisome in the USA where it is now the most common form of cancer and the second leading cause of cancer deaths in males (Carter and Coffey, 1990; Carter BS *et al,* 1990a). These alarming statistics combined with an expanding population at risk for the disease have created the impression that prostate cancer should be of special concern with respect to investigative efforts of both the clinical course of the disease and the molecular and cellular mechanisms implicated in its progression. For the greatest clinical impact of research efforts, it is beneficial to address specific areas where additional information would help in clinical decisions and contribute to the development of more rational therapy. We have formulated three general questions that define specific areas of investigation which we regard as of particular importance in prostate cancer.

1. What are the mechanisms responsible for genetic differences in the rate of progression?
2. What are the molecular events associated with progression?
3. What is the molecular basis for selection and/or adaptation following castration?

What are the mechanisms responsible for genetic differences in the rate of progression? In view of the dearth of molecular information about prostate cancer and the intrinsic complexity and lack of understanding of genetic predisposition to cancer in general, to answer this question is a formidable task. However, the importance of new information in this area is obvious. The natural history of prostate cancer represents an intriguing variation of the multistep process of carcinogenesis (McNeal, 1969; Whitmore, 1984; Scardino, 1989; Carter and Coffey, 1990; Carter BS *et al*, 1990a; Carter HB *et al*, 1990). Histological analyses of many necropsy specimens throughout the world have revealed a class of small sized subclinical prostate cancers (reviewed in Carter and Coffey, 1990; Carter BS *et al*, 1990a; Carter HB *et al*, 1990; Whitmore, 1990). These lesions, often referred to as latent or incidental prostate cancer, are very common, affecting nearly one-third of all men over the age of 50. Curiously, the number of new cases of clinically manifest prostate cancer (about 100 000 cases per year in the USA) represents only a small fraction of latent prostate cancer. This discrepancy indicates that life threatening prostate cancer results from low frequency progression of the common small sized, but clinically insignificant, form of the disease and not the inexorable progression of most small tumours. Interestingly, both genetic and environmental factors seem to be associated with the frequency of conversion of latent to clinically significant prostate cancer. Although most studies suggest that the prevalence of latent prostate cancer discovered at necropsy is similar in all countries and across different racial groups, the incidence of and mortality from clinically important prostatic cancer differ greatly (Franks, 1954; Akazaki and Stemmermann, 1973; Breslow *et al*, 1977; Yatani *et al*, 1982; reviewed in Carter and Coffey, 1990; Carter BS *et al*, 1990a; Meikle and Smith, 1990). In addition, familial aggregation of prostate cancer has been clearly documented in several studies (Gianferrari *et al*, 1956; Morganti *et al*, 1956; Wool, 1960; Cannon *et al*, 1983; Meikle *et al*, 1985; Steinberg *et al*, 1990; reviewed in Carter BS *et al*, 1990a). Overall, the clinical data suggest that the rate limiting step for the development of clinically important prostate cancer involves the ability of the malignant cell to overcome an apparent biological equilibrium with respect to normal surrounding tissue and that the rate of this process is determined by the complex superimposition of heritable and environmental factors. The clinical importance of identifying the genes responsible for genetic predisposition to prostate cancer is apparent.

What are the molecular events associated with progression? Which events promote progression? How do they do it? Presuming that the transition from latent to clinical prostate cancer represents specific genetic alterations, the identification of these genetic alterations or related abnormalities in gene expression, in addition to providing an understanding of the molecular mechanism of the disease, could reveal important clinical tools. As has been documented in colon carcinoma (reviewed in Fearon and Vogelstein, 1990), specific genetic alterations progressively accumulate, leading to increasingly advanced carcinomas. Such genetic changes, including both the acquisition of dominant transforming oncogenes and the loss of growth suppressor genes, have in some cases been resolved at the molecular level (eg *ras* and *p53*), but many putative growth suppressor genes have been detected only as a loss of specific chromosomal regions. In human prostate cancer, activated oncogenes and raised proto-oncogene activities (eg *ras* and *myc*) have been detected (reviewed in Thompson, 1990). Early studies also show that allelic loss is a common event in prostate cancer, and therefore the loss of growth suppressor genes is probably implicated in the progression of the disease (Brothman *et al,* 1990; Carter BS *et al,* 1990c). Studies demonstrating the loss of retinoblastoma gene expression in human prostate cancer and suppression of tumorigenicity of human prostate carcinoma cells by replacing a mutated retinoblastoma gene support this notion (Bookstein *et al,* 1990a,b). In general, however, there is no consensus about the predominant genetic alterations in the progression of prostate cancer. Although it is possible that the acquisition of specific dominantly acting oncogenes or the loss of specific growth suppressor genes is not consistently associated with the development of prostate cancer, other activities such as the expression of specific growth factors and their receptors may represent the culmination of diverse sets of genetic alterations and thus prove to be more common than specific genetic alterations, particularly in the early stages of the disease. These specific growth factor activities may provide clinically useful markers.

What is the molecular basis for selection and/or adaptation following castration? Castration therapy is used widely to induce a temporary remission of advanced prostate cancer (Catalona and Scott, 1986). The success of castration therapy even in such a limited capacity has generated considerable interest and spawned much clinical and basic research. The focus of many clinical studies has been the development of more complete androgen ablation with the view to extend remission of the disease. So far, this approach has resulted in tangible but limited success (Crawford *et al,* 1989; Gittes, 1991). Basic research has focused mainly on understanding the exquisite sensitivity of the prostate to androgens with respect to growth and cytodifferentiation as well as possible molecular and cellular mechanisms by which prostate cancer cells continue to progress in an androgen depleted environment. The castrated male rat model (Coffey and Williams-Ashman, 1968) has provided important information about the androgenic regulation of specific genes. Steady state mRNA levels for transforming growth factor-β1 (TGF-β1) (Kyprianou and Isaacs, 1989), c-*myc* (Quarmby *et al*, 1987; Buttyan *et al*, 1988) and c-*fos* (Buttyan *et al*, 1988) are strikingly increased in the normal rat ventral prostate following castration. This mRNA accumulation either precedes or directly coincides with the loss of luminal epithelial cells, which is known to occur as an active programme of cell death (Buttyan *et al*, 1988; Kyprianou and Isaacs, 1988). In one study of the effects of castration on androgen responsive PC-82 human prostatic adenocarcinoma xenografts, it was shown that TGF-β1 mRNA levels were raised in carcinomas grown in castrated nude mice (Kyprianou *et al*, 1990). Since this study also showed that widespread apoptosis was induced in cancer cells after castration and that this cytopathology accompanied increased TGF-β1 expression, a close parallel between this androgen responsive prostate cancer and normal rat prostate was established. Interestingly, raised c-*myc* mRNA levels are also found in human prostate cancer (Fleming *et al*, 1986; Buttyan *et al*, 1987), and increased TGF-β1 mRNA is associated with experimentally induced mouse prostate cancer (Merz *et al*, 1991). Although the relation between androgen regulated gene expression and the therapeutic effects of androgen ablation on human prostate cancer is not clear, it is possible that castration induced gene expression is implicated in recurrent prostate cancer.

Two possible mechanisms could explain clinical relapse in most prostate cancer patients who initially respond to hormone ablation: (a) the selection and expansion of androgen insensitive clones and (b) the adaptation of androgen sensitive cells to an androgen depleted environment (Isaacs and Coffey, 1981; Isaacs *et al*, 1982). Evidence for clonal selection is substantial but indirect, involving the use of DNA ploidy analysis and/or growth kinetics as markers for distinct clonal subtypes (Isaacs *et al*, 1982). Part of the difficulty in identifying the mechanism(s) in the continuation of initially steroid sensitive tumour growth following hormone ablation is the use of growth exclusively in defining hormone sensitivity and the possibility that both clonal selection and adaptive changes occur simultaneously. Further progress in understanding recurrent prostate cancer may require the experimental separation of clonal selection from adaptation within the context of prostate cancer cells. By studying each process separately, unambiguous, clinically relevant information may emerge.

Mouse Prostate Reconstitution: Conceptual Considerations, Technical Aspects, Advantages and Applications

Initial investigations of the molecular and cellular mechanisms that underlie the initiation and progression of prostate cancer suggested the involvement of various polypeptide growth factors, dominantly acting oncogenes and loss of growth suppressor functions (reviewed in Thompson, 1990). Substantial amounts of growth factors from the fibroblast growth factor and TGF-β families, as well as TGF-α and epidermal growth factor, along with their cognate receptors, are found in normal prostate. Androgenic steroids seem to regulate the expression of some of these growth factors and growth factor receptors and may induce growth and differentiation via these pathways. Raised proto-oncogene and activated oncogene activities have been detected in human prostate cancer—predominantly increased expression of *myc* (Fleming *et al*, 1986; Buttyan *et al*, 1987) and, to a lesser extent, expression of activated *ras* (Peehl *et al*, 1987; Carter BS *et al*, 1990b). Important cell-cell interactions must also be considered when both normal and abnormal prostate growth is analysed. Specifically, mesenchymal-epithelial interactions clearly underlie the initial growth and morphogenesis of the gland and seem to play a part in homeostasis in the mature prostate.

In addition to the known molecular and cellular biology of the normal prostate and of prostate cancer, the salient features of tumorigenesis as it occurs in vivo should also be considered in models of prostate cancer. The initiating molecular alterations (eg somatic mutations) occur in single or very few cells surrounded by tissue that is otherwise normal. This important feature in the early dynamics of prostate carcinogenesis may be the critical, rate limiting step in view of the disparity between the incidence of latent and clinically manifest prostate cancer. It follows from these observations that paracrine activities are implicated in overcoming the natural barriers to the malignant growth of transformed prostate epithelial cells. Thus, perturbation of the normal spatial and organizational barrier, perhaps by the inappropriate or increased expression of growth modulators, acting in a paracrine fashion, may be a critical element of progression in human prostate cancer and must therefore be accommodated in relevant models for the disease.

To investigate the mechanisms of progression in prostate cancer, we designed a mouse model system that incorporates the current understanding of human prostate cancer and many of the important elements of tumorigenesis in general (Thompson *et al*, 1989). In developing the mouse prostate reconstitution (MPR) model, we exploited the ability of the fetal mouse urogenital sinus (UGS) to undergo morphogenesis and differentiation into mature prostate after grafting under the renal capsule of adult isogenic male hosts (Cunha *et al*, 1983; Neubauer *et al*, 1983; Thompson *et al*, 1986; Mills *et al*, 1987). Exogenous genes were introduced into dissociated UGS cells (both urogenital sinus mesenchyme [UGM] derived mesenchymal cells and urogenital sinus epithelium [UGE] derived epithelial cells) with defective recombinant retrovirus stocks devoid of detectable amounts of replication competent helper viruses (Thompson *et al*, 1989). After transfer of the cells into a collagen matrix and overnight incubation in vitro, MPRs are grafted under the renal capsule. Morphogenesis and functional differentiation are achieved in both mock infected and non-oncogenic virus infected MPRs after 4 weeks growth. Initial studies with retroviruses that contain either the v-Ha-*ras* or the v-*gagmyc* (MC29) oncogenes alone showed that the *ras* oncogene induces a grossly dysplastic phenotype with a strong angiogenesis component in the mesenchymal compartment and a focally hyperplastic phenotype in the epithelial compartment. The *myc* oncogene alone induced predominantly focal epithelial hyperplasia. The *ras* and *myc* oncogenes introduced in combination via a single retrovirus, *Zipras/myc*9, induced predominantly carcinomas (Thompson *et al*, 1989).

To investigate the mechanisms of progression in prostate cancer, we have modified the MPR model system. The expanded MPR model system offers unique experimental advantages. The possibility of introducing genes specifically into the epithelial compartment while leaving the adjacent mesenchyme unaltered presents an opportunity to study the direct effects of transforming genes on the epithelium under conditions where the mesenchymal cells are either normal or also transformed. This approach also allows for the study of paracrine activities implicated in carcinogenesis under in vivo conditions (Merz *et al*, 1991). It is also possible to manipulate the ratio of transformed to normal cells by use of retroviral supernatants of various titres. These indices are critical for creating in vivo conditions that mimic the rare initiating events of tumorigenesis such as somatic mutations. This model system also facilitates the analysis of multiple experiments sufficient for statistical analysis. This potential, combined with the biological property of retroviruses to integrate essentially "at random" into the genome of target cells, validates the use of this model to study discrete oncogene specific phenotypic alterations superimposed onto various genetic backgrounds.

The properties of the MPR model are well suited to address important questions in prostate cancer. Organ specific localization of cancer inducing oncogenes and the potential for multiple independent experiments over short time periods offer considerable advantage for experimental studies of genetic differences in the progression of prostate cancer. The restricted introduction of cancer inducing oncogenes into prostate mesenchyme and epithelium allows for the analysis of important paracrine activities involved in malignant disease. In addition, the ability to create primary prostate cancers, determine their clonal status by the analysis of unique virus-cell DNA junction fragments and transplant the cancer cells into both normal intact and castrated hosts is a novel approach for studying the response of prostate cancer to androgen deprivation.

INVESTIGATION OF THE MECHANISMS OF PROGRESSION IN ONCOGENE INDUCED PROSTATE CANCER USING THE MOUSE PROSTATE RECONSTITUTION MODEL

Genetic Factors in the Progression of Prostate Cancer

The initial studies that reported *ras+myc* induced carcinogenesis with the mouse prostate reconstitution model system were carried out with tissues obtained from inbred C57BL/tan mice (Thompson *et al*, 1989). This strain is a coat colour variant of C57BL/6 isolated in London in 1958 and subsequently maintained as an inbred mouse strain (Rowlatt *et al*, 1969). Present studies are being carried out with inbred C57BL/6 and Balb/c strains. Two Moloney murine leukaemia virus based retroviral vectors, BAGα (Price *et al*, 1987) as a non-oncogenic control virus and *Zipras/myc*9 (Thompson *et al*, 1989), which carries both the v-Ha-*ras* and the v-*gagmyc* oncogenes, were used to explore the possibility that the C57BL/6 mouse and the Balb/c mouse respond differently from the *ras+myc* tumour induction protocol. Defective retrovirus stocks produced with ψ-2 cells (Mann *et al*, 1983) were tested for the presence of helper virus with a highly sensitive assay (Rowe *et al*, 1970) before use.

Total UGS cells obtained from both C57BL/6 and Balb/c fetuses were infected with high titre ($>10^5$ colony or focus forming units/ml) BAGα or *Zipras/myc*9 supernatants reconstituted together in collagen, grafted into isogenic adult male hosts and allowed to grow in vivo for 4 weeks. The phenotypic alterations induced by the *ras* and *myc* oncogenes were examined by haematoxylin and eosin and immunohistochemical staining of sections from fixed, paraffin embedded tissues (Fig. 1). BAGα infected MPRs derived from both C57BL/6 (Fig. 1A) and Balb/c tissues (not shown) demonstrated normal prostate morphology. *Zipras/myc*9 infected MPRs produced profoundly different, strain specific phenotypic alterations. Rapidly growing, poorly differentiated adenocarcinomas were seen in greater than 90% of individual experiments with *Zipras/myc*9 infected C57BL/6 MPRs (Fig. 1B and see Table 1). In contrast, the same protocol produced predominantly non-malignant focal hyperplasias with the Balb/c strain (Fig. 1C and see Table 1). One of the hyperplastic Balb/c MPRs contained a focus that was morphologically atypical and resembled a premalignant condition (Fig. 1D). In one exceptional case, a poorly differentiated malignant carcinoma was produced as a result of *Zipras/myc*9 infection (see Table 1). This carcinoma was morphologically indistinguishable from C57BL/6 carcinomas (see Fig. 1B) shown previously to be remarkably similar in all cases (Merz *et al*, 1991). The *ras+myc* induced Balb/c carcinoma was also positive for cytokeratin expression (data not shown), demonstrating a pattern that was also characteristic of *ras+myc* induced C57BL/6 carcinomas (Merz *et al*, 1991).

It was possible to compare the proportion of UGS cells that could be initially infected in control BAGα infections of C57BL/6 versus Balb/c by the analysis of β-galactosidase positive cells in histological sections of MPRs harvested 48–72 hours postgrafting (Thompson *et al*, 1989). In total UGS infections with C57BL/6 as well as Balb/c tissues, positive β-galactosidase staining was seen in about 0.1% of the cells. These values are in agreement with results from previous studies with C57BL/tan mice (Thompson *et al*, 1989). Positive staining was never seen in normal mouse prostate or mock infected MPR tissue sections included as controls.

Taken together, these studies suggest genetic differences in susceptibility to *ras+myc* induced carcinogenesis in the reconstituted mouse prostate model. Experiments in progress may well answer many critical questions that remain with respect to the apparent strain specific response shown here. Hopefully, the MPR model can be used to derive information that will be clinically useful

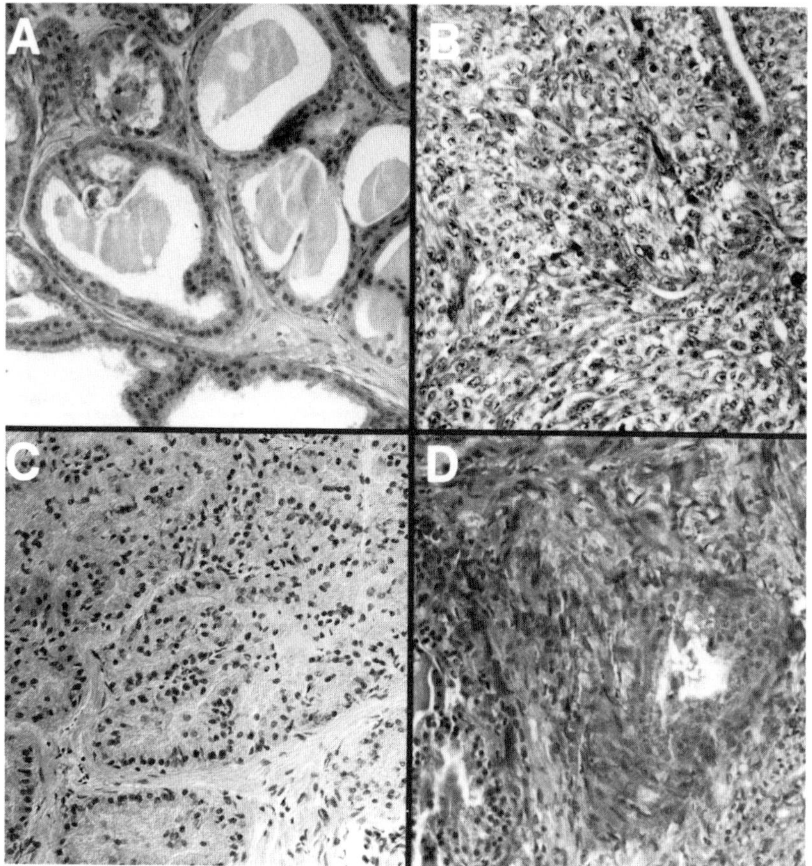

Fig. 1. Morphological characterization of *ras+myc* induced MPRs derived from C57BL/6 and Balb/c tissues. (A) Control BAGα infected C57BL/6 MPR. Note the presence of well formed prostatic acini with smooth luminal surfaces and abundant prostatic secretions. Haematoxylin and eosin (H&E) × 250. Results of BAGα infected Balb/c MPRs were similar (not shown). (B) Anaplastic carcinoma induced by *ras+myc* infection of UGS derived from C57BL/6. Note the lack of glandular organization and the presence of nuclear pleomorphism. H&E × 250. (C) Hyperplasia induced by *ras+myc* infection of UGS derived from Balb/c. Note the presence of intraluminal epithelial proliferation without evidence of malignancy. H&E × 250. (D) Focal dysplasia induced by *ras+myc* infection of UGS derived from Balb/c. Note the extension of hyperplastic epithelial cells. H&E × 250

in distinguishing those at higher risk of developing rapidly progressing, clinically important prostate cancer.

Transforming Growth Factor-β and Malignancy

In the expanded MPR model, C57BL/6 mice were used for compartment restricted infection of enzymatically dissociated total UGS or isolated UGE with high titre BAGα or *Zipras/myc*9 supernatants (Merz *et al*, 1991). The

TABLE 1. Comparative summary of *ras* + *myc* activities in reconstituted mouse prostate derived from C57BL/6 and Balb/c tissues

Virus	Strain	No.	Phenotype
BAGα	C57BL/6	36	36 normal
BAGα	Balb/c	25	25 normal
*Zipras/myc*9	C57BL/6	31	29 carcinomas 1 focal epithelial hyperplasia 1 normal
*Zipras/myc*9	Balb/c	19	18 focal epithelial hyperplasia 1 carcinoma

For each organ reconstitution, 1.5×10^6 UGS cells were infected with high titre retrovirus stocks (1×10^6 to 3×10^6 colony or focus forming units/ml) at a multiplicity that did not exceed 1. Phenotypic alterations were evaluated hematoxylin/eosin stained tissue sections, and carcinomas were verified by positive cytokeratin staining in >95% of the cell population

phenotypic alterations induced by the compartmentalized activities of the *ras* and *myc* oncogenes were examined (see Table 2). BAGα infected total UGS MPRs demonstrated normal prostate morphology (Fig. 2A). *Zipras/myc*9 infected total UGS MPRs produced rapidly growing, poorly differentiated adenocarcinomas in greater than 90% of individual experiments (Fig. 2C). Immunohistochemical staining with anti-cytokeratin sera showed that every carcinoma examined was positive for cytokeratin expression (not shown). In *Zipras/myc*9 infected UGE MPRs, predominantly non-malignant focal epithelial hyperplasias were seen (see Table 2). These hyperplasias were produced in greater than 90% of individual experiments and were characterized

TABLE 2. Comparative summary of compartmentalized *ras* + *myc* activities in C57BL/6 reconstituted mouse prostate

Virus	No.	UGE	UGM	Phenotype
BAGα	36	+	+	36 normal
*ras/myc*9	31	+	+	29 carcinomas
				1 focal epithelial hyperplasia 1 normal
BAGα	17	+	−	17 normal
*ras/myc*9	17	+	−	15 focal epithelial hyperplasia 1 carcinoma[a] 1 focal carcinoma

The reconstitution protocol and phenotype characterization are described in Table 1. The infected compartments are indicated
[a]Non-invasive towards kidney, hypovascular

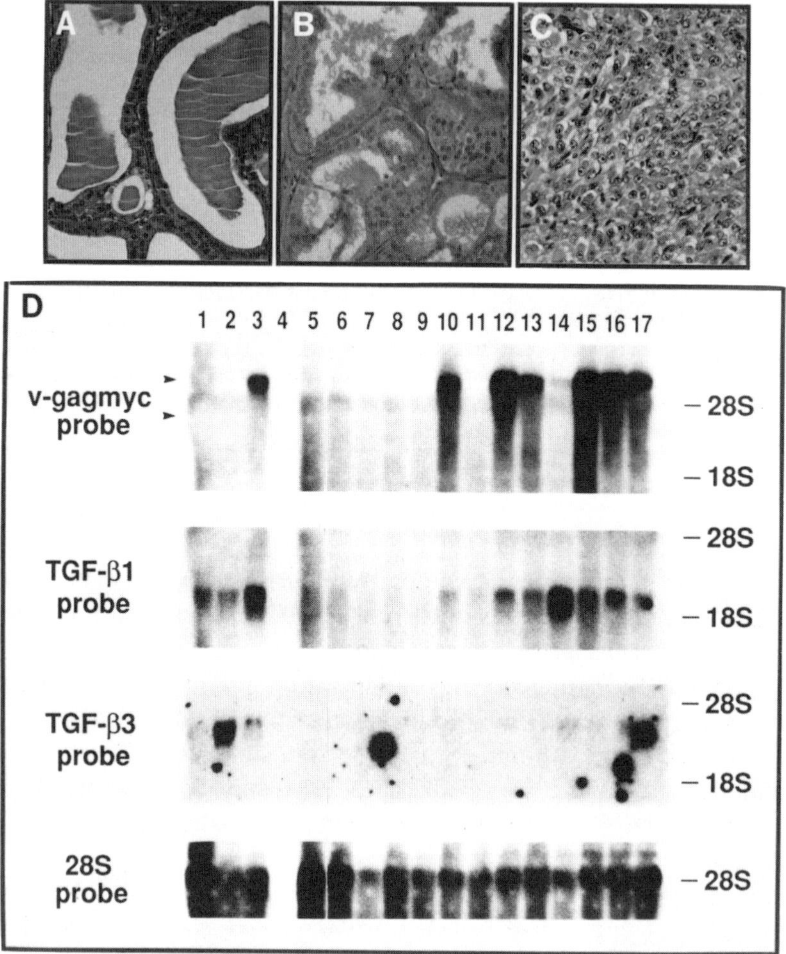

Fig. 2. Morphological characterization and northern analysis of C57BL/6 total (UGE + UGM) and restricted UGE infections. (A–C) H&E stained tissue sections; magnification, ×250. (A) Infection of the total UGS derived from the C57BL/6 mouse with a control (BAGα) retrovirus; (B) infection of the C57BL/6 UGE only with a retrovirus (*Zipras/myc9*) carrying the *myc* and *ras* oncogenes; (C) infection of the C57BL/6 total UGS with the *Zipras/myc9* retrovirus; (D) expression of *Zipras/myc9* virus and endogenous TGF-β1 and TGF-β3 in MPRs. Total cellular RNAs from MPR tissues were analysed by northern analysis, which included sequential probing and stripping with ^{32}P-labelled 28S ribosomal sequences (lower panel), v-*gagmyc* sequences (upper panel), TGF-β1 sequences (second panel from top) and TGF-β3 sequences (second panel from bottom). Samples include normal adult ventral prostate (lane 1), uninfected NIH3T3 cells (lane 2), *Zipras/myc9* infected NIH3T3 cells (lane 3) BAGα infected restricted UGE MPRs (lane 5), BAGα infected total UGS MPRs (lanes 6 and 7), *Zipras/myc9* infected restricted UGE MPRs that produced focal epithelial hyperplasia (lanes 8, 9 and 11), an exceptional case where a malignant carcinoma was produced by *Zipras/myc9* restricted UGE infection (lane 10) and malignant carcinomas produced by total infection with *Zipras/myc9* (lanes 12–17)

by pronounced intraluminal bridging and multilayered epithelium (Fig. 2B). Malignant cells were seen in two *Zipras/myc9* infected UGE MPRs (see Table 2), indicating that these lesions represented premalignant conditions.

We used northern blot analysis to determine if mRNA levels for specific members of the TGF-β family were induced in *Zipras/myc*9 infected total UGS and UGE MPRs. Blots were probed initially with labelled 28S rRNA sequences to ensure comparable loading and transfer (Fig. 2D, bottom panel) and then stripped and reprobed with labelled v-*gagmyc* sequences that detect both the genomic and subgenomic viral RNAs (Fig. 2D, top panel). Viral RNA was not detected in BAGα infected UGE or total UGS MPRs. High levels of virus specific RNAs were seen in all carcinomas from UGS infections with *Zipras/myc*9. High viral RNA levels were also seen in the carcinoma that developed from a *Zipras/myc*9 infected UGE MPR but not in *Zipras/myc*9 infected UGE MPRs that resulted in focally hyperplastic phenotypes. When the blot was stripped and reprobed with labelled TGF-β1 sequences, raised levels were seen only in *Zipras/myc*9 infected total UGS carcinomas (lanes 12–17) and the single case (lane 10) of complete carcinoma that developed from a *Zipras/myc*9 infected UGE MPR. One focal epithelial hyperplasia (lane 11) demonstrates TGF-β1 mRNA levels intermediate to those in carcinomas and those in BAGα infected controls. The pattern of TGF-β3 mRNA levels showed a close correspondence to that of TGF-β1 and supports a positive correlation of raised TGF-β1 and TGF-β3 mRNA levels with the transition from a hyperplastic to a malignant phenotype.

The role of TGF-β1 in carcinogenesis is complex. Transforming growth factor-β1 is generally thought to inhibit the growth of normal epithelial cells (Moses *et al*, 1985; Roberts *et al*, 1985). Although cultured malignant epithelial cells secrete TGF-β1, it appears that in most cases, malignant cell lines have lost their responsiveness to TGF-β1. Curiously, a recent study has shown that under some conditions, TGF-β1 can stimulate the growth of transformed rat prostate epithelial cells (Shain *et al*, 1990). Although it has been argued that an abrogation of growth inhibition by TGF-β1 could result in an exaggerated growth response to other mitogenic factors, this type of reasoning would not lead to the conclusion that increased levels of TGF-β1 would further enhance proliferative responses. However, biological activities of TGF-β1, other than those involved directly in cell growth, might be able to provide a selective advantage to the *ras+myc* initiated prostatic epithelial cells. Some of the known biological activities of TGF-β1 may directly influence the transformed epithelial cell towards a more malignant phenotype. For example, TGF-β1 has been shown under specific conditions to promote angiogenesis (Roberts *et al*, 1986), enhance cell motility (Myrdal *et al*, 1986), induce stromal cell proliferation (Moses *et al*, 1985; Roberts *et al*, 1985, 1986), increase extracellular matrix deposition (Ignotz and Massagué, 1986; Roberts *et al*, 1986) and regulate the expression of genes implicated in the turnover of the extracellular matrix (reviewed in Rizzino, 1988; Mummery and van den Eijnden-van Raaji, 1990). It can be argued that all of these activities may support morphogenesis and differentiation within the context of normal development or alternatively support the invasive behaviour and sustained growth of cancer.

Recent studies showing that TGF-β1 is permissive for the development of tumours in Rous sarcoma virus infected chickens (Sieweke *et al*, 1990) and that TGF-β1 can directly increase the invasive and metastatic potential of a mammary adenocarcinoma cell line (Welch *et al*, 1990) support a role for TGF-β1 in malignant progression.

Response of Prostate Cancer to Androgen Ablation

To establish a clonal prostate adenocarcinoma, we infected dissociated C57BL/6 UGS with helper virus free *Zipras/myc*9 at high titres (>10^5 focus forming units/ml). The tumour was recovered after an 8-week, rather than a 4-week, growth period in isogenic intact adult male hosts. Two small (3 mm^3) pieces obtained from different quadrants of the primary tumour were grafted subcutaneously into intact male hosts (one piece per animal), and the tumours were allowed to grow for an additional 2 weeks. After this growth period when the tumours had achieved substantial size, one tumour was recovered and quickly frozen in liquid nitrogen for further isolation of DNA and RNA. The other tumour was reduced to a single cell suspension and inoculated subcutaneously into the flank area of both intact and castrated (7 days post-surgery) adult male hosts. Three weeks after inoculation, growth was similar in the intact and castrated groups, indicating that the tumour was not dependent on androgens (data not shown). Haematoxylin/eosin staining confirmed that all of the carcinomas were pleomorphic, anaplastic tumours, similar to those analysed previously (see Fig. 1B) and positive for cytokeratin expression.

Integration patterns of *Zipras/myc*9 proviruses in multiple tumour DNAs showed that the carcinoma cell populations of both the intact and castrated groups were the progeny of the same *Zipras/myc*9 infected cell (data not shown). These results suggest that subsequent analysis of gene expression may reflect responsive/adaptive changes in the hormonal environment within a clonal cell population. Alternatively, patterns of gene expression specific to the castrated group may reflect unique properties of selected androgen insensitive cells. It is also possible that responsive changes to hormones as well as selection are involved, ie cells capable of responsive/adaptive changes are selected in an androgen depleted environment.

RNAs extracted from tumours recovered after 3 weeks growth in intact and castrated hosts were analysed by northern blotting. Representative data are shown in Fig. 3. The filter was probed initially with 28S ribosomal sequences followed by sequential stripping and probing with cDNA fragments specific for TGF-β1 and TGF-β3. Transforming growth factor-β1 mRNA levels in carcinomas grown in castrated hosts were increased about twofold compared with those grown in intact animals. A prominent species of about 2.5 kb was detected. Transforming growth factor-β3 was detected as a single band of approximately 3.5 kb. The pattern of expression of TGF-β3 was similar to that of TGF-β1, showing an increase in mRNA levels of about twofold. The complexity of TGF-β activity in carcinogenesis is further supported by Fig. 3

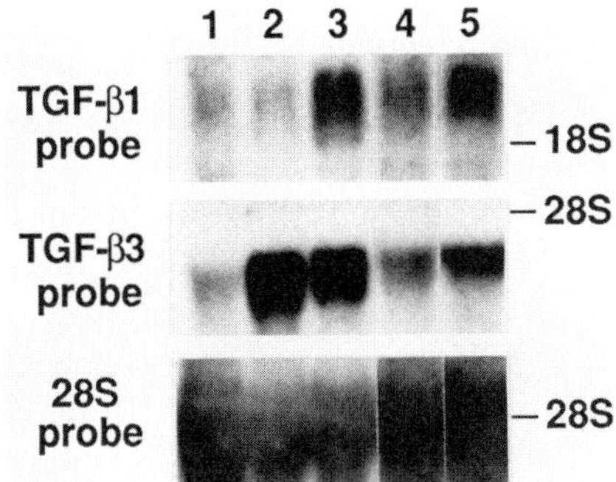

Fig. 3. Northern analysis of clonal *ras+myc* induced C57BL/6 carcinomas after castration therapy. Expression of endogenous TGF-β1 and TGF-β3 in *ras+myc* induced C57BL/6 carcinomas grown subcutaneously in normal, intact or castrated male hosts. Total cellular RNAs from carcinomas were analysed by northern analysis, which included sequential probing and stripping with ^{32}P-labelled 28S ribosomal sequences (lower panel), TGF-β1 sequences (upper panel) and TGF-β3 sequences (middle panel). Samples include normal adult C57BL/6 ventral prostate (lane 1), uninfected NIH3T3 cells (lane 2), *Zipras/myc9* infected NIH3T3 cells (lane 3), clonal *ras+myc* induced carcinomas grown in normal intact male hosts (lane 4) and clonal *ras+myc* induced carcinomas grown in castrated male hosts (lane 5)

(as well as Fig. 2D), which demonstrates an interesting effect on expression of TGF-β1 and TGF-β3 in *Zipras/myc9* infected NIH3T3 cells. Transformation of NIH3T3 cells increases the levels of TGF-β1 mRNAs but decreases the expression of TGF-β3 (cf. lanes 2 and 3 in Fig. 3).

The castration induced increase in TGF-β1 expression in *ras+myc* induced carcinomas parallels previous results in castration induced, involuting normal rat ventral prostate and regressing human prostate cancer xenografts (Kyprianou and Isaacs, 1989; Kyprianou *et al*, 1990). In these studies, steady state TGF-β1 mRNA levels increased concomitantly with increased cell death but declined 1–2 weeks following castration, indicating that the induction was transient. The increased TGF-β1 mRNA present in the androgen deprived mouse prostate adenocarcinoma, although less than the maximum acute response following castration in normal rat ventral prostate was seen 3 weeks postcastration, indicating that the induction can be sustained over longer periods in clonal oncogene induced mouse prostate cancer compared with normal rat ventral prostate or human prostate cancer xenografts. The transiently increased TGF-β1 expression in castration induced involuting rat ventral prostate and human prostate cancer xenografts is probably associated with the cells undergoing apoptosis.

In our studies, we found no evidence that increased cell death occurred in the castrated group relative to the intact group. However, it seems that the epithelial cell subtype that undergoes apoptosis in the castration induced involuting normal rat prostate, human prostate cancer xenografts and viable androgen deprived clonal mouse prostate cancer cells described here shares a similar genetic programme.

It is notable that mRNA levels for both TGF-β1 and TGF-β3, shown previously to be raised in association with the transition from the hyperplastic to malignant phenotype (Merz *et al*, 1991; see Fig. 2), are also increased by castration. It is possible that increased expression of these genes in primary carcinomas represents an initial lack of response and/or an escape from androgen regulation. This question is currently under investigation in our laboratory. The underlying molecular mechanisms for the response of TGF-β1 and TGF-β3 to castration may be direct or possibly mediated by the AP-1 complex shown previously to be directly involved in the positive autoregulation of TGF-β1 (Kim *et al*, 1990).

SUMMARY

The mouse prostate reconstitution model exploits the ability of the fetal urogenital sinus to differentiate into a mature prostate when grafted under the renal capsule of an adult isogenic male host. By use of a recombinant retroviral vector, the *ras* and *myc* oncogenes are introduced singly or in combination into the fetal urogenital sinus—resulting in distinct phenotypes of prostatic pathology: dysplasia (caused by *ras*), hyperplasia (caused by *myc*) and frank carcinomas (caused by a combination of *ras*+*myc*). This unique experimental model creates in vivo conditions that mimic the natural initiation and progression of cancer. An expanded MPR protocol allows restricted retrovirus infection of the mesenchyme or epithelial compartments to evaluate paracrine activities. It enables almost unparalleled flexibility in addressing fundamental questions in prostate cancer. We have identified genetic variance in the susceptibility to tumour induction between two different strains of mice (mimicking the observation of racial variability in the predisposition to clinical prostate cancer). The MPR model supports data from other tumour models and implicates TGF-β1 and TGF-β3 as being strongly associated with tumour progression. Finally, with this model, we have established clonal prostate adenocarcinomas to study directly the affects of castration on gene expression. Not only are TGF-β1 and TGF-β3 mRNA levels increased in association with malignancy but they are also further enhanced by castration treatment. Based on these experimental studies, we believe that TGF-β1 and TGF-β3 expression strongly influences the progression of prostate cancer. This information will hopefully impact on the development of more effective therapy for this important malignancy.

Acknowledgements

We thank Elizabeth Hopkins for technical assistance. This work was supported by a grant from the National Institutes of Health (CA-50588) and in part by the Veterans Administration.

References

Akazaki K and Stemmermann GN (1973) Comparative study of latent carcinoma of the prostate among Japanese in Japan and Hawaii. *Journal of the National Cancer Institute* **50** 1137–1144

Bookstein R, Rio P, Madreperla SA *et al* (1990a) Promoter deletion and loss of retinoblastoma gene expression in human prostate carcinoma. *Proceedings of the National Academy of Sciences of the USA* **87** 7762–7766

Bookstein R, Shew J-Y, Chen P-L, Scully P and Lee W-H (1990b) Suppression of tumorigenicity of human prostate carcinoma cells by replacing a mutated RB gene. *Science* **247** 712–715

Breslow N, Chan CW, Dhom G *et al* (1977) Latent carcinoma of the prostate at autopsy in seven areas. *International Journal of Cancer* **20** 680–688

Brothman AR, Peehl DM, Patel AM and McNeal JE (1990) Frequency and pattern of karyotypic abnormalities in human prostate cancer. *Cancer Research* **50** 3795–3803

Buttyan R, Sawczuk IS, Benson MC, Siegal JD and Olsson CA (1987) Enhanced expression of the c-myc proto-oncogene in high-grade human prostate cancers. *The Prostate* **11** 327–337

Buttyan R, Zakeri Z, Lockshin R and Wolgemuth D (1988) Cascade induction of c-fos, c-myc and heat shock 70K transcripts during regression of the rat ventral prostate. *Molecular Endocrinology* **2** 650–657

Cannon L, Bishop D, Skonick M, Hunt S, Lyon J and Smart C (1983) Genetic epidemiology of prostate cancer in the Utah Mormon genealogy. *Cancer Surveys* **1** 47–69

Carter BS, Carter HB and Isaacs JT (1990a) Epidemiologic evidence regarding predisposing factors to prostate cancer. *The Prostate* **16** 187–197

Carter BS, Epstein JI and Isaacs WB (1990b) ras gene mutations in human prostate cancer. *Cancer Research* **50** 6830–6833

Carter BS, Ewing CM, Ward WS *et al* (1990c) Allelic loss of chromosomes 16q and 10q in human prostate cancer. *Proceedings of the National Academy of Sciences of the USA* **87** 8751–8755

Carter HB and Coffey DS (1990) The prostate: an increasing medical problem. *The Prostate* **16** 39–48

Carter HB, Piantadosi S and Isaacs JT (1990) Clinical evidence for and implications of the multistep development of prostate cancer. *Journal of Urology* **143** 742–746

Catalona WJ and Scott WW (1986) Carcinoma of the prostate, In: Walsh PC, Gittes RF, Perlmutter AD and Stamey TA (eds). *Campbell's Urology*, 5th ed, pp 1463–1534, WB Saunders, Philadelphia

Coffey DS and Williams-Ashman HG (1968) Polymerization of deoxyribonucleotides in relation to androgen-induced prostate growth. *Archives of Biochemistry and Biophysics* **124** 184–198

Crawford ED, Eisenberger MA, McLeod DG *et al* (1989) A controlled trial of leuprolide with and without flutamide in prostatic carcinoma. *The New England Journal of Medicine* **321** 419–424

Cunha GR, Fujii H, Neubauer BL, Shannon JM, Sawyer L and Reese BA (1983) Epithelial-mesenchymal interactions in prostatic development II Morphological observations of prostatic induction by urogenital sinus mesenchyme in epithelium of the adult rodent urinary bladder. *Journal of Cell Biology* **96** 1662–1670

Fearon ER and Vogelstein B (1990) A genetic model for colorectal tumorigenesis. *Cell* **61** 759–767

Fleming WH, Hamel A, MacDonald R *et al* (1986) Expression of the c-myc proto-oncogene in human prostatic carcinoma and benign prostatic hyperplasia. *Cancer Research* **46** 1535–1538

Franks LM (1954) Latent carcinoma of the prostate. *Journal of Pathology and Bacteriology* **68** 603–616

Gianferrari L, Arrigoni G, Cresseri A, Lovati G and Morganiti G (1956) Richerch genetiche e clinico-statistiche sulle neoplasie della prostata. *Acta Genticae Medicae et Gemellologiae* **5** 224–233

Gittes RF (1991) Carcinoma of the prostate. *The New England Journal of Medicine* **324** 236–245

Ignotz RA and Massagué J (1986) Transforming growth factor-β stimulates the expression of fibronectin and collagen and their incorporation into the extracellular matrix. *Journal of Biological Chemistry* **261** 4337–4345

Isaacs JT and Coffey DS (1981) Adaptation versus selection as the mechanism responsible for the relapse of prostate cancer to androgen ablation therapy as studied in the R-3327-H adenocarcinoma. *Cancer Research* **41** 5070–5075

Isaacs JT, Wake N, Coffey DS and Sandberg AA (1982) Genetic instability coupled to clonal selection as a mechanism for tumor progression in the Dunning R-3327 rat prostatic adenocarcinoma system. *Cancer Research* **42** 2353–2361

Kim S, Angel P, Lafyatis R *et al* (1990) Autoinduction of transforming growth factor β1 is mediated by the AP-1 complex. *Molecular and Cellular Biology* **9** 1255–1262

Kyprianou N and Isaacs JT (1988) Activation of programmed cell death in the rat ventral prostate after castration. *Endocrinology* **122** 552–562

Kyprianou N and Isaacs JT (1989) Expression of transforming growth factor-β in the rat ventral prostate during castration-induced programmed cell death. *Molecular Endocrinology* **3** 1515–1522

Kyprianou N, English HF and Isaacs JT (1990) Programmed cell death during regression of PC-82 human prostate cancer following androgen ablation. *Cancer Research* **50** 3748–3753

Mann R, Mulligan RC and Baltimore D (1983) Construction of a retrovirus packaging mutant and its use to produce helper-free defective retrovirus. *Cell* **33** 153–159

McNeal JE (1969) Origin and development of carcinoma of the prostate. *Cancer* **23** 24–34

Meikle AW and Smith JA (1990) Epidemiology of prostate cancer. *Urologic Clinics of North America* **17** 709–718

Meikle W, Smith J and West D (1985) Familial factors affecting prostatic cancer risk and plasma steroid levels. *The Prostate* **6** 121–128

Merz VW, Miller GJ, Krebs T *et al* (1991) Elevated TGF-β1 and β3 mRNA levels are associated with ras + myc-induced carcinomas in reconstituted mouse prostate: evidence for a paracrine role during progression. *Molecular Endocrinology* **5** 503–513

Mills JS, Needham M, Thompson TC and Parker MG (1987) Androgen-regulated expression of secretory protein synthesis in mouse ventral prostate. *Molecular and Cellular Endocrinology* **53** 111–118

Morganti G, Gianferrari L, Cresseris A, Arrigoni G and Lovati G (1956) Recherches clinico-statisque et genetiques sur les neoplasies de la prostate. *Acta Genetica Statistica Medica* **6** 304–305

Moses HL, Tucker RF, Leof EB, Coffey RJ Jr, Halper J and Shipley GD (1985) Type-β transforming growth factor is a growth stimulator and growth inhibitor, In: Feramisco J, Ozanne B and Stiles C (eds). *Cancer Cells*, Vol 3, pp 65–71, Cold Spring Harbor Laboratory, Cold Spring Harbor, New York

Mummery CL and van den Eijnden-van Raaij AJM (1990) Growth factors and their receptors in differentiation and early murine development. *Cell Differentiation and Development* **30** 1–18

Myrdal SE, Twarzdzik DR and Auersperg N (1986) Cell-mediated coaction of transforming growth factors: incubation of type β with normal rat kidney cells produces a soluble activity that prolongs the ruffling response to type α. *Journal of Cell Biology* **102** 1230–1234

Neubauer BL, Chung LWK, McCormick KA, Tauchi O, Thompson TC and Cunha GR (1983) Epithelial-mesenchymal interactions in prostatic development II Biochemical observations of prostatic induction by urogenital sinus mesenchyme in epithelium of the adult rodent urinary bladder. *Journal of Cell Biology* **96** 1671–1676

Peehl DM, Wehner N and Stamey TA (1987) Activated Ki-*ras* oncogene in human prostate adenocarcinoma. *The Prostate* **10** 281–289

Price J, Turner D and Cepko C (1987) Lineage analysis in the vertebrate nervous system by retrovirus medicated gene transfer. *Proceedings of the National Academy of Sciences of the USA* **84** 156–160

Quarmby VE, Beckman Jr WC, Wilson EM and French FS (1987) Androgen regulation of c-*myc* messenger ribonucleic acid levels in rat ventral prostate. *Molecular Endocrinology* **1** 865–874

Rizzino A (1988) Transforming growth factor-β: multiple effects on cell differentiation and extracellular matrices. *Development Biology* **130** 411–422

Roberts AB, Anzano MA, Wakefield LM, Roche NS, Stern DF, Sporn MB (1985) Type beta transforming growth factor: a bifunctional regulator of cellular growth. *Proceedings of the National Academy of Sciences of the USA* **82** 119–123

Roberts AB, Sporn MB, Assoian RK *et al* (1986) Transforming growth factor type b: rapid induction of fibrosis and angiogenesis *in vivo* and stimulation of collagen formation *in vitro*. *Proceedings of the National Academy of Sciences of the USA* **83** 4167–4171

Rowe WP, Pugh WE and Hartley JG (1970) Plaque assay techniques for murine leukemia viruses. *Virology* **42** 1136–1139

Rowlatt C, Franks LM, Sheriff MU and Chesterman FC (1969) Naturally occurring tumors and other lesions of the digestive tract in untreated C57BL mice. *Journal of the National Cancer Institute* **43** 1353–1364

Scardino PT (1989) Early detection of prostate cancer. *Urologic Clinics of North America* **16** 635–655

Shain SA, Lin AL, Koger JD, Karaganis AG (1990) Rat prostate cancer cells contain functional receptors for transforming growth factor-β. *Endocrinology* **126** 818–825

Sieweke MH, Thompson HL, Sporn MB, Bissell MJ (1990) Mediation of wound-related Rous sarcoma virus tumorigenesis by TGF-β. *Science* **248** 1656–1660

Steinberg GD, Carter BS, Beaty TH, Childs B and Walsh PC (1990) Family history and risk of prostate cancer. *The Prostate* **17** 337–347

Thompson TC (1990) Growth factors and oncogenes in prostate cancer. *Cancer Cells* **2** 345–354

Thompson TC, Cunha GR, Shannon JM and Chung LWK (1986) Androgen-induced biochemical responses in epithelium lacking androgen receptors: characterization of androgen receptors in the mesenchymal derivative of urogenital sinus. *Journal of Steroid Biochemistry* **25** 627–634

Thompson TC, Southgate J, Kitchner G and Land H (1989) Multistage carcinogenesis induced by *ras* and *myc* oncogenes in a reconstituted organ. *Cell* **56** 917–930

Welch DR, Fabra A, Nakajima M (1990) Transforming growth factor β stimulates mammary adenocarcinoma cell invasion and metastatic potential. *Proceedings of the National Academy of Sciences of the USA* **87** 7678–7682

Whitmore WF Jr (1984) Natural history and staging of prostate cancer. *Urologic Clinics of North America* **11** 205–219

Whitmore WF Jr (1990) Natural history of low-stage prostatic cancer and the impact of early detection. *Urologic Clinics of North America* **17** 689–697

Wool FC (1960) An investigation of the familial aspects of carcinoma of the prostate. *Cancer* **13** 739–744

Yatani R, Chigusa I, Akazaki K, Stemmermann GN, Welsh RA and Correa P (1982) Geographic pathology of latent prostatic carcinoma. *International Journal of Cancer* **29** 611–616

The authors are responsible for the accuracy of the references.

Regulation of Differentiation and Growth of Normal Adult and Neoplastic Epithelia by Inductive Mesenchyme

GERALD R CUNHA[1] • NORIO HAYASHI[2] • Y C WONG[3]

[1]*Department of Anatomy, University of California, San Francisco, California 94143;*
[2]*Mie University Medical School, Department of Urology, 2-174 Edobashi, Tsu, Mie, 514, Japan;*
[3]*University of Hong Kong, Department of Anatomy, Hong Kong*

Introduction
Responsiveness of adult epithelial cells to mesenchymal inductors
Relevance of epithelial-stromal interactions to cancer
Summary

INTRODUCTION

Mesenchyme is critical to the development of the integumental (Kratochwil, 1987; Sawyer, 1983), urinary (Ekblom, 1984), gastrointestinal (Kedinger *et al*, 1986), skeletal (Hall, 1987) and urogenital systems (Cunha, 1976a; Cunha *et al*, 1980a, 1983b; Chung *et al*, 1984). Mesenchyme induces specific patterns of epithelial morphogenesis (Bernfield *et al*, 1984; Haffen *et al*, 1987; Kratochwil, 1987) and is involved in the regulation of epithelial proliferation (Chung and Cunha, 1983; Shannon and Cunha, 1984; Sugimura *et al*, 1986). Mesenchyme induced development culminates in the emergence of specific types of epithelial cytodifferentiation and the expression of tissue specific secretory proteins (Kedinger *et al*, 1986). The unique feature of male sex gland development is that the overall organogenetic process is regulated by androgens (Cunha *et al*, 1987) and that mesenchymal-epithelial interactions are clearly of importance postnatally. This latter fact raises the possibility that emerging or established carcinomas might also be affected in biologically important ways by inductive mesenchymes.

This chapter will explore the responsiveness of adult epithelial cells to mesenchymal inductors and the implications of this concept to carcinogenesis, focusing specifically on studies in which the differentiation and tumorigenesis of the Dunning prostatic tumour have been altered by various mesenchymes.

Cancer Surveys Volume 11: *Prostate Cancer*

RESPONSIVENESS OF ADULT EPITHELIAL CELLS TO MESENCHYMAL INDUCTORS

For some time, adult connective tissue stroma has been considered to be a permissive matrix that physically supports and maintains epithelial structure and function. In addition, it has been thought that adult epithelial differentiation is immutable. The role of epithelial-stromal interactions in adulthood has thus received little attention. However, recent studies demonstrate that adult epithelial cells remain responsive to the inductive influences from connective tissue.

Developmental plasticity of adult epithelial cells was recognized initially as mesenchyme induced changes in adult epidermal differentiation (Billingham and Silvers, 1968; Spearman, 1974; Karring *et al*, 1975; Bernimoulin and Schroeder, 1980; Mackenzie and Hill, 1984). However, since mesenchyme induced changes in the epidermis only involved minor changes in epidermal thickness and patterns of keratinization, the importance of these findings was not immediately apparent. In the mammary gland and prostate, adult epithelial cells respond to appropriate stromal inductors by undergoing ductal branching morphogenesis and extensive growth. For example, when a small number of adult mammary epithelial cells are introduced into a gland free mammary fat pad, a mammary ductal network will proliferate from the transplanted epithelium to eventually fill the entire fat pad (Daniel and DeOme, 1965; Daniel *et al*, 1965; Hoshino, 1978). Transplantation of embryonic mesenchymes into the adult mammary gland also elicits de novo ductal morphogenesis, thus demonstrating that adult epithelial cells can respond to embryonic inductors (Sakakura *et al*, 1979b). By the same token, recombination of a small fragment of an adult prostatic duct with urogenital sinus mesenchyme (UGM) induces adult prostatic epithelium to undergo extensive proliferation and ductal morphogenesis (Norman *et al*, 1986; Hayashi N and Cunha GR, unpublished). These morphogenetic and growth promoting effects of embryonic and adult connective tissues on adult mammary and prostatic epithelium are permissive inductions since the newly induced tissue architecture maintains its original mammary or prostatic phenotype. This conclusion is, however, an oversimplification in the prostatic system because although the basic prostatic phenotype is preserved, functional expression of the epithelium is altered. For example, when adult ventral prostatic epithelium is induced by UGM, the resultant prostatic tissue expresses secretory proteins unique to both the dorsal and ventral lobes of the prostate, for example DP1, M-40 and C3 (Cunha GR *et al*, unpublished). This mesenchyme induced change in adult prostatic function further emphasizes the responsiveness of adult epithelial cells to their connective tissue environment.

Instructive induction of adult epithelial cells, wherein mesenchymal or stromal cells elicit a complete change in epithelial morphology and differentiation, has also been reported (Sugimura *et al*, 1986; Dudek and Lawrence, 1988). The profound changes in morphogenesis, cytodifferentiation and function elicited by UGM in epithelium of the adult urinary bladder (BLE) pro-

TABLE 1. Epithelial characteristics in prostate, urinary bladder and heterotypic tissue recombinants[a]

Type of analysis or feature	Specimen		
	bladder	prostate	UGM + BLE
Histology	transitional	glandular	glandular
Electron microscopy	non-secretory; asymmetric membrane	secretory; symmetric membrane	secretory; symmetric membrane
Histochemistry			
alkaline phosphate	+	–	–
alcian blue	–	+	+
non-specific esterase	– or ±	+	+
Prostate antigens	–	+	+
Prostatic secretory proteins	–	+	+
Androgen receptors	–	+	+
Androgen dependent			
DNA synthesis	–	+	+
Protein synthesis[b]	bladder	prostate	prostate like

[a]Based on data from Cunha *et al* (1980b, 1983b), Neubauer *et al* (1983), Donjacour *et al* (1988) and Takeda *et al* (1990)
[b]Analysis with two-dimensional gels

vides one of the most striking examples of a mesenchyme induced alteration in adult epithelial differentiation. In this model, embryonic UGM elicited prostatic differentiation in adult BLE, which entailed the morphogenesis of a branched ductal network, a striking stimulation and androgen regulation of epithelial proliferation, the differentiation of a simple columnar secretory epithelium, the expression of epithelial androgen receptors and the expression of prostate specific secretory proteins (Cunha *et al*, 1983a; Neubauer *et al*, 1983; Sugimura *et al*, 1986; Donjacour *et al*, 1988; Takeda *et al*, 1990). Unfortunately, it was not possible to determine whether the full spectrum of prostatic secretory proteins were expressed or whether the induced changes only represented a partial expression of the prostatic phenotype because of too few probes to the many secretory proteins representing the various lobes of the prostate. Despite suggestions that the UGM + adult BLE tissue recombinant system represents only partial expression of the prostatic epithelial phenotype (Suematsu *et al*, 1988; Takeda *et al*, 1990), it is evident that the changes elicited in adult BLE by UGM are indicative of profound changes in epithelial differentiation (Table 1). To establish definitively if mesenchyme induced change in adult epithelial phenotype represents a complete change in functional expression, a new induction system was developed whose endpoint is the differentiation of seminal vesicle tissue.

In studies using embryonic Wolffian duct epithelium as the target, mesenchyme of the seminal vesicle (SVM) was shown to induce seminal vesicle (SV) differentiation in epithelium of the middle and upper Wolffian duct (prospective ductus deferens and epididymis, respectively). Because of the fairly simple

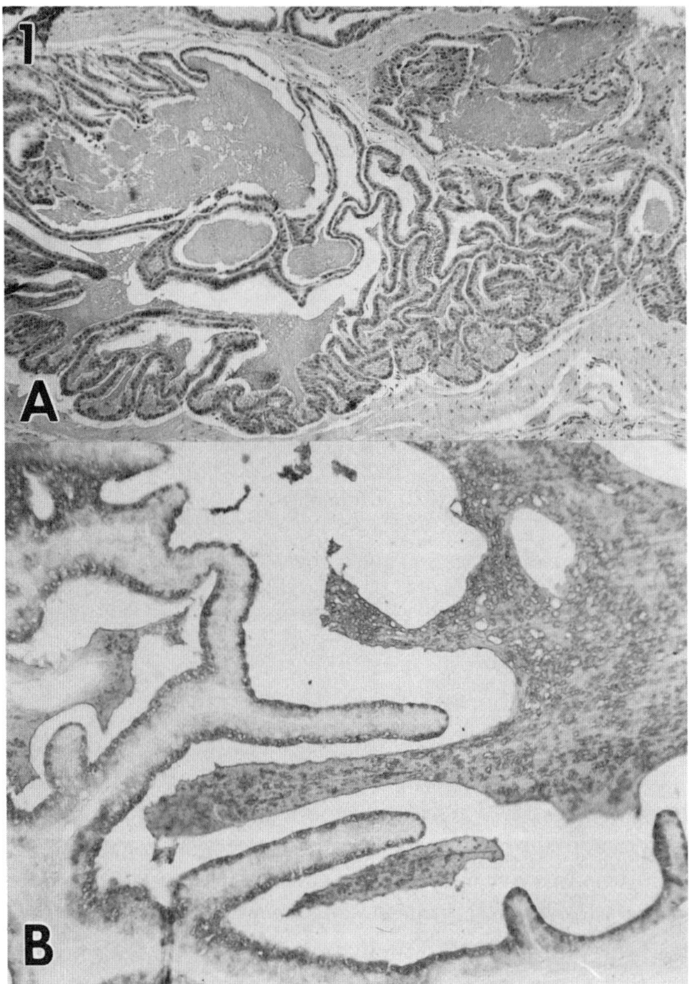

Fig. 1. SVM induces SV development in adult URE. Neonatal rat SVM + adult mouse URE tissue recombinants were grown in male athymic hosts for 1 month. Note the characteristic complex morphology of seminal vesicle (A) and the expression of mouse SV secretory proteins (B) as detected by immunocytochemical staining (×250)

and well characterized secretory proteins of the SV (Higgins and Parker, 1980; Fawell and Higgins, 1986; Fawell *et al*, 1987), the induced embryonic Wolffian duct was shown to express the full complement of SV secretory proteins (Higgins *et al*, 1989a,b). Since the embryonic Wolffian ducts give rise to the epithelia of the epididymis, SV, ureter and ductus deferens, this system has been used to determine whether adult epithelial cells from these Wolffian duct derivatives can be induced by mesenchyme to undergo complete morphological and functional change. In these studies, neonatal SVM induced adult epithelial cells from the ureter (URE), epididymis (EPE) or ductus deferens (DDE) to express SV morphogenesis and cytodifferentiation (Fig. 1) and produce the complete spectrum (Fig. 2) of major SV secretory proteins

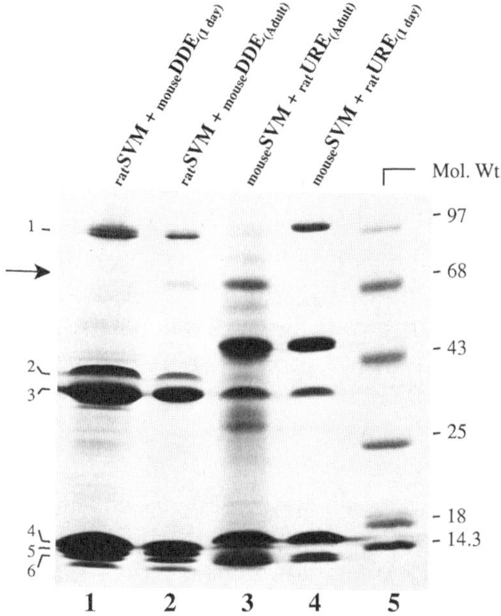

Fig. 2. Gel electrophoretic analysis of secretory proteins of SVM + DDE and SVM + URE recombinants. Tissue recombinants prepared with mouse epithelium (lanes 1 and 2) express mouse SVS proteins (1–6), whereas tissue recombinants prepared with rat epithelium (lanes 3 and 4) express rat SVS proteins (I–V). Note albumin (arrow), an unavoidable contaminant in the tissue recombinants. Lane 3 is somewhat overloaded to show faintly rat SV protein I

(Cunha *et al*, 1988, 1991; Turner *et al*, 1989). In SVM + URE recombinants, epithelial cytodifferentiation was profoundly changed from an androgen receptor deficient urothelium to a simple columnar secretory epithelium, which expressed both androgen receptor and SV secretory proteins (Cunha *et al*, 1991). It is likely that the expression of androgen receptor preceded, and is a prerequisite for, the synthesis of SV secretory proteins since during normal SV development, epithelial androgen receptors appear 2–3 days postpartum (Shima *et al*, 1990; Cooke *et al*, 1991), whereas SV secretory proteins are not detected until day 10 (Fawell and Higgins, 1986). The profound change in epithelial cytodifferentiation and function in SVM + URE recombinants is directly comparable to the induction of prostatic differentiation in the adult BLE by UGM (Cunha *et al*, 1983b; Neubauer *et al*, 1983). Here, too, a stratified androgen receptor deficient urothelium differentiated into an androgen receptor positive simple columnar secretory epithelium. Such profound changes in epithelial cytodifferentiation are accompanied by major reprogramming of biochemical and functional expression.

Two interpretations of these findings have been considered to account for these mesenchyme induced changes in adult epithelial differentiation. The induction of fully functional SV tissue from adult URE, EPE and DDE might indicate that the determined, fully differentiated adult epithelial cells first dedifferentiated and then were reprogrammed to express the SV phenotype.

Alternatively, these adult epithelia might contain undetermined and undifferentiated stem cells that were the source of the induced SV tissue. Although such undifferentiated stem cells have been observed or postulated in many organs, histological, ultrastructural and immunocytochemical observations of adult epithelia demonstrate that stem cells constitute an exceedingly small percentage of the total epithelial cell number. This being so, it is evident that if stem cells were the source of SV differentiation in SVM + URE recombinants, the induced SV tissue should have appeared focally in scattered sites throughout the adult epithelia. This was not observed in preliminary time course studies of SVM + URE recombinants grown for 6–12 days in vitro. Instead, investigations have shown that the conversion of URE (originally organized as a simple tubular structure) into the complex, folded and branched SV mucosa occurred globally throughout the tissue recombinant (Cunha et al, 1991). Thus, the alternate mechanism, dedifferentiation and subsequent reprogramming, is favoured. Since adult epithelial cells are clearly capable of expressing alternative phenotypes when associated with inductive mesenchymes, this suggests that the stability of adult epithelial differentiation in intact glandular organs must be due to ongoing influences of the adult stroma.

Adult epithelial cells in situ express qualitatively distinct histotypes and maintain their characteristic histodifferentiation even in rapidly renewing tissues, thus attesting to the stability of the differentiated state. Functional differentiation of some epithelia, for example from mammary gland and liver, can be maintained by various extracellular matrices without the need for living stromal cells (Reid and Jefferson, 1984; Bissell and Hall, 1987). However, for other epithelia, adult stromal cells have been implicated in the maintenance of adult epithelial differentiation since experimental recombination of adult epithelium with heterotypic stromas can lead to profound changes in adult epithelial cytodifferentiation and function (Billingham and Silvers, 1968; Spearman, 1974; Karring et al, 1975; Bernimoulin and Schroeder, 1980; Cunha et al, 1980b, 1983a, 1985, 1991; Briggaman, 1982; Neubauer et al, 1983; Mackenzie and Hill, 1984; Sakagami et al, 1984; Dudek and Lawrence, 1988). Although all of these studies emphasize the responsiveness of postnatal epithelial cells to inductive mesenchyme, they do not prove that adult stromal cells have inductive properties. However, adult vaginal stroma can induce neonatal uterine epithelium to express vaginal differentiation (Cunha, 1976b), and adult mammary stroma (the fat pad) can induce mammary development in both adult and fetal mammary epithelial cells (Daniel and DeOme, 1965; Daniel et al, 1965; Hoshino, 1978; Sakakura et al, 1979a). Likewise, adult dermal cells have region specific inductive activities (Billingham and Silvers, 1968; Oliver, 1968; Spearman, 1974; Karring et al, 1975; Ibrahim and Wright, 1977; Bernimoulin and Schroeder, 1980; Briggaman, 1982; Jahoda et al, 1984; Mackenzie and Hill, 1984). Finally, neonatal uterine and vaginal mesenchymes, after culture for 1–2 months, have proved to retain their ability to induce responsive epithelia instructively and permissively (Cooke et al, 1987).

Thus, adult stromal cells do seem capable of functioning as either permissive or instructive inductors.

RELEVANCE OF EPITHELIAL-STROMAL INTERACTIONS TO CANCER

The continued importance of epithelial-stromal interactions in adulthood raises the possibility that emerging or established carcinomas might also be regulated by their connective tissue environment. Indeed, embryonic mammary mesenchyme can induce mammary carcinoma cells to express a more orderly histodifferentiation and a lowered growth rate (DeCosse *et al*, 1973, 1975). Similarly, basal cell carcinomas, when grown in association with normal stroma, differentiate normally with an apparent loss of their malignant properties (Cooper and Pinkus, 1977), and human colon carcinoma cells differentiate and form glandular structures in response to embryonic rat intestinal mesenchyme (Fukamachi *et al*, 1986, 1987). As a counterpart to the UGM + adult BLE tissue recombinants described above, UGM can elicit adenocarcinomatous differentiation from transitional carcinoma cells of the urinary bladder (Fujii *et al*, 1982). These findings encouraged us to examine the effect of certain inductive mesenchymes from the urogenital tract on the differentiation of the Dunning prostatic adenocarcinoma.

The R-3327 Dunning rat prostatic tumour (DT) arose in the dorsal prostate of a 22 month old retired male rat breeder of the Copenhagen strain (Dunning, 1963) and has been maintained by serial transplantation into male hosts for almost 30 years. The parental DT is classified as a papillary adenocarcinoma that is histologically similar to certain human prostatic adenocarcinomas for which the DT and its many sublines have been used as an animal model (Isaacs, 1987).

The experimental model for examining the influence of mesenchymal inductors on the Dunning prostatic adenocarcinoma is illustrated in Fig. 3. Various mesenchymes from embryonic and neonatal rat organ rudiments were associated with 0.5 mm^3 fragments of the DT and grown in male nude mouse hosts for 1 month. Such tissue recombinants were designated primary combinants and were examined histologically after 1 month of growth to assess epithelial differentiation.

Grafts of DT alone maintained the stable homogeneous histopathological phenotype characteristic of the DT and formed tumours composed of small ducts lined by one or more layers of undifferentiated squamous or cuboidal epithelial cells as described previously (Isaacs, 1987). In UGM + DT, SVM + DT or bulbourethral gland mesenchyme (BUG-M) + DT recombinations, the mesenchyme induced the undifferentiated DT epithelial cells to differentiate into tall columnar secretory epithelial cells organized into enlarged cystic ducts (Hayashi and Cunha, 1989; Hayashi *et al*, 1990). These induced epithelial cells were highly differentiated, non-pleomorphic and polarized with basally located nuclei and supranuclear clear zones (Fig. 4). Interspersed between these more

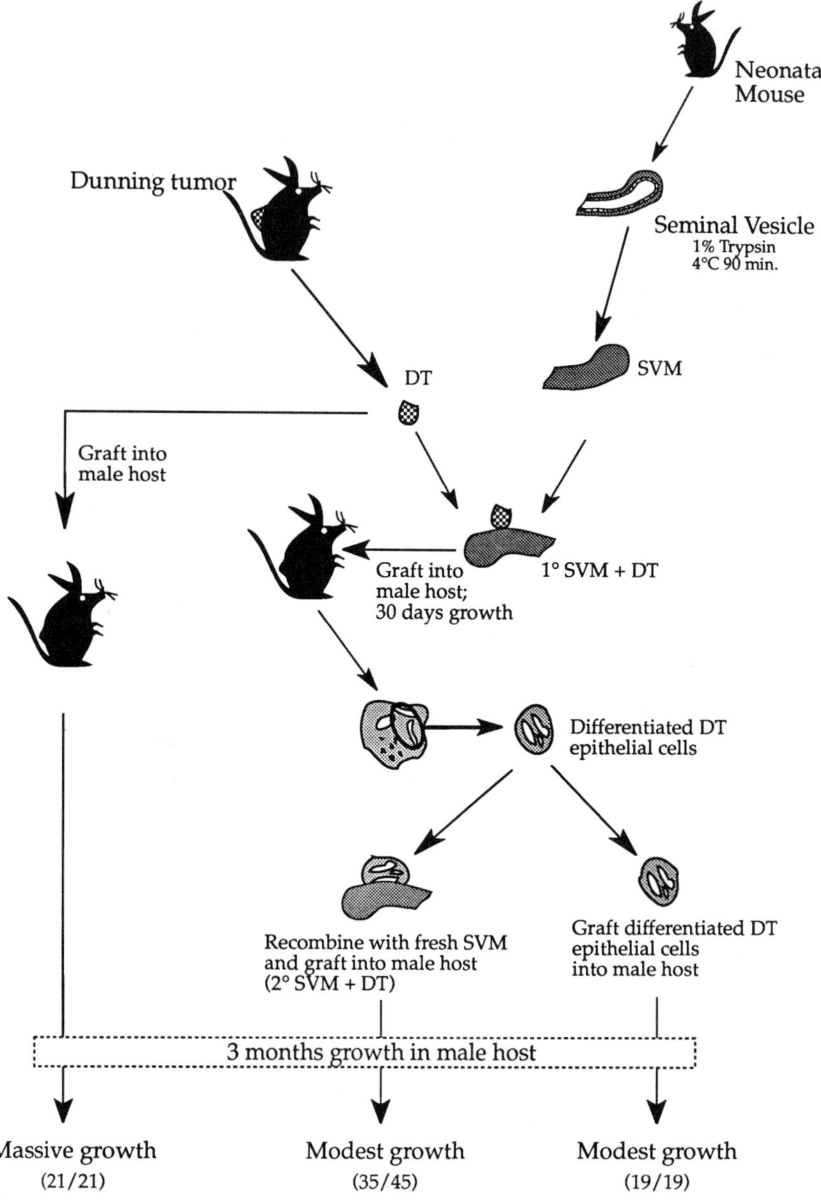

Fig. 3. Experimental protocols for examining the effect of mesenchyme on the DT

normal ducts were regions that continued to express the histopathology characteristic of the parental DT. In some regions, ducts lined with the undifferentiated cells of the DT were in direct continuity with the more highly differentiated epithelial cells (Fig. 5), suggesting that the highly differentiated cells arose from the undifferentiated epithelial cells of the DT. In contrast to the differentiating effects of UGM, SVM and BUG-M, DT grown in associa-

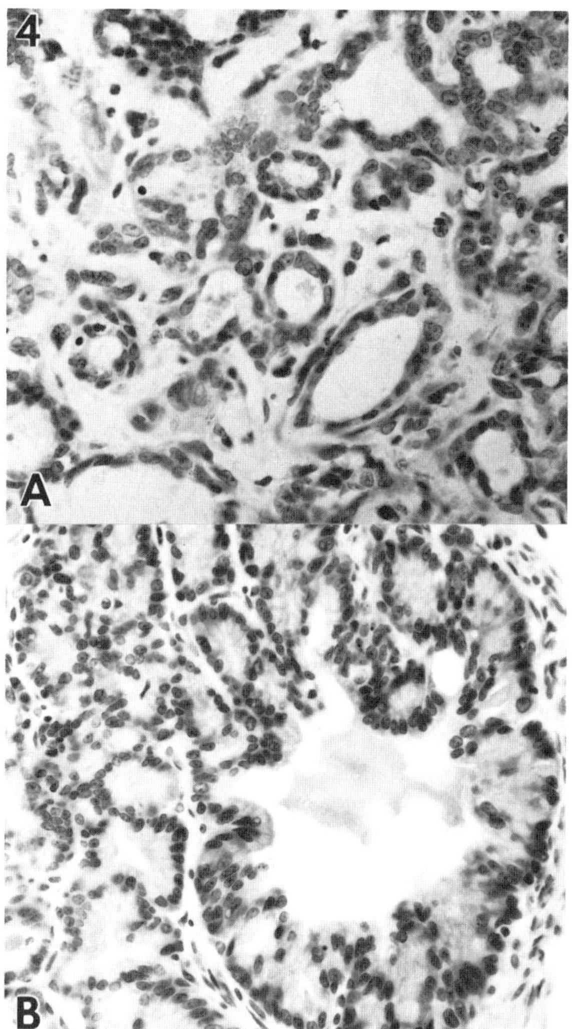

Fig. 4. Sections of grafts of a 0.5 mm^3 cube of Dunning tumour (A) and a tissue combinant (B) composed of the 18 day old fetal rat urogenital sinus mesenchyme + Dunning tumour grown for 1 month in a male host. The DT (A) is composed of small tubules lined with undifferentiated squamous to cuboidal cells, whereas UGM + DT tissue combinations (B) contain large tubules lined with tall columnar epithelial cells (×200)

tion with mesenchyme of the neonatal urinary bladder continued to express the typical DT phenotype (Table 2).

To determine whether the mesenchyme induced change in DT histodifferentiation was coupled to changes in neoplastic growth, the resultant large fluid filled ducts of primary SVM + DT recombinants were excised, cut into 1 mm segments and either grafted to new hosts or combined with fresh mesenchyme to generate secondary SVM + DT recombinants; these were in turn grafted under the renal capsule of a secondary male host (see Fig. 3). Generally, a secondary host was grafted with three 1 mm^3 pieces of the original DT on

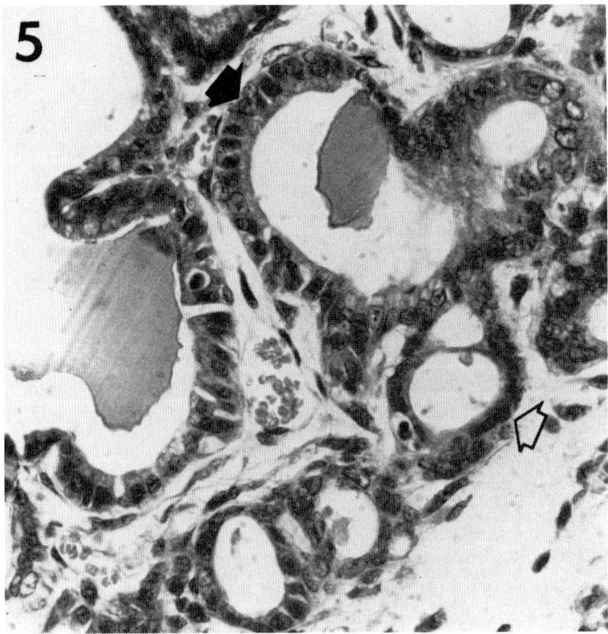

Fig. 5. A recombinant composed of neonatal SVM + DT grown for 1 month as described in Fig. 4 showing undifferentiated epithelial cells (open arrow) characteristic of the DT in direct continuity with tall, highly differentiated epithelial cells (closed arrow) (×250)

one kidney and an equal number of either secondary SVM + DT recombinants or differentiated DT ducts derived from primary SVM + DT recombinants on the contralateral kidney. Secondary hosts were maintained for 3 months. Grafts of cystic ducts of differentiated DT epithelial cells derived from primary SVM + DT recombinants exhibited modest growth, whereas secondary SVM + DT recombinants prepared with differentiated DT epithelial cells

TABLE 2. Simple columnar cytodifferentiation of DT epithelium in tissue combinations with UGM, SVM, BUG-M and BLM[a]

Tissue grafted	No. of grafts	Columnar cytodifferentiation response	Proportion of responding (%)
Control (UGM)	28	0	0[b]
UGM + DT	80	70	88[c]
Control (SVM)	22	0	0[b]
SVM + DT	60	50	83[c]
Control (BUG-M)	10	0	0[b]
BUG-M + DT	17	14	82[c]
Control (BLM)	16	0	0[b]
BLM + DT	27	0	0[c]

[a]From Hayashi *et al* (1990). Abbreviations as per text
[b]Control were recovered as undifferentiated fibromuscular tissues
[c]Unresponsive combinations showed original DT histology

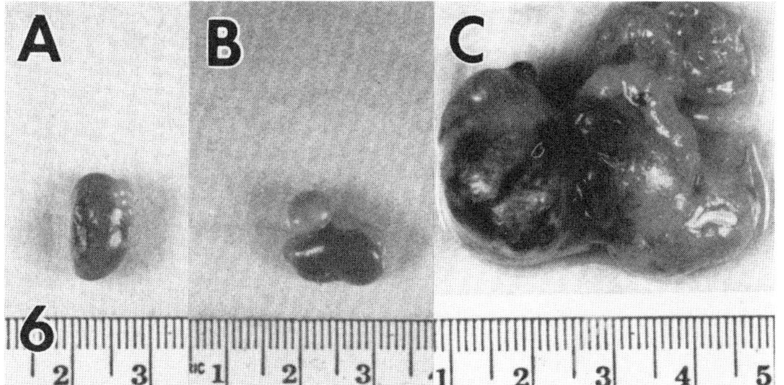

Fig. 6. Gross appearance of grafts grown for 3 months under renal capsule. Grafts of 2°SVM + DT recombinants (A) and of differentiated DT epithelial cells derived from 1°SVM + DT recombinants (B) have grown modestly. Note that the four grafts of the parental DT have grown into a single tumourous mass that obscures the host's kidney (C). (×32)

derived from primary SVM + DT recombinants grew little if at all (Fig. 6). In contrast, after 3 months of in vivo growth in a male host, the three 1 mm^3 grafts of the parental DT completely overgrew the host's kidney, forming a single large tumourous mass weighing 5–7 g. The apparent reduction in growth rate and loss in tumorigenesis of the SVM induced DT epithelial cells was associated with an eightfold reduction in [^{3}H]thymidine labelling index (Fig. 7) (Hayashi and Cunha, in press). The tall columnar epithelial cells of primary and secondary SVM + DT recombinants expressed a secretory phenotype as judged by both light microscopy (Fig. 8) and electron microscopy (Fig. 9). Secretory proteins collected from the lumina of secondary SVM + DT

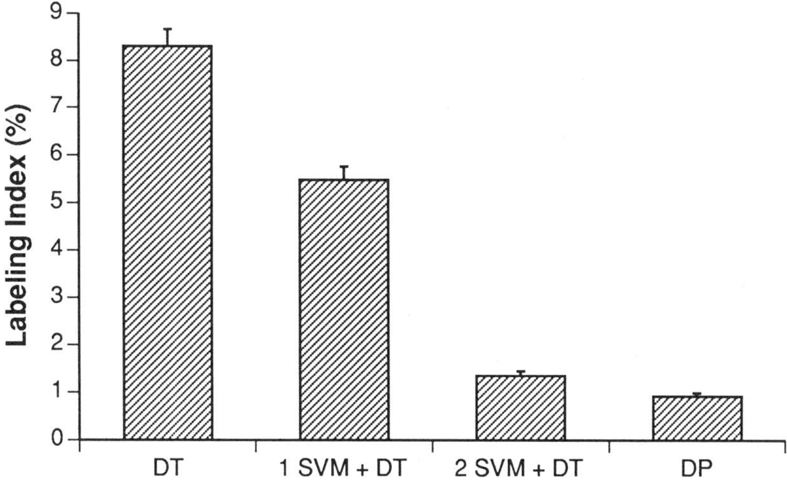

Fig. 7. [^{3}H]Thymidine labelling index of the various grafts after 1 month (dorsal prostate [DP] and 1°SVM + DT recombinants) or 3 months (DT and 2°SVM + DT recombinants) of in vivo growth. Labelling index of 2°SVM + DT recombinants was significantly reduced relative to that of the parental DT

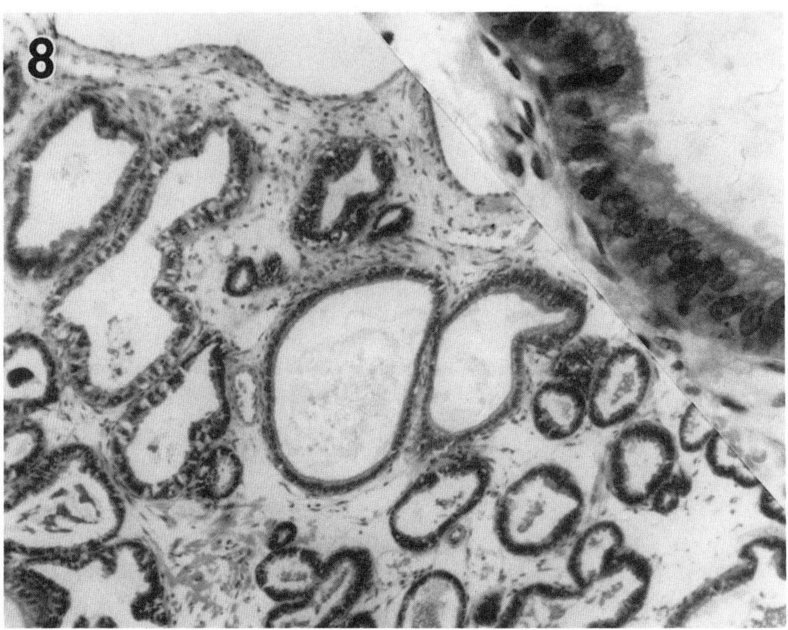

Fig. 8. Histological sections of 2°SVM + DT recombinants grown for 3 months in vivo. Note the maintenance of tall columnar epithelial cells (×100 and ×320)

recombinants, when analysed by SDS-PAGE, demonstrated the presence of a novel set of secretory proteins (42, 38 and 15 kDa) that were different from those of primary SVM + DT recombinants, dorsal prostate, SV, SVM or DT. Whether these secretory proteins are other previously described prostatic secretory proteins is unclear (Hayashi N and Cunha GR, unpublished).

The rationale for this inquiry comes from the the pioneering studies of Pierce, who proposed the idea that cancer is a caricature of differentiation (Pierce *et al*, 1978). According to Pierce, the type of neoplasm is related to the differentiation state of the target epithelial cell at initiation of carcinogenesis. It has been postulated that for any cancer, an embryonic field is capable of exerting profound regulatory influences. The participation of embryonal carcinoma cells in normal murine development with complete loss of tumorigenesis after their injection into the mouse blastocyst is cited as a prime example supporting this theory (Mintz, 1978). Whether this idea is also germane to the more common carcinomas in humans and animals is uncertain since earlier reports of mesenchyme induced regulation of epithelial neoplasia have not been pursued sufficiently (DeCosse *et al*, 1973, 1975; Cooper and Pinkus, 1977; Fujii *et al*, 1982; Fukamachi *et al*, 1986, 1987). The Dunning tumour model presented (Hayashi and Cunha, 1989, in press; Hayashi *et al*, 1990) and recently confirmed (Chung *et al*, 1990) now provides a suitable model for the continued exploration of the role of mesenchyme in epithelial neoplasia.

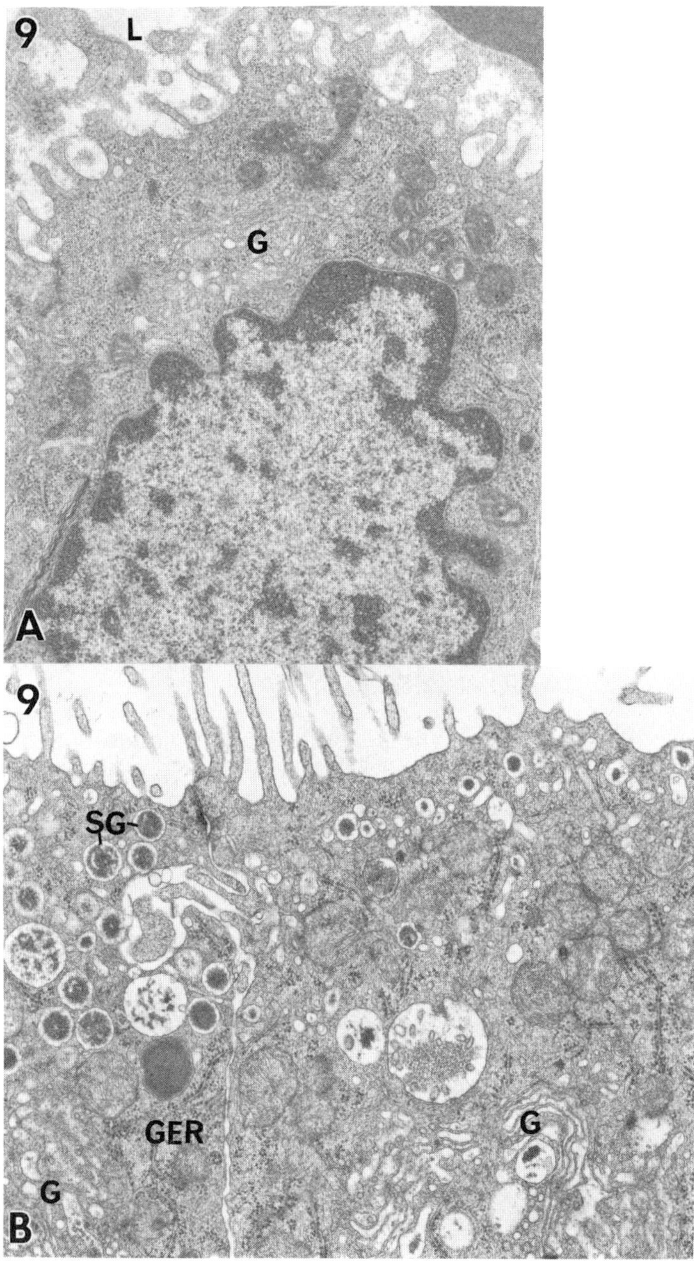

Fig. 9. (A) Electron micrograph of the parental DT showing the apical surface of an epithelial cell. Note the small Golgi (G) apparatus and absence of secretory granules (L = lumen, ×21 225). (B) Electron micrograph of a UGM + DT recombinant grown for 4 weeks in a male host. Apical cytoplasm of three tall columnar epithelial cells showing a well developed GER and the presence of apical secretory granules (SG). Also note the large Golgi apparatus (G) in these cells (×21 225)

On the basis of the developmental biology of the male genital tract (Cunha *et al*, 1987), mesenchyme should have regulative activity on prostatic carcinoma cells. Since UGM and SVM can induce profound changes in phenotypic expression in adult epithelia of the urinary bladder, ureter, ductus deferens and epididymis (Cunha *et al*, 1983a, 1991; Turner *et al*, 1989), it is evident that in adulthood, the connective tissue environment could influence emerging and established carcinomas. Our studies on the DT clearly indicate that various mesenchymes can regulate both the differentiation and growth properties of both normal and neoplastic prostatic epithelial cells (Norman *et al*, 1986; Hayashi and Cunha, 1989, in press; Hayashi *et al*, 1990).

The mechanism by which mesenchyme regulates epithelial morphogenesis, differentiation and growth remains unknown both for normal and for abnormal development (carcinogenesis). Communication between epithelium and stroma is certainly multifactorial, involving extracellular matrix, soluble growth or differentiation factors and angiogenesis factors. Fortunately, the reproducibility and versatility of the mesenchyme + DT model reported here provides many promising avenues for the study of the regulation of neoplastic growth. Further investigation of the paracrine mediators that are implicated in these cell-cell interactions will surely expand our knowledge of the carcinogenic process and may lead to new therapeutic strategies.

SUMMARY

Since adult epithelial cells from the urogenital tract are unquestionably capable of expressing alternative phenotypes when induced by embryonic or neonatal mesenchymes, we examined the effect of certain inductive mesenchymes on the differentiation and growth of the DT by growing 0.5 mm^3 fragments of the DT in association with mesenchyme from various embryonic and neonatal rat organ rudiments. Whereas grafts of DT alone contained narrow ducts lined with undifferentiated epithelial cells characteristic of the DT, the DT derived epithelium of UGM + DT, SVM + DT or BUG-M + DT recombinations differentiated into tall columnar secretory epithelial cells organized into large cystic ducts. These mesenchyme induced changes in histodifferentiation of the DT cells were coupled to a loss of tumorigenesis since the mesenchyme induced highly differentiated DT cells never formed tumours. This reduction in growth rate and loss in tumorigenesis of mesenchyme induced DT epithelial cells was accompanied by a reduction in [^{3}H]thymidine labelling index and the expression of a secretory phenotype as demonstrated by both light microscopy and electron microscopy. These findings demonstrate that the connective tissue environment can have profound regulative effects on both normal and neoplastic epithelial cells.

Acknowledgements

This study has been supported in part by National Institutes of Health grants DK-32157, CA-05388, CA-49996 and HD17491.

References

Bernfield MR, Banerjee SD, Koda JE and Rapraeger AC (1984) Remodeling of the basement membrane as a mechanism of morphogenetic tissue interactions, In: Trelstad RL (ed). *The Role of Extracellular Matrix in Development*, pp 545–596, Alan R Liss, New York

Bernimoulin J-P and Schroeder HE (1980) Changes in the differentiation pattern of oral mucosal epithelium following heterotopic connective tissue transplanation in man. *Pathological Research and Practice* **166** 290–312

Billingham R and Silvers WK (1968) Dermoepidermal interactions and epithelial specificity, In: Fleischmajer R and Billingham RE (eds). *Epithelial-mesenchymal interactions*, pp 252–266, Williams and Wilkins, Baltimore

Bissell MJ and Hall HG (1987) Form and function in the mammary gland: the role of extracellular matrix, In: Neville MC and Daniel CW (eds). *The Mammary Gland: Development, Regulation, and Function*, pp 97–146, Plenum Press, New York

Briggaman R (1982) Epidermal-dermal interactions in adult skin. *Journal of Investigative Dermatology* **79** 21s–24s

Chung LWK and Cunha GR (1983) Stromal-epithelial interactions II Regulation of prostatic growth by embryonic urogenital sinus mesenchyme. *Prostate* **4** 503–511

Chung LWK, Matsuura J and Runner MN (1984) Tissue interactions and prostatic growth. *Biology of Reproduction* **31** 155–165

Chung L, Zhau H and Ro J (1990) Morphologic and biochemical alterations in rat prostatic tumors induced by fetal urogenital sinus mesenchyme. *Prostate* **17** 165–174

Cooke PS, Fujii DK and Cunha GR (1987) Vaginal and uterine stroma maintain their inductive properties following primary culture. *In Vitro Cellular Developmental Biology* **23** 159–166

Cooke PS, Young P and Cunha GR (1991) Androgen receptor expression in developing male reproductive organs. *Endorcinology* **126** 2867–2873

Cooper M and Pinkus H (1977) Intrauterine transplantation of rat basal cell carcinoma: a model for reconversion of malignant to benign growth. *Cancer Research* **37** 2544–2552

Cunha GR (1976a) Epithelial-stromal interactions in development of the urogenital tract. *International Review of Cytology* **47** 137–194

Cunha GR (1976b) Stromal induction and specification of morphogenesis and cytodifferentiation of the epithelia of the Mullerian ducts and urogenital sinus during development of the uterus and vagina in mice. *Journal of Experimental Zoology* **196** 361–370

Cunha GR, Chung LWK, Shannon JM and Reese BA (1980a) Stromal-epithelial interactions in sex differentiation. *Biology of Reproduction* **22** 19–43

Cunha GR, Lung B and Reese B (1980b) Glandular epithelial induction by embryonic mesenchyme in adult bladder epithelium of Balb/c mice. *Investigative Urology* **17** 302–304

Cunha GR, Fujii H, Neubauer BL, Shannon JM, Sawyer LM and Reese BA (1983a) Epithelial-mesenchymal interactions in prostatic development I Morphological observations of prostatic induction by urogenital sinus mesenchyme in epithelium of the adult rodent urinary bladder. *Journal of Cell Biology* **96** 1662–1670

Cunha GR, Shannon JM, Taguchi O, Fujii H and Chung LWK (1983b) Epithelial-mesenchymal interactions in hormone-induced development, In: Sawyer RH and Fallon JF (eds). *Epithelial-Mesenchymal Interactions in Development*, pp 51–74, Praeger Scientific Press, New York

Cunha GR, Bigsby RM, Cooke PS and Sugimura Y (1985) Stromal-epithelial interactions in adult organs. *Cell Differentiation* **17** 137–148

Cunha GR, Donjacour AA, Cooke PS *et al* (1987) The endocrinology and developmental biology of the prostate. *Endocrine Reviews* **8** 338–363

Cunha GR, Higgins SJ and Young PF (1988) Seminal vesicle mesenchyme induces the expression of the seminal vesicle functional cytodifferentiation in adult epithelia. *Journal of Cell Biology* **107** 178a

Cunha GR, Young P, Higgins SJ and Cooke PS (1991) Neonatal seminal vesicle mesenchyme induces a new morphological and functional phenotype in the epithelia of adult ureter and ductus deferens. *Development* **111** 145–158

Daniel CW and DeOme KB (1965) Growth of mouse mammary glands *in vivo* after monolayer culture. *Science* **149** 634–636

Daniel CW, DeOme KB, Young JT, Blair PB and Faulkin LJ (1965) The *in vivo* life span of normal and neoplastic mouse mammary glands: a serial transplantation study. *Proceedings of National Academy of Sciences of the USA* **61** 53–60

De Cosse J, Gossens CL and Kuzma JF (1973) Breast cancer: induction of differentiation by embryonic tissue. *Science* **181** 1057–1058

DeCosse JJ, Gossens CL, Kuzma JF and Unsworth BR (1975) Embryonic inductive tissues that cause histological differentiation of murine mammary carcinoma in vitro. *Journal of the National Cancer Institute* **54** 913–921

Donjacour AA, Cunha GR and Higgins SF (1988) Detection of specific prostatic proteins in an epithelium that lacks androgen receptors. *Endocrinology* **122 (Supplement)** 502

Dudek RW and Lawrence IEJ (1988) Morphologic evidence of interactions between adult ductal epithelium of pancreas and fetal foregut mesenchyme. *Diabetes* **37** 891–900

Dunning WF (1963) Prostate cancer in the rat. *National Cancer Institute Monograph* **12** 351–370

Ekblom P (1984) Basement membrane proteins and growth factors in kidney differentiation, In: Trelstad RL (ed). *The Role of Extracellular Matrix in Development*, pp 173–206, Alan R Liss, New York

Fawell SE and Higgins SJ (1986) Tissue distribution, developmental profile and hormonal regulation of androgen-responsive secretory proteins of rat seminal vesicles studied by immunocytochemistry. *Molecular and Cellular Endocrinology* **48** 39–49

Fawell SE, MacDonald CJ and Higgins SJ (1987) Comparison of seminal vesicle secretory proteins of rodents using antibody and nucleotide probes. *Molecular Cellular Endocrinology* **50** 107–114

Fujii H, Cunha GR and Norman JT (1982) The induction of adenocarcinomatous differentiation in neoplastic bladder epithelium by an embryonic prostatic inductor. *Journal of Urology* **128** 858–861

Fukamachi H, Mizuno T and Kim YS (1986) Morphogenesis of human colon cancer cells with fetal rat mesenchymes in organ culture. *Experientia* **42** 312–315

Fukamachi I, Mizuno T and Kim YS (1987) Gland formation of human colon cancer cells combined with foetal rat mesenchyme in organ culture: an ultrastructural study. *Journal of Cell Science* **87** 615–621

Haffen K, Kedinger M and Simon-Assmann P (1987) Mesenchyme-dependent differentiation of epithelial progenitor cells in the gut. *Journal of Pediatric Gastroenterology and Nutrition* **6** 14–23

Hall BK (1987) Tissue interactions in the development and evolution of the vertebrate head, In: Maderson PFA (ed). *Development and Evolution of the Neural Crest*, pp 215–260, John Wiley & Sons, New York

Hayashi N and Cunha GR (1989) Changes in histodifferentiation of the Dunning rat prostatic adenocarcinoma elicited by mesenchyme. *Cancer Research* **30** 52

Hayashi N and Cunha GR Mesenchyme-induced changes in the neoplastic characteristics of the Dunning prostatic adenocarcinoma. *Cancer Research* **51** (in press)

Hayashi N, Cunha GR and Wong YC (1990) Influence of male genital tract mesenchymes on differentiation of Dunning prostatic adenocarcinoma. *Cancer Research* **50** 4747–4754

Higgins SF and Parker MC (1980) Androgenic regulation of generalized and specific responses in accessory sexual tissues in the male rat, In: Litwak G (ed). *Biochemical Actions of Hormones*, pp 287–309, Academic Press, New York

Higgins SJ, Young P, Brody JR and Cunha GR (1989a) Induction of functional cytodifferentiation in the epithelium of tissue recombinants I Homotypic seminal vesicle recombinants. *Development* **106** 219–234

Higgins SJ, Young P and Cunha GR (1989b) Induction of functional cytodifferentiation in the epithelium of tissue recombinants II Instructive induction of Wolffian duct epithelia by neonatal seminal vesicle mesenchyme. *Development* **106** 235–250

Hoshino K (1978) Mammary transplantation and its histogenesis in mice, In: Yokoyama A, Mizuno H and Nagasawa H (eds). *Physiology of Mammary Glands,* pp 163–228, University Press, Baltimore

Ibrahim L and Wright EA (1977) Inductive capacity of irradiated dermal papillae. *Nature* **265** 733–734

Isaacs JT (1987) Development and characteristics of the available animal model systems for the study of prostatic cancer, In: Coffey DS, Bruchovsky N, Gardner Jr WW, Resnick MI and Karr JP (eds). *Current Concepts and Approaches to the Study of Prostate Cancer,* pp 513–576, Alan R Liss, New York

Jahoda CAB, Horne KA and Oliver RF (1984) Induction of hair growth by implantation of cultured papilla cells. *Nature* **311** 560–562

Karring T, Lang NP and Löe H (1975) The role of gingival connective tissue in determining epithelial differentiation. *Journal of Periodontal Research* **10** 1–11

Kedinger M, Simon-Assmann PM, Lacroix B, Marxer A, Hauri HP and Haffen K (1986) Fetal gut mesenchyme induces differentiation of cultured intestinal endodermal and crypt cells. *Developmental Biology* **113** 474–483

Kratochwil K (1987) Tissue combination and organ culture studies in the development of the embryonic mammary gland In: Gwatkin RBL (ed). *Developmental Biology: a Comprehensive Synthesis,* pp 315–334, Plenum Press, New York

Mackenzie IC and Hill WM (1984) Connective tissue influences on patterns of epithelial architecture and keratinization in skin and oral mucosa. *Cell and Tissue Research* **235** 551–559

Mintz B (1978) Genetic mosaicism and in vivo analyses of neoplasia and differentiation, In: Saunders G (eds). *Cell Differentiation and Neoplasia,* pp 27–56, Raven Press, New York

Neubauer BL, Chung LWK, McCormick KA, Taguchi O, Thompson TC and Cunha GR (1983) Epithelial-mesenchymal interactions in prostatic development II Biochemical observations of prostatic induction by urogenital sinus mesenchyme in epithelium of the adult rodent urinary bladder. *Journal of Cell Biology* **96** 1671–1676

Norman JT, Cunha GR and Sugimura Y (1986) The induction of new ductal growth in adult prostatic epithelium in response to an embryonic prostatic inductor. *Prostate* **8** 209–220

Oliver RF (1968) The regeneration of vibrissae: a model for the study of dermal-epidermal interactions, In: Fleischmajer R and Billingham RE (eds). *Epithelial-mesenchymal Interactions,* pp 267–279, Williams & Wilkins, Baltimore

Pierce G, Shikes R and Fink L (1978) *Cancer: A Problem of Developmental Biology,* Prentice Hall, New Jersey

Reid LM and Jefferson DM (1984) Cell culture studies using extracts of extracellular matrix to study growth and differentiation in mammalian cells, In: Mather JP (ed). *Mammalian Cell Culture,* pp 239–280, Plenum Press, New York

Sakagami Y, Inaguma Y, Sakakura T and Nishizuka Y (1984) Intestine-like remodeling of adult mouse glandular stomach by implanting fetal intestinal mesenchyme. *Cancer Research* **44** 5845–5849

Sakakura T, Nishizuka Y and Dawe CJ (1979a) Capacity of mammary fat pads of adult C31/HeMs mice to interact with fetal mammary epithelium. *Journal of the National Cancer Institute* **63** 733–736

Sakakura T, Sakagami Y and Nishizuka Y (1979b) Persistence of responsiveness of adult mouse mammary gland to induction by embryonic mesenchyme. *Developmental Biology* **72** 201–210

Sawyer RH (1983) The role of epithelial-mesenchymal interactions in regulating gene expression during avian scale morphogenesis, In: Sawyer RH and Fallon JF (eds). *Epithelial-mesenchymal Interactions in Development,* pp 115–146, Praeger, New York

Shannon JM and Cunha GR (1984) Characterization of androgen binding and deoxyribonucleic acid synthesis in prostate-like structures induced in testicular feminized (Tfm/Y) mice. *Biology of Reproduction* **31** 175–183

Shima H, Tsuji M, Young PF and Cunha GR (1990) Postnatal growth of mouse seminal vesicle is dependent on 5a-dihydrotestosterone. *Endocrinology* **127** 3222–3233

Spearman RIC (1974) Alteration of keratinization in mouse ear epidermis in recombinant grafts with tail dermis. *Acta Anatomy* **89** 195–202

Suematsu N, Takeda H and Mizuno T (1988) Glandular epithelium induced from urinary bladder epithelium of the adult rat does not show full prostatic cytodifferentiation. *Zoological Science* **5** 385–395

Sugimura Y, Cunha GR and Bigsby RM (1986) Androgenic induction of deoxyribonucleic acid synthesis in prostatic glands induced in the urothelium of testicular feminized (Tfm/y) mice. *Prostate* **9** 217–225

Takeda H, Suematsu N and Mizuno T (1990) Transcription of prostatic steriod binding protein (PSBP) gene is induced by epithelial-mesenchymal interaction. *Development* **110** 273–282

Turner T, Young P and Cunha GR (1989) Seminal vesicle induction of adult mouse epididymal epithelium by newborn mouse and rat seminal vesicle mesenchyme. *Journal of Cell Biology* **109** 69a [Abstract]

The authors are responsible for the accuracy of the references.

Reciprocal Mesenchymal-Epithelial Interaction Affecting Prostate Tumour Growth and Hormonal Responsiveness

LELAND W K CHUNG[1] • MARTIN E GLEAVE[1] • JER-TSONG HSIEH[1]
SUNG-JOON HONG[2] • HAIYEN E ZHAU[1]

[1]*Urology Research Laboratory, University of Texas M D Anderson Cancer Center, Houston, Texas 77030;* [2]*Department of Urology, Yonsei University College of Medicine, Seoul, Korea*

INTRODUCTION

The role of mesenchymal-epithelial interaction in the pathogenesis of prostate cancer and benign prostate hyperplasia (BPH) has been appreciated at the histomorphological level ever since the pioneer studies of Moore (1943) and Franks (1954). To characterize the functional significance of the mesenchyme and epithelium in prostatic growth, Franks *et al* (1970) devised an ingenious in vitro system by mechanically separating the stromal from the epithelial compartments of human BPH specimens. They observed that DNA synthesis in the epithelium is dependent on the presence of adjacent stromal and myoepithelial cells. However, in recent years, more extensive investigations of the in vivo and in vitro mechanisms of mesenchymal-epithelial interaction be-

Cancer Surveys Volume 11: *Prostate Cancer*
© 1991 Imperial Cancer Research Fund. 0-87969-368-1/91. $3.00 + .00

came possible for two reasons. Firstly, overwhelming evidence in the literature suggests that embryonic induction, as observed by Spemann in 1901, must be operative in normal and neoplastic development of the prostate gland. It is assumed that the mesenchymal and epithelial components from the prostate gland interact with each other in vivo through short range signals that determine the developmental outcome of the interacting tissue compartments. Our laboratory (Chung *et al*, 1981, 1984) and others (Cunha *et al*, 1983; Neubauer *et al*, 1986) have employed the concept of embryonic induction and have defined the directive roles of fetal urogenital sinus mesenchyme (UGM) in prostatic epithelial growth and hormonal responsiveness. Recently, we have extended this effort to determine further the reciprocal interaction between the mesenchymal (fibroblast) and epithelial cells and the possible cellular and molecular bases of such interaction (Chang and Chung, 1989; Chung *et al*, 1989; Camps *et al*, 1990). Secondly, improved tissue culture methods and growth conditions have allowed the establishment of relevant prostatic cell lines (Horoszewicz *et al*, 1983; Isaacs *et al*, 1986; Chung *et al*, 1989; Kaighn *et al*, 1989) or strains (Peehl *et al*, 1988; Merchant, 1990) that have been subjected to detailed and precise molecular and biochemical analyses. By employing these improved cell culture and molecular biological methods, many laboratories have obtained valuable information about the regulation of prostate cancer and BPH growth and progression (Kabalin *et al*, 1989; Ramaekers *et al*, 1989; Story *et al*, 1989; Camps *et al*, 1990).

In this chapter, we focus on two areas. Firstly, we analyse investigations that used tissue-tissue recombination techniques to determine which tissue compartment influences prostatic epithelial growth and mediates hormonal responsiveness. Secondly, we expand this discussion to include our more recent studies using the cell-cell interaction model to delineate the mechanisms and bidirectionality of mesenchymal-epithelial interaction. We emphasize growth factors, extracellular matrix and the neuroendocrine network that are likely to serve as important mediators between mesenchymal (or fibroblast) and epithelial cells. We also present here a novel experimental model of human prostate cancer and the evidence to support the concept that it is through aberrant cell-cell interaction rather than the intrinsic genetic changes of a single cell type alone that may be the principal mechanism leading to prostate tumorigenesis.

RECOMBINATION MODELS FOR STUDYING TISSUE-TISSUE AND CELL-CELL INTERACTION

Since the pioneer studies in 1901 by Spemann and Grobstein (1953) on embryonic induction, extensive and impressive developmental studies have been performed by various laboratories in an attempt to elucidate the mechanisms of morphogenesis and functional differentiation in the development of kidney, salivary gland, skin, mammary gland, pancreas, lung, tooth, testis and male and female reproductive tracts (Grobstein, 1956; Bernfield *et al*, 1972; Levine *et al*, 1973; Cunha, 1976; Sengel, 1976; Burwen and Pitelka, 1980; Hilfer, 1983; Kollar, 1983; Skinner and Fritz, 1985). As depicted in Fig. 1a, the success of many of these studies was due in part to the technical improvement that allowed the mesenchymal and epithelial tissue components to be separated cleanly from embryonic organs and the subsequent success in recombining and observing the occurrence of morphogenesis and cytodifferentiation in recombinants grafted in competent hosts in vivo. The ability to analyse unequivocally the developmental outcome of the tissue recombinants by reliable biochemical, molecular, immunochemical and histomorphological techniques has also contributed to the success of these studies.

Using the tissue-tissue interaction model, we and others have made the following observations: (a) Prostatic morphogenesis and functional differentiation can occur in tissue recombinants composed of the inductive fetal UGM and a competent embryonic (Chung *et al*, 1981; Chung and Cunha, 1983) or adult (Chung *et al*, 1984; Thompson and Chung, 1986) epithelium; fetal UGM also induces the outgrowth of prostatic bud and its branching morphogenesis in tissue explants grown in organ culture (Lasnitzki and Mizuno, 1980). (b) Fetal UGM may be the primary target for androgenic steroid, accelerating the growth of prostatic epithelium (Chung and Cunha, 1983) and mediating its hormonal responsiveness (Cunha and Chung, 1981). (c) Mesenchymal-epithelial interactions occur during embryonic life and continue through adulthood; during embryonic development, such interaction is crucial and will determine the ultimate sizes of the adult organs and their morphogenetic and hormonal responsiveness in adulthood (Rajfer and Coffey, 1978; Chung and MacFadden, 1980); in the adult, moreover, mesenchymal (stromal)-epithelial interaction may be required to maintain growth and differentiative (secretory) functions of the prostate gland (Neubauer *et al*, 1986; Guthrie *et al*, 1990). (d) Although adult prostate tissue does not regenerate and is incapable of inducing prostate growth, it responds strongly to inductive influences exerted by fetal UGM both in vivo as tissue recombinants (Chung and Cunha, 1983) and in situ as tissue implants directly into the host prostate gland (Chung *et al*, 1984); fetal UGM is a potent inducer capable of exerting a directive action by reprogramming the histomorphological (Chung *et al*, 1990; Hayashi *et al*, 1990) and biochemical (Chung *et al*, 1990) expression of selected rat prostatic tumours in vivo. (e) We have found that both β-adrenergic receptor and androgen receptor pathways are required to activate certain androgen responsive genes in the rat ventral prostate gland (Guthrie *et al*, 1990). Neuroendocrine networks residing primarily in the mesenchyme (Higgins and Gosling, 1989) and testosterone metabolizing enzymes residing primarily in the epithelium (Chang and Chung, 1989) are thought to interact reciprocally, thus establishing a tight metabolic cooperation between these tissue types.

Because mesenchymal and epithelial tissues are known to contain many morphologically and functionally distinct cell types, our laboratory has developed a cell-cell interaction model using biochemically and morphologically

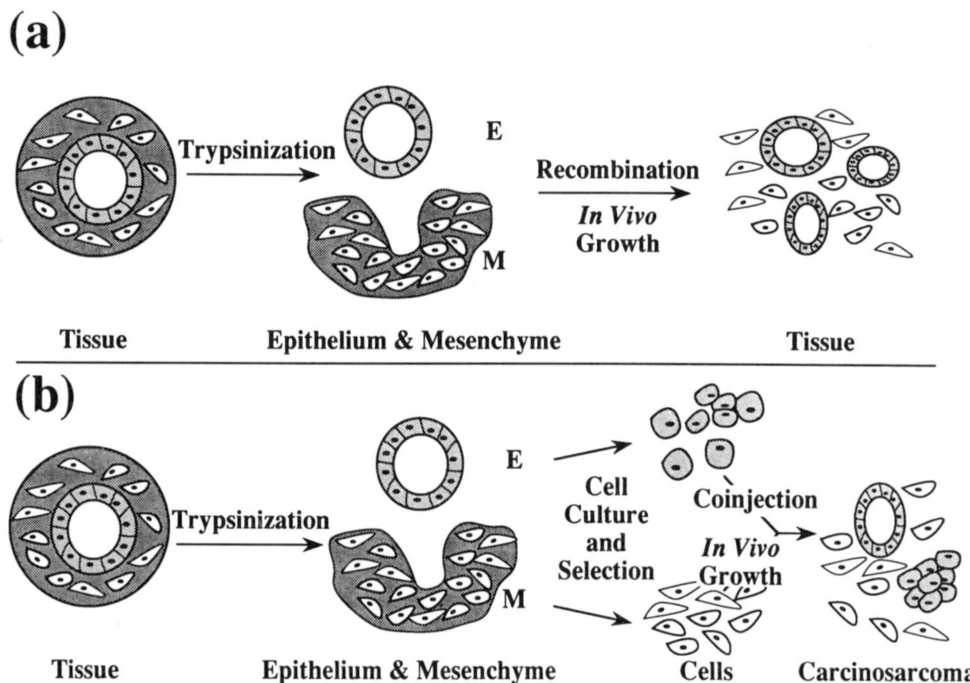

Fig. 1. Mesenchymal-epithelial interaction models: (a) Tissue-tissue interaction model; (b) cell-cell interaction model. (a) Fetal UGS separated by trypsinization to form fetal UGM (M) and fetal UGE (E) tissues. Neither fetal UGM nor fetal UGE can grow alone but on recombination of these tissues can grow under the renal capsules of a sexually mature male syngeneic or athymic host and undergo prostatic development (Cunha, 1976; Chung *et al*, 1981). (b) Respective mesenchymal and epithelial components cultured in vitro to generate cell lines or strains; the cells can be coinjected in male hosts to observe tumour formation (Chung *et al*, 1989). We have expanded this cell-cell interaction model to examine the reciprocal interaction between mesenchymal (or fibroblast) and epithelial cells derived from both embryonic and adult tissues (Camps *et al*, 1990; Gleave *et al*, 1991a)

well defined cell types from the prostate gland in an effort to understand the cellular and molecular basis of mesenchymal-epithelial interaction. Figure 1b illustrates that morphologically and biochemically well characterized prostatic fibroblast and epithelial cell lines established from both embryonic and adult prostate glands can be easily inoculated together in vivo (Chung *et al*, 1989; Camps *et al*, 1990) or cocultured in vitro (Camps *et al*, 1990; Djakiew *et al*, 1990) to study the likely pathways leading to mesenchymal (fibroblast)- epithelial interaction. This cell-cell interaction model is convenient, reproducible and more amenable to mechanistic study. Using this model system, we have made the following observations: (a) Interactions between fibroblast and epithelial cells in vivo appear to be reciprocal and can occur between species, but no interaction occurs between fibroblasts or between epithelial cells of similar cell lineages from the same species. (b) Fetal mesenchymal and adult fibroblast cell lines established from human and rat prostatic tissues accelerate the growth of non-tumorigenic human epithelial cells to form solid tumours in vivo (Camps *et al,* 1990). Our results indicate that mesenchymal and fibroblast cell lines or strains differentially affect human prostatic epithelial tumour growth and progression (Camps *et al,* 1990; Chung *et al,* 1991; Gleave *et al,* 1991a). (c) A mesenchymal cell line derived from fetal rat UGM (rUGM) confers androgen sensitivity on the growth of androgen receptor negative and androgen unresponsive human prostatic (PC-3) and bladder (WH) epithelial cell lines in vivo (Chung *et al,* 1991). A fibroblast cell line derived from adult rat prostate gland also conferred androgen induced growth response on rat prostate epithelial cells in vivo (Chung *et al,* 1988). (d) We noted that both growth factors and extracellular matrices may serve as important modulators for mesenchymal-epithelial interaction (Gleave *et al,* 1991a). Under appropriate inoculation conditions, non-tumorigenic epithelial cells can be induced to form solid tumours by conditioned media collected from the inductive mesenchymal cells (Gleave *et al,* 1991a) or by the extracellular matrix components that are known to be expressed abundantly by cultured prostatic mesenchymal cells (Freeman *et al,* 1991).

The cell-cell interaction model described above offers distinct advantages for the investigation of cellular and molecular mechanisms mediating mesenchymal-epithelial interaction. However, because the established epithelial cell lines often lose their cell polarity and cease to express organ specific markers, efforts must be made to combine this approach with an improved bicameral cell culture method (Djakiew *et al,* 1990) and a tissue-tissue recombination approach to gain further insight into the physiological significance of cell-cell interaction. Alternatively, we (Gleave *et al,* 1991a,b; Marengo S and Chung LWK, unpublished) and others (Stephenson R, Dinney C, Zhau H, Killion J and Fidler I, unpublished) have explored the possibility of injecting prostatic cells along with other biologically relevant growth factors directly into the host animals or their prostate gland to evaluate the host organ microenvironment on the growth and subsequent biological behaviours of prostatic cells in vivo.

INTERACTION BETWEEN MESENCHYMAL AND EPITHELIAL TISSUES

Mesenchyme Mediated Epithelial Growth and Hormonal Responsiveness

The prostate gland, an exquisitely androgen sensitive organ, requires testicular androgen for development and functional maintenance. To determine the precise target tissue(s) for androgen action, several laboratories have pursued the original concept developed by Drews (1975) that focuses specifically on the question of direct as opposed to indirect (ie mesenchymally mediated) effect of testosterone on the differentiation of the epithelial tissues associated with the reproductive tracts. We constructed heterotypic tissue recombinants consisting of the fetal UGM derived from wild type (androgen receptor positive) mice with a competent urinary bladder epithelium derived from testicular feminized (Tfm/y, androgen receptor deficient) mice in an effort to determine androgen induced responses (Cunha and Chung, 1981; Thompson *et al*, 1986). We observed that despite the lack of androgen receptors in the responding epithelium, characteristic androgen induced DNA synthesis and protein profiles were detected in the test tissue recombinants, suggesting that the epithelial response to androgen is mediated by its primary action on the mesenchyme. The conclusion that androgen mediates its effect (rather than acts directly) on the growth and differentiation of Tfm/y epithelial cells via the mesenchyme is consistent with the original results of Drews (1975), Kratochwil and Schwartz (1976) and Drews and Drews (1975, 1977). In addition, similar observations suggesting an indirect action of androgen on the responding epithelium was reported by Lasnitzki and Mizuno (1980) using an organ culture system to evaluate the outgrowth of prostatic buds and the growth stimulation of the preputial gland (Hannappel and Drews, 1981). The demonstration, by means of autoradiographic studies, that androgen receptors are localized in the mesenchyme and not in the epithelium of the developing murine urogenital sinus corroborates this concept (Shannon and Cunha, 1983; Takeda *et al*, 1985). Furthermore, in the X inactivation of intersex chromosome mosaic mouse model, in which the development of both male and female reproductive tracts occurs simultaneously, the morphogenesis of the characteristic male organs appears adjacent to surrounding connective tissues that contain androgen receptors (Schleicher *et al*, 1988). Takeda *et al* (1985) noted that androgen receptors were present in the mesenchyme during early urogenital sinus development but disappeared from this cellular compartment and appeared in the epithelium during postnatal development. In the adult prostate, androgen receptors, as determined by means of autoradiography, are present mostly in the epithelium, with only a few labelled cells being associated with the connective tissue (Schleicher *et al*, 1985).

Because mesenchyme appears to be the primary androgen target tissue, the possible role of mesenchyme in prostate growth was addressed by means of two approaches. Firstly, tissue recombinants consisting of varying ratios of fetal UGM and fetal urogenital sinus epithelium (UGE) are constructed, and the resultant growth and morphogenesis of the recombinants are monitored in syngeneic hosts. Secondly, fetal UGM or intact fetal urogenital sinus (UGS) is introduced directly into the host prostate, and the resultant growth of the chimaeric prostate gland is analysed. With the first approach, Chung and Cunha (1983) and Neubauer *et al* (1986) demonstrated conclusively that it is the mesenchyme and not the epithelium that determines the growth potential of the murine prostate. As few as several hundred epithelial cells are required to develop a complete mouse prostate gland, provided that the equivalent of a whole mouse prostate mesenchyme was present in the tissue recombinant. These results were confirmed with the second approach outlined above, whereby fetal UGM and not fetal UGE was shown to be capable of inducing adult host prostate overgrowth in a mesenchymal dose dependent manner (Chung *et al*, 1984). Intact fetal UGS was also induced by the host ventral prostate gland (VP) to express a rat VP specific protein, prostatic binding protein (PBP), when implanted and contributed to chimaeric prostate organ growth in intact male hosts (Thompson and Chung, 1986). These results suggest that fetal UGM or UGS is the driving force for additional prostate growth but is influenced by the host organ microenvironment to express PBP. It is therefore conceivable that human benign hyperplastic prostatic (BPH) growth may be attributed to growth elicited by reactivation of the embryonic growth potential within the adult prostate gland, as suggested by McNeal (1978). Our results also raised the possibility that the restriction placed on the growth of the adult prostate gland is not absolute but arbitrary. Fetal mesenchymal driving forces can effectively remove the constraint and promote additional proliferative response of the normal adult prostate epithelium.

To address the question of whether human BPH may be attributable to the regenerative growth of both glandular and stromal elements in response to an inductive cue from "embryonic" cells present in the aging prostate, Jarow and Isaacs (1989) implanted human BPH tissues directly into the rat VP of immunodeficient animals and observed no overgrowth of the host prostate gland. However, these results must be interpreted with caution. Firstly, the degree of viability of human BPH implants in athymic rat VP needs to be critically assessed. The lack of host VP growth in response to the BPH implant may be due to a diminished metabolic activity of human BPH tissue graft in the host VP. Secondly, human BPH is an extremely slow growing, benign condition, presumably because of the presence of a low level of growth factors; therefore, a much longer observation period may be necessary to observe any solid tissue growth.

Mesenchyme Mediated Differentiation of Rat Prostatic Adenocarcinoma

The concept of regulation of cancer cell differentiation has aroused interest and prompted debate by research workers in both genetics and epigenetics. There is little doubt that genetic changes have occurred in a normal cell during multistep malignant transformation (Fearon and Vogelstein, 1990; Stanbridge and Nowell, 1990). However, it is equally clear that the lifting of certain physiological and selective pressure constraints can reverse the expression of previously malignant phenotypes and restore the cell to its normal phenotype (Pierce, 1983; Rubin *et al*, 1990). This latter concept has profound implications, considering that the interaction between a tumour cell and its host microenvironment can be interrupted with drugs (eg suramin), which can be therapeutically beneficial.

Because fetal UGM possesses broad specificity in its ability to interact with various fetal and adult tissues and is capable of influencing the histomorphology of the transitional cell carcinoma of the urinary bladder through short range tissue interaction (Fujii *et al*, 1982), we tested the ability of fetal UGM to affect the growth, histomorphology and biochemical characteristics of the rat prostatic tumours (Chung *et al*, 1990). When four types of androgen responsive and androgen unresponsive rat Dunning and Nb prostatic tumours were tested, fetal UGM was found to affect the differentiation of some of these tumours selectively (Chung *et al*, 1990). The induction of prostatic tumour differentiation by fetal UGM appears to be androgen receptor mediated because mesenchyme lacking androgen receptors (eg neonatal urinary bladder mesenchyme) fail to induce glandular morphogenesis and secretory functions within the androgen responsive Dunning R-3327 tumour (Hayashi *et al*, 1990). Thus, it appears that fetal UGM in the presence of androgenic steroids may influence differentiation of some rat prostatic tumours. However, it remains undefined whether this inductive influence of fetal UGM on the differentiation of rat prostatic cancer is permanent and inversely related to the malignant potential of the responding tumour epithelium.

This model of mesenchyme mediated prostatic cancer differentiation supports the concept that fetal UGM is a powerful embryonic inducer capable of reprogramming the phenotypic expression of selected rat prostate cancers either by removing epigenetic constraints or by activating embryonic differentiation programmes within tumour tissues. Our results are consistent with the reports of many inductive systems whereby embryonic tissues can, through close contact, induce differentiation in embryonal carcinoma (Mintz and Illmensee, 1975; Pierce *et al*, 1984), breast cancer (DeCosse *et al*, 1973; Sakakura *et al*, 1981), neuroblastoma (Podesta *et al*, 1984), colon cancer (Fukamachi *et al*, 1986) and leukaemia (Gootwine *et al*, 1982). Potential mechanisms of induction of cancer cell differentiation are discussed below.

Characteristics of Mesenchymal-Epithelial Tissue Interaction

The salient features of mesenchymal-epithelial interaction that lead to prostate growth and differentiation involve: (a) Mesenchyme mediated induction of epithelial growth and differentiation, which requires the presence of androgen receptors in the mesenchyme. A composite interaction model involving the delivery of long range endocrine factors (eg testosterone) plus a short range contact dependent communications network (eg local growth factors and extracellular matrix) is the most likely mechanism of mesenchymal-epithelial interaction in the prostate (Chang and Chung, 1989; Camps *et al*, 1990). (b) Close contact between live mesenchyme and epithelium are required for induction of prostatic growth and morphogenesis (Chung *et al*, 1984). Numerous attempts to place membrane filter barriers between mesenchyme and epithelium have failed to uncover significant promotion of prostatic growth or morphogenesis in the apposed cells, implying that cell-cell contact (possibly through extracellular matrix and growth factor pathways) may be necessary for prostatic growth and development. (c) Because of the lack of well defined tissue specific markers and the absence of well characterized androgen responsive genes in the mesenchyme, there has been little evidence to suggest that epithelium directs mesenchyme differentiation. However, using a cell-cell recombination model (Camps *et al*, 1990; Chung *et al*, 1991; Gleave *et al*,

1991a,b), we have demonstrated reciprocal mesenchymal-epithelial interaction in the prostate. (d) Although various tissue recombination models have successfully recreated the three dimensional architecture of the prostate gland and its morphogenic and secretory functions, tissue recombinants grown under the renal capsular or subcutaneous site do not express the key androgen regulated secretory protein, PBP (Guthrie *et al*, 1990). Failure to express PBP is unlikely to be due to the possible regional differences in prostatic segments used for the study of tissue recombination or to luminal pressure induced atrophy. Expression of PBP was not observed in any tissue recombinants constructed from fetal UGM and dissected rat prostatic segments from terminal vesicles to proximal ducts (Neubauer *et al*, 1986). Rat VP implants, when maintained as renal grafts, usually regressed and ceased to produce secretory proteins, including the PBP. However, PBP expression by rat VP renal implants can be restored with exogenous androgen and/or a β-adrenergic agonist, isoproterenol (Guthrie *et al*, 1990). Under these conditions, we observed evidence of increased secretory and protein synthetic activity by the rat VP renal implants. Because rat VP renal implants, when grafted under a number of the body sites, specifically lose their β-adrenergic (but not androgen) receptors (which can be restored by exogenous androgen administration) (Guthrie *et al*, 1990), we propose that a tight coupling between androgen and neurotransmitters may be required for the expression of PBP in rat VP. This proposal is relevant to the tissue recombination model because the rat tissue recombinants (eg fetal UGM + fetal UGE) consistently failed to express PBP, but when the intact fetal UGS was implanted directly into the host VP gland, the chimaeric prostate gland expressed amounts of PBP comparable to those found in the normal intact rat VP gland (Thompson and Chung, 1986). These results suggest that the organ microenvironment, possibly the connection of vascular and neuroendocrine networks within the prostate, may be crucial for the expression of secretory functions of the gland.

INTERACTION BETWEEN MESENCHYMAL AND EPITHELIAL CELLS

Reciprocal Acceleration of Mesenchymal and Epithelial Tumour Growth In Vivo

To understand the cellular and molecular bases of mesenchymal-epithelial interaction in the prostate, our laboratory has developed a cell-cell recombination model to define the reciprocal interaction between epithelial and fibroblast cells, to determine the direct interaction of androgen with the mesenchymal cells that confer androgen induced growth responsiveness on the epithelium and to assess the involvement of growth factors and extracellular matrix as paracrine regulators for prostate growth and differentiation (Fig. 1b).

We induced carcinosarcomas in syngeneic and athymic animals by inoculating them simultaneously with cells from a tumorigenic rat prostate fibroblast cell line and a non-tumorigenic epithelial cell line (Chung *et al*, 1989). In this study, we obtained evidence that cellular interaction mediated by paracrine factors rather than by cell fusion is the most likely mechanism to explain the tumour forming capability of the interacting epithelial cells within the tumour fibroblast microenvironment. Subsequently, we noted that the growth of non-tumorigenic prostatic epithelial cells was stimulated (or accelerated) when these cells were injected subcutaneously together with non-tumorigenic prostatic or non-prostatic fibroblasts (Gleave *et al*, 1991a,b). The use of this fibroblast-epithelial interaction model is an efficient technique for growing various non-tumorigenic human epithelial cell lines in athymic mice from organs including prostate, breast, bladder and kidney (Camps *et al*, 1990). In this study, we provided further evidence that fibroblast and epithelial interaction in vivo is bidirectional. We observed that even lethally irradiated fibroblasts can elicit a tumorigenic response from a non-tumorigenic epithelial cell line (Camps *et al*, 1990), which suggests the possible importance of growth factors (lethally irradiated cells are known to produce growth factors) and the extracellular matrix (ECM) in prostate tumour growth in vivo.

To address further the questions of whether tumorigenic prostate fibroblasts can induce normal prostatic epithelial cells to participate in tumour formation and, conversely, whether normal prostatic fibroblasts influence the tumorigenicity and growth rate of marginally tumorigenic prostatic epithelial cells, we inoculated tumorigenic prostate fibroblasts, the NbF-1 cells, directly into syngeneic Nb rat VP gland and observed that the normal prostatic epithelium did not participate in prostatic tumorigenesis. The inoculated NbF-1 formed clearly demarcated fibrosarcoma, which spread randomly within the loosely packed fibromuscular stroma but failed to induce the normal rat VP glandular epithelium to participate in tumour formation. These results suggest that tumorigenic prostatic fibroblasts do not confer tumorigenicity on their adjacent normal epithelium. As a second approach, we inoculated a non-tumorigenic dose of human prostatic epithelial cancer cell line, LNCaP (1×10^6 cells per subcutaneous site), directly into the mouse dorsolateral prostate gland and observed that LNCaP tumours formed in 50% of the mice. Histologically, they were carcinomas and were composed of human prostate cancer cells, as evidenced by the presence of *Alu* repetitive DNA sequences and prostate specific antigen (PSA) in the tumours. These results suggest that even in normal prostatic cells, the fibroblasts can possibly induce immortalized but marginally tumorigenic human prostate cancer epithelial cells to participate in tumorigenesis.

The significance of fibroblast-epithelial interaction in human prostate cancer growth and progression was substantiated by the demonstration that fibroblasts differ in their ability to accelerate prostate cancer growth (Gleave *et al*, 1991b). The marginally tumorigenic human LNCaP prostatic cancer cell line can be accelerated to form carcinomas in male athymic mice when inoculated together with either non-tumorigenic prostate or bone fibroblasts (Fig. 2a), but the non-tumorigenic human lung (CCD-16) and mouse embryonic

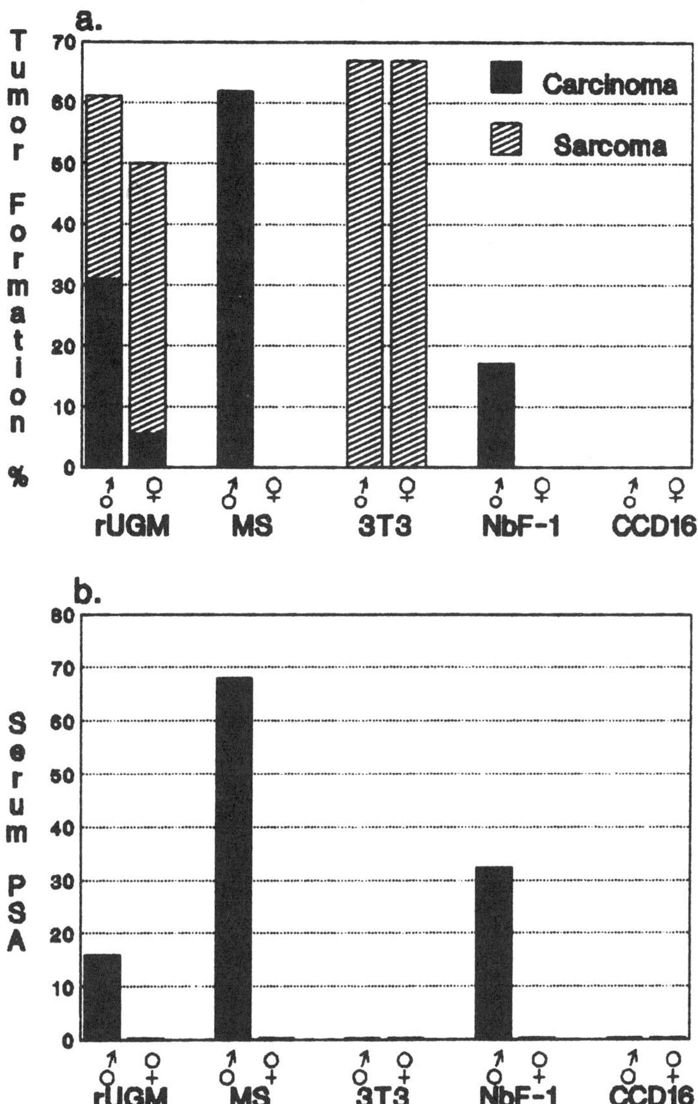

Fig. 2. Establishment of an animal model for human prostatic LNCaP tumour. (a) Coinoculation of prostatic (rUGM and NbF-1) and bone (MS) mesenchymal or fibroblast cells with LNCaP epithelial cells in male athymic mice could induce prostate carcinoma formation; in contrast, embryonic fibroblasts (3T3) and human lung fibroblasts (CCD-16) were ineffective. These tumours secrete prostate specific antigen (PSA), a known human prostate cancer marker, in sera of adult male hosts (b) (Gleave *et al*, 1991a)

fibroblasts (3T3) were ineffective (Fig. 2a). The formation of LNCaP carcinomas was paralleled by elevations in the serum PSA concentration (Fig. 2b). Furthermore, in this study, Gleave *et al* (1991b) noted that the LNCaP tumours grew preferentially in the male hosts. In most instances, chimaeric LNCaP tumours did not form in the female rats, but the coinoculated non-tumorigenic fibroblasts formed sarcomas. These results demonstrate that in

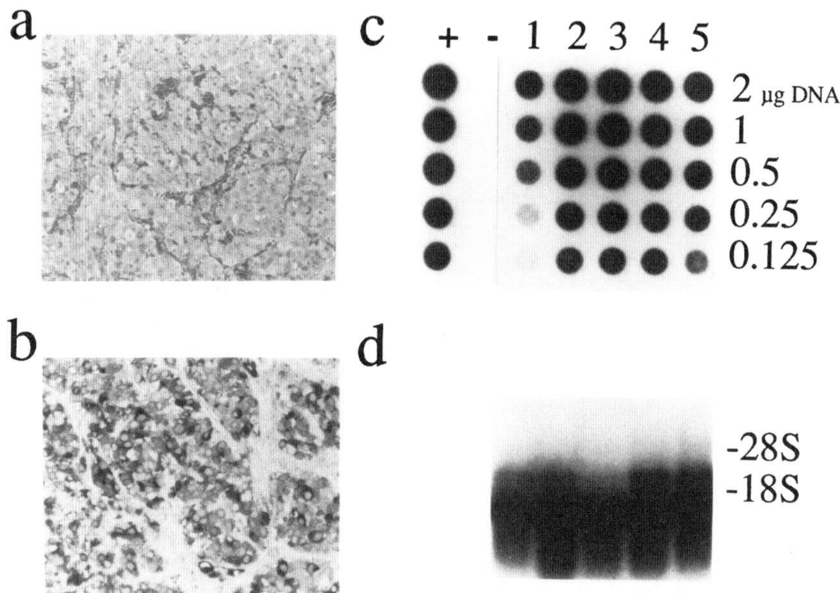

Fig. 3. Histomorphology, PSA expression and the presence of *Alu* repetitive DNA sequence in MS-LNCaP chimaeric tumours. (a) Highly angiogenic MS/LNCaP chimaeric tumour, which stains positive for PSA (b). The tumours were found to contain human *Alu* repetitive DNA sequence (c) and expressed abundant PSA mRNA (1.6 kb), as evidenced by northern blot hybridization (d)

the presence of androgenic steroid in male hosts, non-tumorigenic prostate and bone fibroblasts accelerated epithelial tumour growth, whereas in castrated male or female hosts, a reciprocal acceleration of fibroblast growth by the epithelial cells to form sarcomas was noted (Fig. 2a).

The fact that human bone fibroblasts accelerated LNCaP tumour growth in vivo implies that fibroblasts may play an important part in promoting prostatic cancer progression and may in part explain the propensity of human prostate cancer to metastasize to bone. The tumour formed from bone fibroblasts and LNCaP epithelial cells in vivo was a highly angiogenic human prostatic adenocarcinoma with minimal fibroblastic component (Fig. 3a). This tumour stained positively for PSA (Fig. 3b). Southern dot blot results showed that the tumours were almost exclusively of human origin, because they contained *Alu* repetitive sequences (Fig. 3c); northern blot results confirmed the presence of 1.6 kb PSA mRNA in the tumour (Fig. 3d). These results, taken together, suggest that fibroblasts provide a supportive role for LNCaP tumour growth in vivo.

This finding raised an interesting question as to the possible functional role of fibroblasts in human prostate cancer growth. It is conceivable that prostatic carcinoma grows through clonal expansion under the influence of its surrounding fibroblasts. The fibroblasts themselves do not have to participate in the expansion of tumour volume, but they may affect the growth rate of neighbouring malignant cells through the release of paracrine growth factors, as was the case in cellular interaction between bone fibroblasts and LNCaP epithelial cells. We have confirmed that conditioned media collected from LNCaP and competent fibroblast cell lines exert a paracrine rather than an autocrine growth stimulatory effect on cell growth in vitro (Gleave *et al*, 1991b).

Our results demonstrate that reciprocal fibroblast-epithelial interaction occurs in vivo and in vitro, the outcome of which, ie fibroblast or epithelial cell derived tumour growth in vivo, is a function of the sex steroid milieu of the host and the sources and the developmental lineage of the interaction between fibroblasts and epithelial cells. Our data indicate that fibroblast-epithelial interactions not only influence the rate of prostatic tumour growth but may also have a critical role in determining the route of human prostate cancer metastasis. Interactions between tumour cells and their surrounding stroma have been observed clinically. In 85% of prostate cancer patients, the predilection of prostate cancer cells to metastasize to bone is accompanied by osteoblastic or stimulatory responses (Jacobs, 1983; Berrettoni and Carter, 1986). In addition, tumour growth may be accompanied by desmoplastic stromal reaction (eg linitis plastica) or, in contrast, by regressive stromal alterations from the production of collagenases or plasminogen activators (reviewed in van den Hooff, 1988).

Mesenchymal Cells Confer Androgen Sensitivity on Epithelial Tumour Growth In Vivo

We established a rat fetal urogenital sinus mesenchymal cell line (rUGM) from 18 day old fetal rat urogenital sinuses. By employing the cell-cell recombination model, we observed that this cell line can confer androgen sensitivity on androgen insensitive human epithelial cell lines, WH, isolated from a human bladder transitional cell carcinoma (Chung *et al*, 1991; Zhau H, Hong S and Chung L, unpublished) and PC-3, a previously established prostatic cancer cell line derived from osseous metastasis.

The basic protocol involves subcutaneous coinoculation of athymic mice with equal numbers of rUGM and either WH or PC-3 cells (1×10^6 cells). In the male hosts, rUGM cells stimulated WH tumour growth 20-fold compared with the chimaeric WH tumours grown in the female hosts (Fig. 4); no sex difference was observed in the growth of WH tumour alone. NIH3T3 cells, not a target for androgenic steroid, failed to confer androgen induced growth responses on WH cells in vivo (Chung *et al*, 1991; Zhau H, Hong S and Chung L, unpublished). Similarly, we observed that rUGM stimulated PC-3 tumour growth in male mice only (Fig. 5); sarcomatoid tumours formed occasionally in the females coinoculated with rUGM and PC-3 cells, as evidenced by the lack of human DNA in these tumours. We found that live rUGM cells were required to confer these androgen induced growth responses on PC-3 and WH cells; cells that had been heated and homogenized were no longer capable of in vivo interaction (Hong S, Zhau H and Chung L, unpublished). The rUGM plus PC-3 chimaeric tumours were transplanted and initially retained their

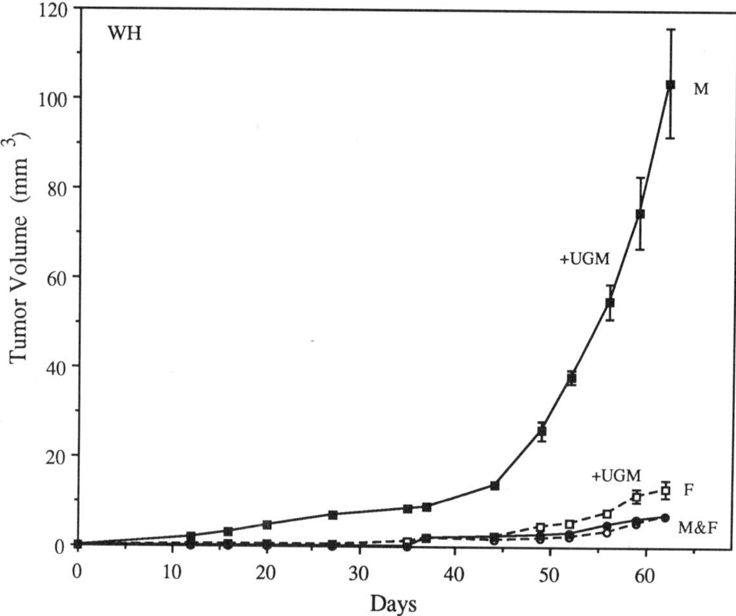

Fig. 4. Fetal UGM derived mesenchymal cells (UGM) confer androgen induced growth response on human bladder epithelial cells (WH) in vivo. Note: UGM accelerated WH tumour growth markedly only in the male host (M). WH cells formed slow growing tumours in both male and female (F) hosts

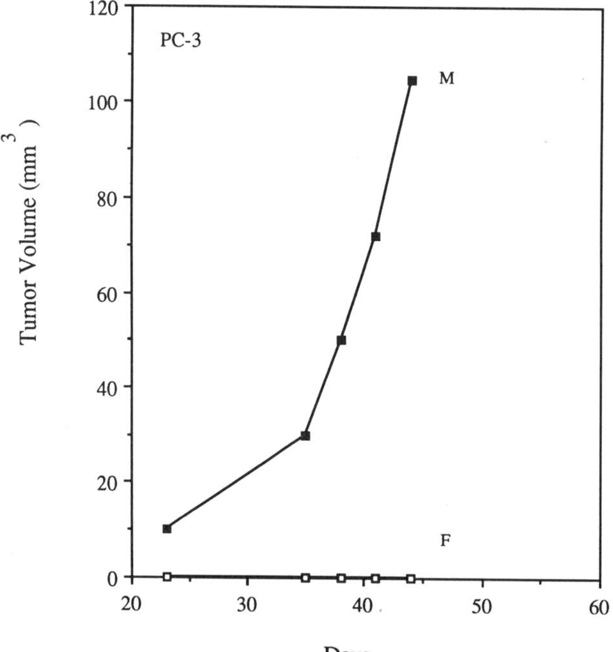

Fig. 5. Fetal UGM cells accelerated the growth of PC-3 tumours in male (M) but not female (F) hosts

sex dependent differences in growth rate. However, we noted that once the chimaeric PC-3 tumours became established, they grew at the same rate in both male and female hosts. In serial passage of the transplanted tumours, mesenchymal cell growth often became dominant. The androgen responsiveness of chimaeric WH + rUGM tumours was further confirmed by the demonstration that the growth of the chimaeric tumours was depressed in castrated hosts but increased when exogenous androgen (eg testosterone propionate) was administered.

Histomorphologically, the WH + rUGM tumours were predominantly carcinomas with a minimal number of mesenchymal cells, an observation that was supported by dot blot hybridization of the tumour DNA using a human specific *Alu* cDNA as a probe. The PC-3 + rUGM tumours were carcinomas in males and sarcomas in females. Transplanted tumours derived from the males behaved histologically as carcinomas in both males and females. These results were further confirmed by dot blot analysis using an *Alu* cDNA probe, which demonstrated that the predominant tumour DNA was derived from human sources. The ability of the established human PC-3 chimaeric tumours to grow equally well in male and female hosts as subcutaneous transplants was probably the result of autocrine stimulation by the epithelial cell derived growth factors whose production was no longer under androgen regulation.

Our results demonstrate that the characteristics of androgen sensitive growth can be conferred on the androgen unresponsive human epithelial cells, WH and PC-3, in vivo by interaction with specific mesenchymal cells. The rUGM cells alone appear to be sufficient to mediate androgen induced mitogenic responses in vivo. Our results agreed with the early in vivo tissue-tissue interaction studies, which clearly demonstrated that androgen mediates rather than acts directly on the responding epithelium. This hypothesis of indirect action of androgen is supported by the following observations: (a) Androgen, when added directly to cultured rat prostatic epithelial cells, either inhibited (Nishi *et al*, 1988; Chang and Chung, 1989) or had no effect (McKeehan *et al*, 1984) on cell growth in vitro. However, when androgen was added to cocultured prostatic fibroblast and epithelial cells in vitro, it exerted a mitogenic action on cultured prostatic epithelial cells (Chang and Chung, 1989), a result consistent with the effect of androgen in vivo. (b) Androgen induced growth of Shionogi epithelial tumour cells in vitro can be neutralized by antibodies prepared against basic fibroblast growth factor (bFGF) or FGF like peptide (Lu *et al*, 1989). In this model, it is likely that growth factors serve as mediators of androgen induced cellular proliferation. (c) Conditioned medium isolated from prostatic stroma contains paracrine factors that elicit a growth stimulatory response on the cultured prostatic epithelium (Chang and Chung, 1989). Prostatic stromal factors also promoted the expression of a differentiation marker, transferrin, by the testicular Sertoli cells (Swinnen *et al*, 1990), which are under tight paracrine regulation by neighbouring peritubular cells (Skinner and Fritz, 1985).

In attempting to determine the possible mechanisms by which rUGM cells and human epithelial cell lines interact, we encountered some logistical problems. For example, coinjecting male hosts with rUGM cells and either WH or PC-3 cells usually produces carcinomas, but coculturing rUGM and WH or PC-3 cells in vitro, even under the influence of androgens, usually results in the dominance of mesenchymal cell proliferation. Also, an in vitro assay cannot assess the biological activities of angiogenic and other host factors. Our attempts to demonstrate direct interaction between rUGM and WH or PC-3 cells in vitro by coculturing them under various conditions have been unsuccessful.

Roles of Growth Factors

The polypeptide growth factors are a diverse and ever expanding gene family with known physiological functions. Growth factor peptides are required in normal mammalian development. Because the aberrant expression of growth factors, growth factor receptor and growth factor related oncogenes can cause hyperplastic and malignant transformation of cells, much attention in recent years has focused on the isolation, characterization and definition of structures and functions of prostatic growth factors, their receptors and the proto-oncogenes closely associated with the pathways of growth factor action (Story *et al*, 1987; Kyprianou and Isaacs, 1988; Mydlo *et al*, 1988; Thompson, 1990; Zhau *et al*, 1991). Focusing on growth factor research in prostate cancer and BPH is attractive and relevant, for several reasons: (a) Both human prostate cancer and BPH are characterized by their ability to proliferate. Up- and downregulation of specific growth factors, growth factor receptors and proto-oncogenes have been demonstrated during the growth of both human and rodent prostate (Traish and Wotiz, 1987, Katz *et al*, 1989), involution (Kyprianou and Isaacs, 1989) and carcinogenesis (Buttyan *et al*, 1988; Zhau *et al*, 1991). (b) Growth factors are expressed by prostatic cells, and the concentrations of growth factors present are sufficient to stimulate cell growth in vitro (Perkel *et al*, 1990). (c) Growth factors and their receptors in the prostate gland are regulated by androgen (Traish and Wotiz, 1987; Kyprianou and Isaacs, 1988); tight coupling between growth factor and ECM pathways has been demonstrated (Chiquet-Ehrismann *et al*, 1989; Gleave *et al*, 1991b) and may profoundly influence the growth and differentiative potential of the prostate cells (Gleave *et al*, 1991a,b; Hsieh *et al*, 1991). (d) Growth factors have been shown to play crucial parts in mammalian development, including morphogenesis, cell growth, migration and invasion.

Two broad categories of locally produced growth factors, the autocrine and paracrine growth factors, have been described. These categories are not mutually exclusive, because some growth factors exhibit bifunctional properties, stimulating the growth of target cells by both autocrine and paracrine pathways (Nonomura *et al*, 1988; Lu *et al*, 1989; Furuya *et al*, 1990). These investigators demonstrated that Shionogi carcinoma 115 (SC-115) cells, an androgen responsive mouse mammary cancer cell line, secrete an FGF like peptide that stimulates the growth of androgen responsive SC-115 cells in an autocrine fashion, but this same growth factor also stimulates the growth of an androgen unresponsive SC-115 subline in a paracrine manner. Connolly and Rose (1990) reported the biosynthesis and secretion of epidermal growth factor (EGF) and transforming growth factor-α (TGF-α) as autocrine growth factors in human prostatic DU-145 and LNCaP cells in culture. Studies by Jacob and Story (1988) indicated that EGF is actively secreted by rat VP when the prostate is perfused with neurotransmitters. Story *et al* (1987), Jacob *et al* (1979) and Lawson (1989) were among the first to isolate and characterize a human prostate derived growth factor (from human BPH) that shared structural homology with bFGF. Begun *et al* (1989) presented evidence that this growth factor may be derived predominantly from the periurethral region of the human prostate gland, where BPH often arises (McNeal, 1990). The role of bFGF in prostatic hyperplasia was further supported by using a transgenic mouse model whereby insertion of an *int-2* gene, a member of the bFGF family, resulted in the development of prostatic hyperplasia in the male and breast enlargement in the female hosts (Muller *et al*, 1990).

Transforming growth factor-β appears to be a predominantly inhibitory factor for the growth of many epithelial cell lines in vitro. Kyprianou and Isaacs (1988) showed an upregulation of TGF-β receptor in the rat VP during the active phase of prostatic regression, implicating the potential role of TGF-β in prostatic cell death upon androgen withdrawal. TGF-β strongly inhibits the growth of the androgen responsive prostate cancer cell line, LNCaP, in vitro (Gleave *et al*, 1991a,b). Using androgen induced growth of SC-115 cells as a model, Yamanishi *et al* (1990) reported that although TGF-β itself has no effect on the growth of SC-115 cells, it inhibited the growth elicited by androgen, presumably by blocking the secretion of an androgen induced bFGF or FGF like peptide; TGF-β did not affect either the affinity or the capacity of receptors for androgen or bFGF. Transforming growth factor-β is a bifunctional growth regulator, stimulating the growth of fibroblasts but inhibiting the growth of epithelial cells (Moses *et al*, 1985). However, TGF-β inhibited the growth of fibroblasts derived from human benign prostatic hyperplasia (Story M, personal communication), and fetal rUGM cells (Gleave M, Hsieh J and Chung L, unpublished) stimulated the growth of rat prostatic epithelial cancer cells (Shain *et al*, 1990) and immortalized human neonatal prostatic epithelial cells (Kaighn *et al*, 1989). Using a mouse prostate reconstitution model, Thompson (1990) proposes that TGF-β derived from mesenchyme may promote the malignant transformation of the *ras* and *myc* transfected prostate epithelial cells (Thompson *et al*, 1989). Moses *et al* (1990) reviewed the mechanism of TGF-β action involving a cascade of intermediary factors such as retinoblastoma (*RB*) and c-*myc* genes.

In addition, a number of other growth factors have also been found in prostate tissues and cells (Connolly and Rose, 1990). Sitaras *et al* (1988) reported that human prostate carcinoma cell lines, DU-145 and PC-3, express both platelet derived growth factors 1 (PDGF-1) and 2 (PDGF-2/c-*sis*) and

PDGF like proteins. Because PDGF receptors are not expressed by the secretory cells, these investigators suggest that PDGF may serve a paracrine role in organizing the ECM of the malignant prostate tissues. Platelet derived growth factor is capable of inducing the expression of c-*fos* (Greenberg and Ziff, 1984) and c-*myc* (Kelly *et al*, 1983); the latter was found to be elevated in human prostate cancer (Fleming *et al*, 1986; Buttyan *et al*, 1987) and may be required for enhanced mitogenic response to PDGF (Nag and Smith, 1989).

The propensity of human prostate cancer to metastasize to bone and the characteristic osteoblastic response induced by the metastasizing human prostatic cells have led to the search for both prostate and bone derived growth factors. Prostatic cancer cell lines seem capable of producing a large number of growth stimulating and inhibiting factors specifically for the growth of osteoblasts and/or bone fibroblasts (Perkel *et al*, 1990). Conversely, a mitogen found in the conditioned media of unstimulated human, rat or bovine bone marrow stimulated specifically human prostatic carcinoma cell line growth (Chackal-Roy *et al*, 1989). This bone marrow derived growth factor may assume an important role in vivo, enhancing a higher growth rate of the metastatic tumours in the bone than their primary tumours (Jacob, 1983; Berrettoni and Carter, 1986). Many known growth factors are tightly bound to bone matrix. Hauschka *et al* (1986) isolated at least four types of bone matrix derived growth factors by using an affinity column chromatography on heparin sepharose. Bashkin *et al* (1989) suggested that the bFGF tightly bound to ECM is prevented from acting on the endothelial cells; however, upon release by heparitinase, which degrades the ECM or displaces bFGF by heparin-like molecules, bFGF can induce local neovascular responses. Thus, it appears likely that specific growth factors presented locally can affect the growth and clonal selection of the prostate tumour cells and contribute to local neovasculization. Growth factors may be the ultimate driving force that determines the rate of prostatic cancer progression, metastatic potential, and the local osteoblastic reactions following prostatic cancer metastasis.

The complexity of interactions between growth factors and target cells can perhaps be placed in perspective. In particular, developmental biology studies investigating the molecular basis of morphogenesis and differentiation have yielded potentially exciting information about the possible action of growth factors in normal and neoplastic prostate development. During early *Xenopus* development, tissue interaction occurs between animal and vegetal poles, which leads to mesoderm differentiation at the tissue-tissue interface. This tissue interaction later determines the body axis of the embryo, an inductive event that can be best reproduced by the combination of FGF and TGF-β. Fibroblast growth factor seems to specify the more ventral mesoderm, whereas the combination of TGF-β and FGF specifies the more dorsal forms. A new member of the TGF-β family, activin B, has recently been shown to be a potent inducer capable of determining the dorsal-ventral axis, and to a significant degree, the anterior-posterior axis. The mRNA for activin B is expressed in the blastula stage of the embryo at the time when the body axis is determined. Thus, the biological properties of activin B share significant degrees of similarity with the proposed Spemann organizer. A prevailing common theme in the study of *Xenopus* and *Drosophila* development and differentiation is that growth factors seem to work in concert as morphogens, and each combination of growth factors seems to be regulated temporally, influencing the development of the organisms in a threshold dependent manner. A gradient of growth factors and their combinations can be created during various stages of embryonic development; multiple threshold response is clearly required for subsequent induction of cell specialization during cell differentiation (Reid, 1990). Because the basic principles underlying cell growth and differentiation are highly conserved throughout evolution, it is conceivable that similar temporal and spatial interaction between growth factors on specific target cells may be operative during prostate growth and neoplastic transformation.

Roles of Extracellular Matrix

Whereas tissue-tissue and cell-cell recombination models demonstrate that mesenchymal and epithelial cells communicate with each other through soluble growth factors (Chang and Chung, 1989; Camps *et al*, 1990; Djakiew *et al*, 1990; Furuya *et al*, 1990), the important role of ECM, by which the cells are in direct contact, cannot be discounted. The ECM is structurally localized between the interphase of mesenchymal and epithelial cells and is comprised of many heterogeneous but interacting proteins such as fibronectin, laminin, collagen IV, vitronectin, tenascin and sulphated proteoglycans. These ECM molecules are known to serve as the substratum for the attachment of both mesenchymal and epithelial cells. The functions of ECM are diverse: regulation of adhesion, migration, proliferation and differentiation of cells (Folman and Moscona, 1978; Hay, 1981; Reddi, 1985). The ECM can mediate its action through direct binding to cell membrane receptors or the integrins of the target cells and evokes signal transduction and cellular responses. By monitoring β-casein expression in hormone responsive mammary cells in culture, Goodman and Rosen (1990) and Schmidhauser *et al* (1990) suggest that an ECM responsive element may regulate transcription. The regulation by ECM must be tissue specific, as reported by Fujita *et al* (1986) for cultured liver cells and Emerman *et al* (1977) for cultured mammary epithelial cells.

The ECM can also act indirectly as follows: (a) It can affect cell morphology, hence its subsequent response to growth factors. Gospodarowicz *et al* (1978) showed that growth factor sensitivity of cultured cells was determined by cell morphology, which was intimately governed by the ECM substratum to which the cells attach. (b) The ECM can be differentially regulated by growth factors (Chakrabarty *et al*, 1988), influencing the growth factor receptor proteoglycan assembly (Hamati *et al*, 1989), forming tight complexes with growth factors (Bashkin *et al*, 1989) and modulating growth factor activities (Gordon *et al*, 1989), all of which alter the response of target cells to local growth factor microenvironment. (c) The ECM can induce cellular differentiation in vivo, which most likely requires the participation of less well defined host factor(s). Reddi and Anderson (1976) showed that mature fibroblasts can be induced to redifferentiate into chondroblasts and chondrocytes when in direct contact with demineralized bone collagen matrix in vivo. Recently, we reported (Gao and Chung, 1990) that exposing a non-tumorigenic rat prostatic epithelial cell line, NbE-1, to selective ECM components in vivo induced the cells to acquire tumorigenic potential; cells derived from the epithelial tumours were tumorigenic when inoculated in vivo in the absence of ECM, suggesting certain irreversible genetic changes induced by exposing NbE-1 cells in vivo with ECM.

The molecular mechanisms of cell-matrix interaction have been extensively investigated. A specific polypeptide sequence such as arginl-glycyl-aspartic acid (RGD) is required by cells for the attachment to fibronectin, laminin, vitronectin and other ECM components. Vukicevic *et al* (1990) reported that laminin derived synthetic peptides YIGSR-NH$_2$ and CSRARKQAASIKVAV-SADR-NH$_2$ promote the differentiation processes between rat primary calvarial bone cells and a mouse osteoblast like cell line to undergo the formation of osteocyte canalicular network in the bone. The latter 19 aminoacid synthetic laminin like peptide enhances metastastic potential of melanoma cells in vivo (Kanemoto *et al*, 1990). Sakamoto *et al* (1991) found that CDPGYIGSR-NH$_2$, similar to a synthetic laminin peptide YIGSR-NH$_2$, inhibited tumour angiogenesis and blocked endothelial cell migration. Thus, it appears that cell-matrix and matrix-matrix interactions are highly specific and that most of these interactions may involve specific regions of the protein and/or glycosamino-glycan domains. Pienta *et al* (1989) comprehensively reviewed the possible significance of cell-matrix interactions, the tensegrity model and the mechanism by which the chemomechanic properties of the cells that are coupled tightly to cell-matrix interactions may exert a profound effect on cell motility and ultimately influence their metastatic potential.

Mechanisms of Fibroblast-Epithelial Cellular Interaction

The reciprocal fibroblast-epithelial interaction in normal and neoplastic growth can be determined by using at least two fundamental mechanisms. Firstly, fibroblast-epithelial interaction is intrinsically driven and involves close metabolic cooperation between these two cell types. Secondly, fibroblast-epithelial interaction is epigenetically driven, evolving from cell differentiation and determination during the courses of cellular interaction and development.

The metabolic cooperation model recognizes the intrinsic differences between fibroblast and epithelial cells and emphasizes that each cell type may contribute dissimilar cellular components essential for eliciting hormone-mediated responses and tumour growth and progression. Figure 6 depicts rat prostatic epithelial cells converting testosterone to 5α-dihydrotestosterone (5α-DHT), which serves as the direct and active mitogen for the growth of

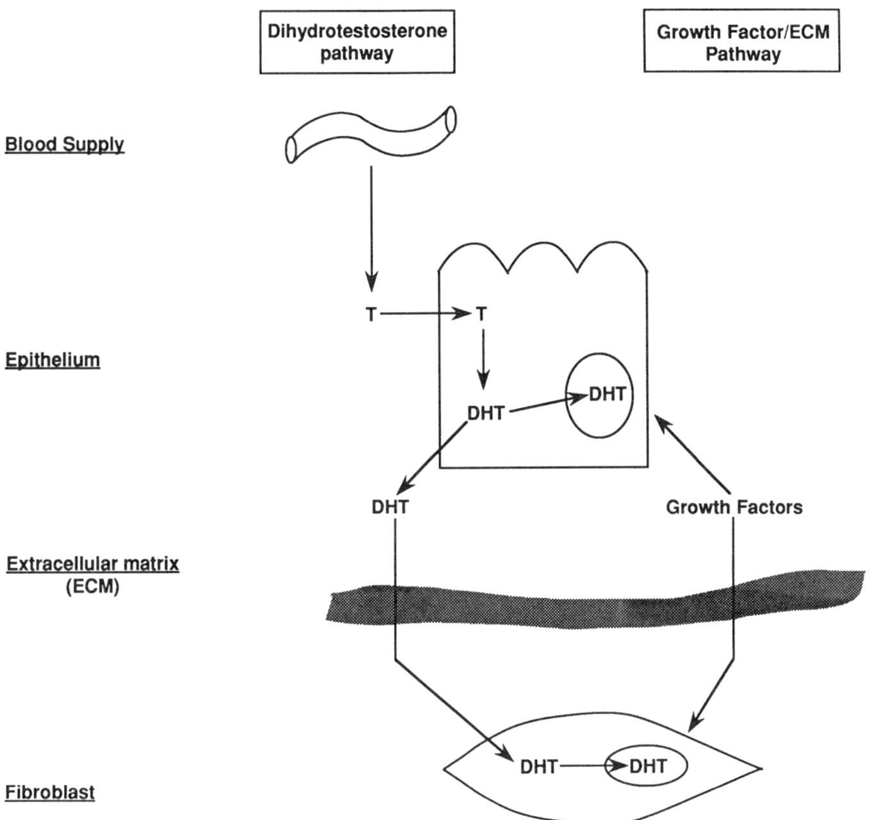

Fig. 6. A model of metabolic cooperation between prostatic epithelial and fibroblast cells. Circulating testosterone is metabolized to 5α-DHT predominantly by the epithelial cells. 5α-DHT acts either on the epithelial cells to promote protein synthesis or on the fibroblasts to promote cell proliferation when these cell types are cocultured. We speculated that growth factors (derived from epithelial or fibroblast cells), extracellular matrix (ECM) and neuroendocrine network (not shown, see Guthrie *et al*, 1990) are intimately involved in the cellular communication and regulation of gene expression by epithelial and fibroblast cells (see Chang and Chung, 1989)

prostatic fibroblasts in vitro. 5α-Dihydrotestosterone stimulates epithelial cell proliferation in vitro only if the epithelial cells are cocultured with prostatic fibroblasts (Chang and Chung, 1989). Specific fibroblast and epithelial cell derived paracrine factors have been reported to stimulate growth and gene expression. Conversely, the growth factors may act indirectly by "homing" the ingrowth of host endothelial cells to form local microvasculature that supports the growth of the chimaeric tumours. The cellular interaction between fibroblast and epithelial cells may also occur through growth factor and ECM exchanges. For example, the growth of LNCaP cells in vivo is dependent on the presence of competent fibroblasts (Gleave *et al*, 1991b). It is likely that growth factors produced by the epithelial cells will signal ECM production by the appropriate fibroblasts. This growth factor and ECM exchanges may be crucial to the maintenance of the growth and differentiative functions of the epithelial cells. This concept seems to also apply to other systems, including the human urinary bladder epithelial tumour model (Chung *et al*, 1991; Zhau H, Hong S and Chung L, unpublished) and the human mammary epithelial cancer model (Chiquet-Ehrismann *et al*, 1989). Finally, ECM may immobilize growth factor(s), produced by either the host or the tumour, that enhance tumour growth. rUGM cells may be involved in bidirectional interaction with the WH or PC-3 cells in vivo through pathways that possibly involve undefined host factors that help to create a microenvironment favourable to promoting chimaeric tumour growth. Cellular interaction with direct cell contact between fibroblasts and epithelial cells could not have occurred in well differentiated normal tissues because of the presence of a physical barrier, the basement membrane, between these two cell types. However, direct fibroblast-epithelial contact occurs during early embryonic development and during tumour invasion and metastasis. Thus, under these physiological and pathological conditions, fibroblasts can interact with epithelial cells through cell surface matrix proteins. Fehon *et al* (1990) demonstrated that during early *Drosophila* development, two epidermal growth factor like transmembrane proteins derived from two non-identical cell types are required to interact to form aggregates that program later epidermal development.

The adaptation and cell differentiation model emphasizes that fibroblast-epithelial interaction is a dynamic rather than a static system. As cellular interaction progresses in vivo, certain clonal selection and adaptation pressure may be placed on the cells for subsequent selection and establishment of appropriate new cell lineages. Furthermore, reciprocal mesenchymal-epithelial interconversion (Toole and Underhill, 1983; Ekblom, 1989), with the possibility of generating new cell lineages, is operative during early development and neoplastic progression. This model stresses the importance of fibroblast-epithelial interaction as an event that is temporally and developmentally regulated. It is assumed that certain genetic changes (eg DNA methylation and rearrangement) may or may not have occurred in response to host microenvironment. Thus, factors involved in this process may be multiple, may appear transiently and can induce subtle but stable and heritable changes.

Several experimental models provide evidence that certain epigenetic factors rather than conventional genetic alterations may be involved in tumour development and progression. Our laboratory (Chung *et al*, 1989) reported that a non-tumorigenic prostatic epithelial cell line (NbE-1) can be induced to participate in carcinosarcoma growth by coinoculation with a tumorigenic fibroblast cell line (NbF-1). Minimal genetic alterations appear to be induced in the NbE-1 cells cloned from the carcinosarcoma, because the cloned cell line remains non-tumorigenic and behaves similarly to its parental cell line, as analysed by flow cytometry. Rubin *et al* (1990) selected tumorigenic NIH3T3 fibroblast clones from non-tumorigenic parental background by depriving serum from the culture medium. They found that this induction of tumorigenic phenotypic expression can be reversed by further passage of the tumorigenic fibroblasts in tissue culture medium containing high concentrations of serum. Tumorigenic phenotypes were much more favourably expressed among the normal cells under conditions of repressed growth (Foulds, 1969); this phenomenon is applicable to the development and progression of human (Franks, 1954) and rodent (Noble, 1977) prostate tumours.

Although interconversion of stroma and epithelium has been recognized as an important step during mouse kidney and chick embryo development, there is no evidence that such conversion may have occurred in the normal development of the prostate gland or during its neoplastic transformation. It is, however, recognized that some cultured rodent prostatic cell lines lose their cytokeratin expression and assume a spindle shape during prolonged culture in vitro. Curiously, such cells often regain their cytokeratin expression when grown as a tumour in vivo. Because cell morphology is influenced by its surrounding ECM substratum, these observations may indicate possible interconversion of epithelial to fibroblast cells. At this time, the significance of this cellular interconversion, if it occurs at all, and its potential implication on the generation of new cell lineage relationship and on tumour development and progression are not clear.

SIGNIFICANCE OF HOST AND TUMOUR MICROENVIRONMENT ON PROSTATE CANCER PROGRESSION

Despite our observation that tumorigenic or non-tumorigenic fibroblasts and normal fetal UGM have marked growth inductive capability and are capable, to some extent, of inducing the differentiation of prostatic tumours, the question remains as to the potential roles and the significance of fibroblasts in prostate cancer growth and progression. Because more than 95% of the human prostate cancers are carcinomas, the question raised is what could be the roles of stroma in prostate carcinoma development and progression. Data from our LNCaP human prostate cancer model have revealed the following possibilities: (a) Stroma may be required to prime the epithelium and promote its expression of tumorigenic behaviour. Once the epithelium has been properly primed, it can progress independently from the influence of stroma. (b) Stroma could induce epithelial tumour metastasis by constant copresence with tumour epithelium. The amount of stroma present in a carcinoma specimen may be insignificant and even undetectable but is nonetheless required to support ECM and crucial growth factors for the continuous growth of tumour epithelium. (c) Stroma of the host organs to which the tumour metastasized may play a permissive role in supporting tumour epithelium growth. Thus, it is possible that prostate stroma is required to initiate metastatic growth, whereas stroma of the host organ to which the prostate cancer has metastasized is required to maintain metastatic growth. This reciprocal stromal-epithelial interaction is consistent with an early "seed and soil" hypothesis proposed by Paget (1889).

In theory, carcinogenesis may involve multiple hits of either mesenchymal or epithelial cell types or both and carcinogenic insults may be cumulative.

Thus, can multistep carcinogenesis of the epithelium be the end result of hits accumulated by the epithelium and its adjacent mesenchyme? In the presence of an inductive mesenchyme, a transformed but non-tumorigenic epithelium can be activated to express full tumorigenic potential including rapid growth, angiogenesis, invasion and possibly cell migration and metastasis. Equally important is the stage(s) of progression of the interacting epithelial and mesenchymal (fibroblast) cells. There is evidence that acceleration of epithelial cell growth in vivo and in vitro by fibroblasts is tumour epithelial cell stage specific. For example, by using a coculture of epithelial and fibroblast cells in vitro, we have shown that normal prostate fibroblasts inhibit normal prostatic epithelial growth (Chang and Chung, 1989), whereas tumorigenic (Chung *et al*, 1989; Camps *et al*, 1990) and non-tumorigenic (Gleave *et al*, 1991a,b) fibroblasts accelerated both tumorigenic and non-tumorigenic epithelial cell growth in vivo. Pritchett *et al* (1989) demonstrated that bladder epithelial cells derived from only highly invasive human bladder cancer responded to stromal induced growth stimulation. These observations raised an extremely important possibility, ie that host and tumour stroma may have an even more important role than previously recognized in promoting tumour growth and metastasis, particularly at the end stage of tumour progression. It is entirely possible that because epithelial cancer cells invade and migrate, thus crossing the basement membrane barrier, they are in contact with the stroma during the end stage of carcinogenesis. This encounter may greatly facilitate the growth of cancer epithelial cells, a hypothesis that requires vigorous testing and that could be of pivotal importance in determining the ultimate outcome of tumour progression.

SUMMARY

A novel cell-cell recombination model was established to test the reciprocal mesenchymal (fibroblast)-epithelial interaction in the prostate gland. Both growth factors and ECM pathways were found to be actively engaged during cellular communications. The application of this cell-cell recombination concept to prostate cancer established a new human prostate cancer animal model in which the tumours actively secrete prostate specific antigen, a known human prostate cancer marker. This review explores the significance of mesenchymal-epithelial interaction in determining prostate hormonal responsiveness and prostate cell transformation and speculates on the potential roles of mesenchymal-epithelial interaction in prostate cancer growth and progression.

Acknowledgements

The authors wish to acknowledge the excellent secretarial and editorial assistance of Carolyn Davis and Dana Evans, respectively. This work was supported in part by a research grant from National Institutes of Health (DK-38649) and the David Bruton Jr. Charitable Trust.

References

Bashkin P, Doctrow S, Klagsbrun M, Svahn CM, Folkman J and Vlodavsky I (1989) Basic fibroblast growth factor binds to subendothelial extracellular matrix and is released by heparitinase and heparin-like molecules. *Biochemistry* **28** 1737–1743

Begun FP, Story MT, Jacobs SC and Lawson RK (1989) Distribution of basic fibroblast growth factor within the prostate. *Journal of Urology* **141** 307A

Bernfield MR, Banerjee SD and Cohn RH (1972) Dependence of salivary epithelial morphology and branching morphogenesis upon acid mucopolysaccharide-protein (proteoglycan) at the epithelial surface. *Journal of Cell Biology* **52** 674–689

Berrettoni BA and Carter JR (1986) Mechanisms of cancer metastasis to bone. *Journal of Bone and Joint Surgery American Journal* **68A** 308–312

Burwen SJ and Pitelka DR (1980) Secretory function of lactating mouse mammary epithelial cells cultured on collagen gels. *Experimental Cell Research* **126** 249–262

Buttyan R, Sawczuk IS, Benson MC, Siegal JD and Olsson CA (1987) Enhanced expression of c-myc protooncogene in high-grade human prostate cancers. *Prostate* **11** 327–337

Buttyan R, Zakeri Z, Lockshin R and Wolgemuth D (1988) Cascade induction of c-fos, c-myc and heat shock 70K transcripts during regression of the rat ventral prostate. *Molecular Endocrinology* **2** 650–657

Camps JL, Chang SM, Hsu TC *et al* (1990) Fibroblast-mediated acceleration of human epithelial tumor growth in vivo. *Proceedings of the National Academy of Sciences of the USA* **87** 75–79

Chackal-Roy M, Niemeyer C, Moore M and Zetter BR (1989) Stimulation of human prostatic carcinoma cell growth by factors present in human bone marrow. *Journal of Clinical Investigation* **84** 43–50

Chakrabarty S, Tobon A, Varani J and Brattain MG (1988) Induction of carcinoembryonic antigen secretion and modulation of protein secretion/expression and fibronectin/laminin expression in human colon carcinoma cells by transforming growth factor-β. *Cancer Research* **48** 4059–4064

Chang SM and Chung LWK (1989) Interaction between prostatic fibroblast and epithelial cells in culture: role of androgen. *Endocrinology* **125** 2719–2727

Chiquet-Ehrismann R, Kalla P and Pearson CA (1989) Participation of tenascin and transforming growth factor-β in reciprocal epithelial-mesenchymal interactions of MCF7 cells and fibroblasts. *Cancer Research* **49** 4322–4325

Chung LWK and MacFadden DK (1980) Sex steroid imprinting and prostate growth. *Investigative Urology* **17** 337–342

Chung LWK and Cunha GR (1983) Stromal-epithelial interactions: II Regulation of prostate growth by embryonic urogenital sinus mesenchyme. *Prostate* **4** 503–511

Chung LWK, Anderson NG, Neubauer BL, Cunha GR, Thompson TC and Rocco AK (1981) Tissue interaction in prostate development, In: Murphy GP, Sandberg AA, Karr JP (eds). *The Prostatic Cell: Structure and Function*, pp 177–203, AR Liss, New York

Chung LWK, Matsuura J and Runner MN (1984) Tissue interactions and prostatic growth: I Induction of adult mouse prostatic hyperplasia by fetal urogenital sinus implants. *Biology of Reproduction* **31** 155–163

Chung LWK, Chang SM, Bell C, Zhau H, Ro JY and von Eschenbach AC (1988) Prostatic carcinogenesis evoked by cellular interaction. *Environmental Health Perspectives* **77** 23–28

Chung LWK, Chang SM, Bell C, Zhau HE, Ro JY and von Eschenbach AC (1989) Coinoculation of tumorigenic rat prostate mesenchymal cells with nontumorigenic epithelial cells results in the development of carcinosarcoma in syngeneic and athymic animals. *International Journal of Cancer* **43** 1179–1187

Chung LWK, Zhau HE and Ro JY (1990) Morphologic and biochemical alterations in rat prostatic tumors induced by fetal urogenital sinus mesenchyme. *Prostate* **17** 165–174

Chung LWK, Hong SJ, Zhau HE *et al* (1991) Fibroblast-mediated human epithelial tumor growth and hormonal responsiveness in vivo, In: Karr JP, Coffey DS, Smith RG, Tindall AJ (eds). *Molecular and Cellular Biology of Prostate Cancer*, pp 91–102, Plenum Press, New York

Connolly JM and Rose DP (1990) Production of epidermal growth factor and transforming growth factor α by the androgen-responsive LNCaP human prostate cancer cell line. *Prostate* **16** 209–218

Cunha GR (1976) Epithelial-stromal interactions in the development of the urogenital tract. *International Review of Cytology* **47** 137–194

Cunha GR and Chung LWK (1981) Stromal-epithelial interaction: I Induction of prostatic phenotype in urothelium of testicular feminized (TFm/y) mice. *Journal of Steroid Biochemistry* **14** 1317–1321

Cunha GR, Chung LWK, Shannon JM, Taguchi O and Fujii H (1983) Hormone-induced morphogenesis and growth: role of mesenchymal-epithelial interactions. *Recent Progress in Hormone Research* **39** 559–598

DeCosse J, Gossens CL and Kuzma JF (1973) Breast cancer: induction of differentiation by embryonic tissue. *Science* **181** 1057–1058

Djakiew D, Tarkington MA and Lynch JH (1990) Paracrine stimulation of polarized secretion from monolayers of a neoplastic prostatic epithelial cell line by prostatic stromal cell proteins. *Cancer Research* **50** 1966–1974

Drews U (1975) Direct and mediated effects of testosterone: the development of intersexes in sex reversed mosaic mice, heterozygous for testicular feminization. *Anatomy and Embryology* **146** 325–340

Drews U and Drews U (1975) Metabolic cooperation between Tfm and wild-type cells in mosaic mice after induction of DNA synthesis. *Cell* **6** 475–479

Drews U and Drews U (1977) Regression of mouse mammary gland anlagen in recombinations of Tfm and wild-type tissues: testosterone acts via the mesenchyme. *Cell* **10** 401–404

Ekblom P (1989) Developmentally regulated conversion of mesenchyme to epithelium. *FASEB Journal* **3** 2141–2150

Emerman JT, Enami J, Pitelka DR and Nandi S (1977) Hormonal effects on intracellular and secreted casein in cultures of mouse mammary epithelial cells on floating collagen membranes. *Proceedings of National Academy of Sciences of the USA* **74** 4466–4470

Fearon ER and Vogelstein B (1990) A genetic model for colorectal tumorigenesis. *Cell* **61** 759–767

Fehon RG, Kooh PJ, Rebay I *et al* (1990) Molecular interactions between the protein products of neurogenic loci Notch and Delta, two EGF-homologous genes in Drosophila. *Cell* **61** 523–534

Fleming WH, Hamel A, MacDonald R *et al* (1986) Expression of c-myc protooncogene in human prostatic carcinoma and benign prostatic hyperplasia. *Cancer Research* **46** 1535–1538

Folkman J and Moscona A (1978) Role of cell shape in growth control. *Nature* **273** 345–349

Foulds L (1969) *Neoplastic Development*, vol 1, p 73, Academic Press, New York

Franks LM (1954) Benign nodular hyperplasia of the prostate: a review. *Annals of the Royal College of Surgeons of England* **14** 92–106

Franks LM (1956) The spread of prostate cancer. *Journal of Pathology and Bacteriology* **72** 603–611

Franks LM, Riddle PN, Carbonell AW and Gey GO (1970) A comparative study of the ultrastructure and lack of growth capacity of adult human prostate epithelium mechanically separated from its stroma. *Journal of Pathology* **100** 113–119

Freeman MR, Song Y, Carson DD, Guthrie PD and Chung LWK (1991) Extracellular matrix and androgen receptor expression associated with spontaneous transformation of rat prostate fibroblasts. *Cancer Research* **51** 1910–1916

Fujii H, Cunha GR and Norman JT (1982) The induction of adenocarcinomatous differentiation in neoplastic bladder epithelium by an embryonic prostatic inductor. *Journal of Urology* **128** 858–861

Fujita M, Spray DC, Choi H *et al* (1986) Extracellular matrix regulation of cell-cell communication and tissue-specific gene expression in primary liver culture. *Progress in Clinical and Biological Research* **226** 333–360

Fukamachi H, Mizuno T and Kim YS (1986) Morphogenesis of human colon cancer cells with fetal rat mesenchymes in organ culture. *Experientia* **42** 312–315

Furuya Y, Sato N, Akakura K, Ichikawa T, Suzuki N and Sato R (1990) Paracrine growth stimulation of androgen-responsive Shionogi carcinoma 115 by its autonomous subline (Chiba subline 2). *Cancer Research* **50** 4979–4983

Gao C and Chung LWK (1990) Role of extracellular matrix in prostatic carcinogenesis. *American Association in Cancer Research Proceedings* **31** 227 [Abstract]

Gleave ME, Hsieh JT, Gao C, von Eschenbach AC and Chung LWK (1991a) Prostate and bone fibroblasts induce human prostate cancer growth in vivo: implications for bidirectional stromal-epithelial interaction in prostate carcinoma growth and metastasis. *Journal of Urology* **145** 213A

Gleave M, Hseih JT, Gao C, von Eschenbach AC and Chung LWK. (1991b) Acceleration of human prostate cancer growth in vivo by factors produced by prostate and bone fibroblasts. *Cancer Research* **51** 3753–3761

Goodman HS and Rosen JM (1990) Transcriptional analysis of the mouse β-casein gene. *Molecular Endocrinology* **4** 1661–1670

Gospodarowicz D, Greensburg G and Birdwell CR (1978) Determination of cellular shape by the extracellular matrix and its correlation with the control of cellular growth. *Cancer Research* **38** 4155–4171

Gootwine E, Webb CG and Sachs L (1982) Participation of myeloid leukemia cells injected into embryo in haematopoietic differentiation in adult mice. *Nature* **299** 63–65

Gordon PB, Choi HU, Conn G *et al* (1989) Extracellular matrix heparan sulfate proteoglycans modulate the mitogenic capacity of acidic fibroblast growth factor. *Journal of Cellular Physiology* **140** 584–592

Greenberg ME and Ziff EB (1984) Stimulation of 3T3 cells induces transcription of the c-fos proto-oncogene. *Nature* **311** 433

Grobstein C (1953) Epithelio-mesenchymal specificity of the morphogenesis of mouse submandibular rudiments in vitro. *Journal of Experimental Zoology* **124** 383–413

Grobstein C (1956) Trans-filter induction of tubules in mouse metanephrogenic mesenchyme. *Experimental Cell Research* **10** 424–440

Guthrie PD, Freeman MR, Liao S and Chung LWK (1990) Regulation of gene expression in rat prostate by androgen and β-adrenergic receptor pathways. *Molecular Endocrinology* **4** 1343–1353

Hamati HF, Britton EL and Carey DJ (1989) Inhibition of proteoglycan synthesis alters extracellular matrix deposition, proliferation and cytoskeletal organization of rat aortic smooth muscle cells in culture. *Journal of Cell Biology* **108** 2495–2505

Hannappel E and Drews U (1981) Stimulation of growth by testosterone via the mesenchyme: recombination of tissues from Tfm and wild-type preputial gland anlagen of mouse embryo. *Cell Tissue Research* **221** 321–332

Hauschka PV, Maurakos AE, Iafrati MD, Soleman SE and Klagsbrun M (1986) Growth factors in bone matrix: isolation of multiple types by affinity chromatography on heparin sepharose. *Journal of Biological Chemistry* **261** 12665–12674

Hay ED (1981) *Cell Biology of Extracellular Matrix*, Plenum Publishing Co, New York

Hayashi N, Cunha GR and Wong YC (1990) Influence of male genital tract mesenchymes on differentiation of Dunning prostatic adenocarcinoma. *Cancer Research* **50** 4747–4754

Higgins JRA and Gosling JA (1989) Studies on the structure and intrinsic innervation of the normal human prostate. *Prostate* (**Supplement**) **2** 5–16

Hilfer SR (1983) Development of terminal buds in the fetal mouse lung. *Scad Electron Microscope* **3** 1387–1401

Horoszewicz JS, Leong SS, Kawinski E *et al* (1983) LNCaP model of human prostatic carcinoma. *Cancer Research* **43** 1809–1818

Hsieh JT, Wang XH, Zhau HE, Liew CC and Chung LWK (1991) Cloning and characterization of the expression of a specific cytokeratin subtype from the rat ventral prostate gland: evidence for a new class of androgen-repressed gene. *Journal of Urology* **145** 330A (abstract)

Isaacs JT, Isaacs WB, Feitz WFJ and Sheres J (1986) Establishment and characterization of seven Dunning rat prostatic cancer cell lines and their use in developing methods for predicting metastatic abilities of prostatic cancer. *Prostate* **9** 261–281

Jacobs SC (1983) Spread of prostate cancer to bone. *Urology* **21** 337–344

Jacob SC and Story MT (1988) Exocrine secretion of epidermal growth factor by the rat prostate: effects of andrenergic agents, cholinergic agents and vosactive intestinal peptide. *Prostate* **13** 79–87

Jacob SC, Pikna D and Lawson RK (1979) Prostatic osteoblastic factor. *Investigative Urology* **17** 195–198

Jarow JP and Isaacs JT (1989) Prostatic growth effects of rat urogenital sinus and human prostatic tissue in the rat. *Prostate* **14** 301–308

Kabalin JN, Peehl DM and Stamey TA (1989) Clonal growth of human prostatic epithelial cells is stimulated by fibroblasts. *Prostate* **14** 251–263

Kaighn ME, Reddel RR, Lechner JF *et al* (1989) Transformation of human neonatal prostate epithelial cells by strontium phosphate transfection with a plasmid containing SV40 early region genes. *Cancer Research* **49** 3050–3056

Kanemoto T, Reich R, Royce L *et al* (1990) Identification of an amino acid sequence from laminin A chain that stimulates metastasis and collagenase IV production. *Proceeding of the National Academy of Sciences of the USA* **87** 2279–2283

Katz AE, Benson GJ, Wise CA *et al* (1989) Gene activity during the early phase of androgen-stimulated rat prostate regrowth. *Cancer Research* **49** 5889–5894

Kelly K, Cochran BH and Stiles CD (1983) Cell specific regulation of c-myc gene by lymphocyte mitogens and platelet-derived growth factor. *Cell* **35** 603–610

Kollar EJ (1983) Epithelial-mesenchymal interactions in the mammalian integument: tooth development as a model for instructive induction, In: Sawyer RH, Fallon JF (eds). *Epithelial-Mesenchymal Interactions in Development*, pp 27–49, Praeger Publishers, New York

Kratochwil K and Schwartz P (1976) Tissue interaction in androgen response of embryonic mammary rudiment of mouse: identification of target for testosterone. *Proceedings of the National Academy of Sciences of the USA* **73** 4041–4044

Kyprianou N and Isaacs JT (1988) Identification of a cellular receptor for transforming growth factor-β in rat ventral prostate and its negative regulation by androgens. *Cancer Research* **123** 2124–2131

Kyprianou N and Isaacs JT (1989) Expression of transforming growth factor-β in the rat ventral prostate during castration-induced programmed cell death. *Molecular Endocrinology* **3** 1515–

Lasnitzki I and Mizuno T (1980) Prostatic induction: interaction of epithelium and mesenchyme from normal wild-type mice and androgen-insensitive mice with testicular feminization. *Journal of Endocrinology* **85** 423–428

Lawson RK (1989) Growth factor and benign prostatic hyperplasia. *World Journal of Urology* **6** 189–193

Levine S, Pictet R and Rutter WJ (1973) Control of cell proliferation and cytodifferentiation by a factor reacting with the cell surface. *Nature* **246** 49–52

Lu J, Nishizawa Y, Tanaka A *et al* (1989) Inhibitory effect of antibody against basic fibroblast growth factor on androgen- or glucocorticoid-induced growth of Shionogi carcinoma 115 cells in serum-free culture. *Cancer Research* **49** 4963–4967

McKeehan WL, Adams PS and Rosser MP (1984) Direct mitogenic effects of insulin, epidermal growth factor, glucocorticoid, cholera toxin, unknown pituitary factors and possibly prolactin, but not androgen or normal prostate epithelial cells in serum-free, primary cell culture. *Cancer Research* **44** 1998–2010

McNeal JE (1978) Origin and evolution of benign prostatic enlargement. *Investigative Urology*

15 340–345

McNeal J (1990) Pathology of benign prostatic hyperplasia insight into etiology. *Urologic Clinic of North America* **17** 477–486

Merchant DJ (1990) Primary explant culture of human prostate tissue: a model for the study of prostate physiology and pathology. *Prostate* **16** 103–126

Mintz B and Illmensee K (1975) Normal genetically mosaic mice produced from malignant teratocarcinoma cells. *Proceedings of the National Academy of Sciences of the USA* **72** 3585–3589

Moore RA (1943) Benign hypertrophy of prostate: a morphological study. *Journal of Urology* **50** 680–710

Mori H, Maki M, Oishi K *et al* (1990) Increased expression of genes for basic fibroblast growth factor and transforming growth factor type β_2 in human benign prostatic hyperplasia. *Prostate* **16** 71–80

Moses HL, Yang EY and Pietenpol JA (1990) TGF-β Stimulation and inhibition of cell proliferation: new mechanistic insights. *Cell* **63** 245–247

Muller WU, Lee FS, Dickson C, Peters C, Pattengale P and Leder P (1990) The int-2 gene product acts as an epithelial growth factor in transgenic mice. *EMBO Journal* **9** 907–913

Mydlo JH, Michaeli J, Heston WDW and Fair WR (1988) Expression of basic fibroblast growth factor mRNA in benign prostatic hyperplasia and prostatic carcinoma. *Prostate* **13** 241–247

Nag A and Smith RG (1989) Amplification, rearrangement and elevated expression of c-myc in the human prostatic carcinoma cell line LNCaP. *Prostate* **15** 115–122

Neubauer BL, Best KL, Hoover DM, Slisz ML, VanFrank RM and Goode RL (1986) Mesenchymal-epithelial interactions as factors influencing male accessory sex organ growth in the rat. *Federation Proceedings* **45** 2618–2626

Nishi N, Matuo Y, Nakamoto T and Wada F (1988) Proliferation of epithelial cells derived from rat dorsolateral prostate in serum-free primary cell culture and their response to androgen. *In Vitro: Cellular Developmental Biology* **8** 778–786

Noble RL (1977) Hormonal control of growth and prognosis in tumors of Nb rats and a theory of action. *Cancer Research* **37** 82–94

Nonomura N, Nakamura N, Uchida N *et al* (1988) Growth stimulatory effect of androgen-induced autocrine growth factor(s) secreted from Shionogi carcinoma 115 cells on androgen-unresponsive cancer cells in a paracrine mechanism. *Cancer Research* **48** 4904–4908

Paget S (1889) The distribution of secondary growths in cancer of the breast. *Lancet* **i** 571–573

Peehl DM, Wong ST and Stamey TA (1988) Clonal growth characteristics of adult human prostatic epithelial cells. *In Vitro: Cellular Developmental Biology* **24** 530–536

Perkel VS, Mohan S, Herring SJ, Baylink DJ and Linkhart TA (1990) Human prostatic cancer cells, PC-3 elaborate mitogenic activity which selectively stimulates human bone cells. *Cancer Research* **50** 6902–6907

Pienta KJ, Partin AW and Coffey DS (1989) Cancer as a disease of DNA organization and dynamic cell structure. *Cancer Research* **49** 2525–2532

Pierce GB (1983) The cancer cell and its control by the embryo: Rous-Whipple Award Lecture. *American Journal of Pathology* **113** 117–124

Pierce GB, Aguilar D, Hood G and Wells RS (1984) Trophectoderm in control of murine embryonal carcinoma. *Cancer Research* **44** 3987–3996

Pritchett TR, Wang JKM and Jones PA (1989) Mesenchymal-epithelial interactions between normal and transformed human bladder cells. *Cancer Research* **49** 2750–2754

Podesta AH, Mullins J, Pierce GB and Wells RS (1984) The neurula stage mouse embryo in control of neuroblastoma. *Proceedings of the National Academy of Sciences of the USA* **81** 7608–7611

Raijfer J and Coffey DS (1978) Sex steroid imprinting of the immature prostate—long term effects. *Investigative Urology* **16** 186–190

Ramaekers FCS, Verhagen APM, Isaacs JT *et al* (1989) Intermediate filament expression and the progression of prostatic cancer as studied in the Dunning R3327 rat prostatic carcinoma system. *Prostate* **14** 323–339

Reddi AH (1985) *Extracellular Matrix: Structure and Function*, Alan R Liss, New York

Reddi AM and Anderson WA (1976) Collagenous bone matrix induced endochondral ossification and hemopoiesis. *Journal of Cellular Biology* **69** 557–572

Reid L (1990) From gradients to axes, from morphogenesis to differentiation. *Cell* **63** 875–882

Rubin AL, Arnstein P and Rubin H (1990) Physiological induction and reversal of focus formation and tumorigenicity in NIH 3T3 cells. *Proceedings of the National Academy of Sciences of the USA* **87** 10005–10009

Sakakura T, Sakagami Y and Nishizuka Y (1981) Accelerated mammary cancer development by fetal salivary mesenchyme isografted to adult mouse mammary epithelium. *Journal of the National Cancer Institute* **66** 953–959

Sakamoto N, Iwahana M, Tanaka NG and Osada Y (1991) Inhibition of angiogenesis and tumor growth by a synthetic laminin peptide, CDPGYIGSR-NH2. *Cancer Research* **51** 903–906

Schleicher G, Stumpf WE, Drews U, Thiedemann KU and Sar M (1985) Differential distribution of ^{3}H dihydrotestosterone and ^{3}H estradiol nuclear binding sites in mouse male accessory sex organs: an autoradiographic study. *Histochemistry* **82** 453–461

Schleicher G, Stumpf WE, Thiedemann K and Drews U (1988) Intersex mice composed of androgen insensitive Tfm and wild-type cells analyzed by ^{3}H dihydrotestosterone autoradiography. *Anatomy and Embryology* **178** 521–528

Sengel (1976) *Morphogenesis of Skin*, Cambridge University Press, London

Shain SA, Lin AL, Koger JD and Karaganis AG (1990) Rat prostate cancer cells contain functional receptors for transforming growth factor-β. *Endocrinology* **126** 818–825

Shannon JM and Cunha GR (1983) Autoradiographic localization of androgen binding in the developing mouse prostate. *Prostate* **4** 367–373

Sitaras NM, Sariban E, Bravo M, Pantazis P and Antoniades HN (1988) Constitutive production of platelet-derived growth factor-like proteins by human prostate carcinoma cell lines. *Cancer Research* **48** 1930–1935

Skinner MK and Fritz IB (1985) Androgen stimulation of Sertoli cell functions is enhanced by peritubular cells. *Molecular and Cellular Endocrinology* **40** 115–122

Stanbridge EJ and Nowell PC (1990) Origins of human cancer revisited. *Cell* **63** 867–874

Story MT, Sasse J, Jacobs SC and Lawson RL (1987) Prostatic growth factor: purification and structural relationship to basic fibroblast growth factor. *Biochemistry* **26** 3843–3849

Story, MT, Livingston B, Baeten L *et al* (1989) Cultured human prostate-derived fibroblasts produce a factor that stimulates their growth with properties indistinguishable from basic fibroblast growth factor. *Prostate* **15** 355–365

Swinnen K, Cailleau J, Heyns W and Verhoeven G (1990) Prostatic stromal cells and testicular peritubular cells produce similar paracrine mediators of androgen action. *Endocrinology* **126** 142–150

Takeda H, Mizuno T and Lasnitzki I (1985) Autoradiographic studies of androgen-binding sites in the rat urogenital sinus and postnatal prostate. *Journal of Endocrinology* **104** 87–92

Thompson TC (1990) Growth factors and oncogenes in prostate cancer. *Cancer Cells* **2** 345–354

Thompson TC and Chung LWK (1986) Regulation of overgrowth and expression of prostatic binding protein in rat chimeric prostate gland. *Endocrinology* **118** 2437–2444

Thompson TC, Cunha GR, Shannon JM and Chung LWK (1986) Androgen-induced biochemical responses in tissues lacking epithelial androgen receptors: characterization of androgen receptors in the mesenchyme of urogenital sinus-derived tissues. *Journal of Steroid Biochemistry* **25** 627–634

Thompson TC, Southgate J, Kitchner G and Land H (1989) Multi-stage carcinogenesis induced by ras and myc oncogenes in a reconstituted organ. *Cell* **56** 917–930

Toole BP and Underhill CB (1983) Regulation of morphogenesis by the pericellular matrix, In: Yamada M (ed). *Cellular Interactions and Development: Molecular Mechanisms*, pp 203–230, John Wiley and Sons, New York

Traish AM and Wotiz HH (1987) Prostatic epidermal growth factor receptors and their regulation by androgen. *Endocrinology* **121** 1461–1467

Van den Hooff A (1988) Stromal involvement in malignant growth. *Advanced Cancer Research* **50** 159–196

Vukicevic S, Luyten FP, Kleinman HK and Reddi AH (1990) Differentiation of canalicular cell processes in bone cells by basement membrane matrix component: regulation by discrete domains of laminin. *Cell* **63** 437–445

Yamanishi H, Nonomura N, Tanaka A *et al* (1990) Roles of transforming growth factor β in inhibition of androgen-induced growth of Shonogi carcinoma cells in serum-free medium. *Cancer Research* **50** 6179–6183

Zhau HE, Wan D, Chung LWK *et al* (1991) Expression of the HER-2/neu protooncogene in human prostate cancer. *Journal of Urology* **145** 348A [Abstract]

The authors are responsible for the accuracy of the references.

Polypeptide Modulators of Prostatic Growth and Development

MICHAEL T STORY

Departments of Urology and Biochemistry, Medical College of Wisconsin, Milwaukee, Wisconsin 53226

INTRODUCTION

Development of the prostate and maintenance of adult structure and function, as well as its pathological disturbances, benign prostatic hyperplasia (BPH) and prostate cancer, are strongly influenced by testicular androgens. There is abundant evidence, however, that androgens are not the only substances capable of influencing these events in prostate. The past decade of investigation has identified several polypeptides that either stimulate or inhibit growth. A list of these factors identified in the prostate, or in cultured cells derived from the prostate, is found in Table 1. Only those factors that have been positively identified by structural analysis and immunoreactivity with antibodies against known growth factors or whose gene transcripts have been identified are included. It is possible that other polypeptide modulators of prostatic growth and development are yet to be identified.

Cancer Surveys Volume 11: *Prostate Cancer*
© 1991 Imperial Cancer Research Fund. 0-87969-368-1/91. $3.00 + .00

TABLE 1. Growth stimulatory and inhibitory factors in prostate

Growth factor	Source	Species	Reference
HBGF			
bFGF	tissue (normal, BPH, cancer)	human	Story *et al* (1987a,b)
			Mydlo *et al* (1988)
			Mori *et al* (1990)
	fibroblasts in vitro		Story *et al* (1989)
	epithelial cells in vitro		Story (this issue)
	tissue	dog	Story (this issue)
	tissue	rat	Jacobs *et al* (1988)
	Dunning R-3327AT-3 tumour		Mansson *et al* (1989)
aFGF	tissue	rat	Katz *et al* (1989)
	epithelial cells in vitro		Mansson *et al* (1989)
	Dunning R-3327AT-3 tumour		Mansson *et al* (1989)
	Dunning R-3327PAP, mesenchymal cells		Mansson *et al* (1989)
KGF	tissue	human	Peehl DM *et al* (unpublished)
	fibroblasts in vitro		Peehl DM *et al* (unpublished)
TGF-β			
TGF-β1	tissue (normal, BPH)	human	Mori *et al* (1990)
	PC-82 xenograft		Kyprianou *et al* (1990)
	PC-3 cell line		Wilding *et al* (1989)
	DU-145 cell line		Wilding *et al* (1989)
	ventral prostate	rat	Kyprianou and Isaacs (1989)
TGF-β2	tissue (normal, BPH)	human	Mori *et al* (1990)
	PC-3 cell line		Ikeda *et al* (1987)
EGF, TGF-α			
EGF	tissue (BPH, cancer)	human	Shaikh *et al* (1990)
			Fowler *et al* (1988)
			Kishi *et al* (1988); Habib (1990)
	prostatic fluid		Gregory *et al* (1986)
	DU-145 cell line		Connolly and Rose (1989)
	tissue	rat	Jacobs *et al* (1988)
	tissue	mouse	Hiramatsu *et al* (1988)
	tissue	guinea pig	Shikata *et al* (1984)
TGF-α	LNCaP cell line	human	Schuurmans *et al* (1988)
	DU-145 cell line		Connolly and Rose (1989)
NGF	tissue	guinea pig	Harper *et al* (1979)
PDGF	DU-145 cell line	human	Sitaras *et al* (1988)
	PC-3 cell line		Sitaras *et al* (1988)

HEPARIN BINDING GROWTH FACTOR FAMILY

Identification in Prostate and Properties

The notion that growth factors were present in prostate came from the work of Jacobs *et al* (1979), who reported that extracts of normal postpubertal prostate, BPH prostate and well differentiated prostate cancer were mitogenic for cultured osteoblasts and fibroblasts. Since prostate cancer is notorious for metastases to bone with osteoblastic proliferation, and since increased stromal to epithelial cell content is a hallmark of BPH, it was postulated that the extracts contained a factor, termed prostate growth factor, that had a role in these disease states of the prostate. Prostate growth factor was subsequently purified to homogeneity from BPH tissue and shown by immunoreactivity (Story *et al*, 1987a) and aminoterminal sequence analysis (Story *et al*, 1987b) to be basic fibroblast growth factor (bFGF). These findings have been confirmed by others (Mydlo *et al*, 1988; Mori *et al*, 1990).

Basic FGF is a member of the heparin binding growth factor family (HBGF). To date, seven members of the HBGF family have been identified (reviewed in Benharroch and Birnbaum, 1990). As the name implies, members of the HBGF family share the common property of binding heparin. Family members share a high degree of structural homology. Basic FGF and acidic FGF (aFGF) share 55% aminoacid sequence homology (Esch *et al*, 1985). The complementary DNA (cDNA) sequences of both factors have been isolated (Jaye *et al*, 1986; Kurokawa *et al*, 1987). The primary translation product of each is a 155 aminoacid polypeptide. Smaller 146 and 131 aminoacid forms of bFGF and 140 and 134 aminoacid forms of aFGF have been described. These truncated forms, which exhibit full biological activity, result from proteolytic cleavage of the precursor molecule. The primary translation products of these factors do not contain sequences usually associated with secretory signals. This apparent lack of a signal peptide for bFGF will be important to considerations of the possible physiological role of this factor in prostate.

Basic FGF has been isolated from a wide variety of normal tissues derived from mesoderm and neuroectoderm, as well as from malignant tissues (reviewed in Gospodarowicz, 1990). It is difficult to compare growth factor levels in various tissues reported in the literature because of the lack of uniformity in assays used by different laboratories. Our analysis, employing a standarized radioimmunoassay specific for bFGF, indicates that human prostate is a rich source of the growth factor. Among tissues that we have analysed, bFGF levels were highest in bovine pituitary. Levels of the growth factor were higher in human prostate than in human placenta, canine and rat prostates and considerably higher than in human kidney and testis. Basic FGF levels in BPH are two to three times higher per mass of tissue than in normal prostate (Story MT, unpublished). A recent report by Mori *et al* (1990) illustrating that bFGF mRNAs were higher in BPH than in normal prostate is consistent with our findings. Nishi *et al* (1988) also reported that the growth factor content of BPH tissue was two to four times higher than that of normal and cancerous prostates. It is likely that the higher level of biological activity found in BPH tissue was due to bFGF. The mitogen was associated with a fraction that bound heparin with high affinity, consistent with the properties of bFGF. Together, these reports provide strong evidence that bFGF is significantly higher in BPH than in normal prostate.

Previous studies demonstrating bFGF in prostate used homogenates prepared from whole tissue. Progress has been made in identifying the population of prostatic cells that synthesize bFGF. Our approach has been to (a) isolate stromal and epithelial cells from prostate, propagate the cells in culture and determine the capacity of the cells to synthesize the growth factor; (b) localize bFGF immunohistochemically in cultured cells and in prostate specimens; and (c) perform northern analysis and in situ hybridization for bFGF transcripts. These studies (Story *et al*, 1989) showed that cell lysates prepared from cultured prostate derived fibroblasts were mitogenic for the same cells in culture. The mitogen competed with radioactively labelled bFGF for binding to antiserum against bFGF. The elution profile of the mitogen from a column of heparin-Sepharose was identical to that of authentic bFGF, and the eluted protein reacted with antiserum against bFGF when analysed by western blotting. Furthermore, prostatic fibroblasts incorporated [^{35}S]methionine into protein that was both precipitated with antiserum against bFGF and of the same molecular weight as authentic bFGF. Recently, bFGF transcripts have been identified in prostatic fibroblasts by northern analysis (Story MT, unpublished). The conclusion is that cultured prostate derived fibroblasts synthesize a growth factor that stimulates their growth and has properties consistent with those of bFGF. Cultured prostatic epithelial cells also appear to synthesize bFGF. However, the level of the growth factor in the epithelial cells appeared much lower than in fibroblasts. Metabolic labelling studies and precipitation of cellular proteins with antiserum against bFGF indicated that epithelial cells have the capacity to synthesize bFGF (Story MT, unpublished). It will be important to determine whether prostatic epithelial cells and prostate cancer cells in vivo express the growth factor.

Immunohistochemical staining of prostate specimens for bFGF with monoclonal antibody developed against bFGF suggests that the stroma is a rich source of bFGF (Story MT, unpublished). Intense staining was seen in the stroma supporting the ascinar ducts. There was also faint staining of some of the epithelial cells. Since immunohistochemical techniques only provide information about the location of the factor and not about the cell population that synthesizes it, in situ hybridization studies will be needed to identify the prostatic cells that synthesize bFGF.

Advances have been made in propagating epithelial cells from human (Peehl and Stamey, 1986; Kozlowski *et al*, 1988) and rodent (McKeehan *et al*, 1984; Taketa *et al*, 1990) prostates. The requirements for in vitro propagation of prostatic epithelial cells differ considerably from the requirements for propagation of the fibroblasts. Stromal cells seem to require serum for propagation in vitro, although growth in serum free medium has recently been reported (Taketa *et al,* 1990). Epithelial cells can be propagated in serum free medium supplemented with selenium, glucocorticoid, cholera toxin, insulin, transferrin, epidermal growth factor (EGF) and bovine pituitary extract (BPE). Bovine pituitary extract contains bioactive and immunoactive FGFs and perhaps other growth factors. Controversy exists as to the requirement for FGF for propagation of prostatic epithelial cells in culture. In this respect, McKeehan *et al* (1987) reported that BPE could be replaced by FGF. Kabalin *et al* (1989) were unable to substitute purified FGF for BPE to support the growth of human prostatic epithelial cells in vitro, but they found that cocultivation of epithelial cells with stromal cells or stromal cell conditioned medium stimulated epithelial cell proliferation.

Epidermal growth factor and insulin are needed for the propagation of prostatic epithelial cells in culture (McKeehan *et al,* 1984; Peehl and Stamey 1986). Peehl DM, Rubin JS, Ron D, Wong ST and Stamey TA (unpublished) found that keratinocyte growth factor (KGF), a member of the HBGF family, was secreted by prostatic fibroblasts. This growth factor is believed to be selectively mitogenic for epithelial cells, and unlike FGFs, KGF has a signal secretory sequence (Finch *et al,* 1989). Peehl's group found that KGF and aFGF could, in part, replace the requirement for EGF for clonal growth of prostatic epithelial cells. Basic FGF was found to be less effective than KGF and aFGF. Keratinocyte growth factor transcripts were detected in prostatic fibroblasts, and KGF activity was found in medium conditioned by these cells. These observations support the notion that factors produced by prostatic fibroblasts regulate growth of the epithelium. Keratinocyte growth factor has characteristics that make it a strong candidate as a mediator of stromal-epithelial interactions in prostate.

Whether aFGF is present in human prostate is not entirely clear. We have suggested that human prostate may contain low levels of aFGF (Story *et al,* 1987a). Nishi *et al* (1988) described a growth factor in extracts of normal prostate whose affinity for heparin-Sepharose was consistent with the known property of aFGF. The factor was said to be absent from BPH prostates. These observations have not been extended nor confirmed by others. Mydlo *et al* (1988) did not detect immunoreactive aFGF in their analysis of HBGFs in human prostate. However, Mori *et al* (1990) indicated that aFGF transcripts were detected in 1 of 12 BPH, but none of 3 normal prostate, specimens analysed.

Controversy also exists regarding the form(s) of HBGFs synthesized by rat prostate. Jacobs *et al* (1988) identified a growth factor in adult rat ventral prostate with high affinity binding for heparin. Western blot analysis, with three different antibodies produced against bFGF synthetic sequences, identified the factor as bFGF. The factor competed with recombinant bovine bFGF for binding to antiserum against bFGF. Additionally, ventral prostate tissue preparations contained two other factors with EGF like properties. One of these was of unusually high molecular weight for EGF, whereas the other resembled EGF in size and immunological reactivity. Matuo *et al* (1987) found two types of growth factors, based on their different affinities for heparin-Sepharose, in rat prostates and in Dunning tumours. The predominant growth factor in dorsolateral prostate was of the low affinity type, whereas the major form of the growth factor in the Dunning tumour was of the high affinity type. The properties of the high affinity factor from the Dunning tumour were consistent with those of aFGF, and the properties of the low affinity type growth factor found in dorsolateral prostate were similar to those of EGF. Mansson *et al* (1989) identified aFGF transcripts in prostates of 6–8 week old rats. The transcripts were said to be specifically expressed by the epithelial cells. Expression of aFGF transcripts declined at 14 weeks of age and was undetectable in 35 week old animals. Basic FGF transcripts were reported to be undetectable in prostates from any age group of rats. Dunning R-3327PAP tumour, composed of a well defined epithelium and stroma, expressed aFGF (HBGF-1) transcripts specifically in the mesenchymal cells, whereas the Dunning R-3327AT-3 variant, which consists of a single cell type, expressed both HBGF-1 and HBGF-2 (bFGF) transcripts. Katz *et al* (1989) reported hybridization of their bFGF cDNA probe with polyadenylated RNA isolated during androgen stimulated regrowth of the rat prostate. It is possible that failure to detect bFGF mRNA in normal rat prostate (Mansson *et al,* 1989) was related to the probe that was used. The investigators used an HBGF-2 cDNA probe with sequence specificity for the bovine sequence, whereas Katz's group used a probe with sequence specificity for the human transcript. Thus, there is immunological and transcriptional evidence indicating that rat prostate expresses bFGF, the major FGF form in human prostate. Additionally, rat prostate may express aFGF, as do Dunning tumour variants. However, it would appear that some differences exist in expression of FGFs by human prostate and rat and Dunning tumours. Thus, it may be misleading if information regarding FGFs is extrapolated from one species to another.

Receptors

Little attention has been given to the identification of HBGF receptors in prostate. To modulate cellular proliferation and differentiation, these growth factors must presumably bind to their cell surface receptor. Information about the population(s) of prostatic cells that express HBGF receptors is important to the understanding of their physiological role in the prostate. Because these growth factors bind heparin, the design of experiments to characterize receptor-ligand interaction has been complicated. However, using either heparin or salt extraction to block high capacity low affinity binding (kDa = 10^{-9} M) believed to be heparin sulphate containing proteoglycan, it has been possible to identify high affinity receptors (kDa = 10^{-11} M) for HBGFs. Indeed, receptors for aFGF and bFGF have been identified on a number of growth factor responsive cells (Kan *et al,* 1988; Neufeld *et al,* 1988; Burrus and Olwin, 1989). Competition for radioactively labelled FGF binding and cross linking studies suggest that aFGF and bFGF cross react with two proteins in the range 110–165 kDa, depending on the species studied. Recently, the cDNAs for both human FGF receptors have been isolated (Dionne *et al*, 1990). The clones, termed *bek* and *flg*, predict mature core proteins of approximately 89 kDa; glycosylation would account for higher molecular weight forms that have been identified. Transfection of mammalian cells with expression vector confirmed that both *bek* and *flg* represent high affinity receptors for aFGF, as well as bFGF.

Studies by Mansson *et al* (1989) have demonstrated HBGF receptors in both epithelial and mesenchymal cells cultured from rat prostate. Additionally, both epithelial and mesenchymal cells of the Dunning tumour R-3327PAP and R-3327AT-3 cells exhibited HBGF receptors. Our studies with cultured human prostatic fibroblasts and epithelial cells indicated that both cell types express high affinity binding sites specific for bFGF (Story MT, unpublished). Incubation with cross linking agent and labelled ligand has identified specific binding proteins in the size range characteristic for the receptor.

A recent report by Bottaro *et al* (1990) has provided evidence for multiple HBGF receptors. They found that mouse epidermal keratinocyte cells, Balb/MK, possessed receptors for KGF. Acidic FGF displaced radioactively labelled KGF binding with 4-fold lower efficiency than KGF. Basic FGF also competed for KGF binding but with 20-fold lower efficiency than KGF, suggesting that these cells possessed related but distinct HBGF receptors. Progress has been reported in cloning the KGF receptor cDNA (Miki *et al*, 1991). Peehl *et al* (unpublished) found that KGF and aFGF could replace the requirement for EGF for clonal growth of prostatic epithelial cells. Basic bFGF was capable of providing some growth stimulation but was less potent than KGF and aFGF. Their findings suggest that the prostatic cells express receptors that recognize preferentially KGF and aFGF over bFGF. As antibodies and nucleotide probes for HBGF receptors become available, it should be possible to identify the prostatic cells that express HBGF receptors and determine whether receptor distribution is altered in BPH and prostate cancer.

Possible Role in Embryonic Development

Development of the prostate from the embryonic urogenital sinus and maintenance of the morphology and secretory function of the adult prostate are dependent on androgen. Castration results in reduction of prostatic weight, cessation of secretory activity and atrophy and death of the prostatic epithelium (Lee, 1981; Coffey, 1986). These events can be restored to the precastrated condition by androgen. Insight into possible mechanisms involved in androgen induced development and maintenance of the prostatic epithelium is found in the work of Cunha and coworkers (reviewed in Cunha, 1984). These investigators showed that fetal development of the prostate is dependent on stromal-epithelial interaction and that mesenchyme and not the epithelium is the target and mediator of androgen induced prostatic glandular development. It is likely that an androgen induced growth factor produced by mesenchyme controls the development of the prostatic epithelium.

Heparin binding growth factors have been implicated as mesenchyme inducers in embryonic development (reviewed in Gospodarowicz, 1990). Basic FGF mRNA and protein have been identified in *Xenopus* oocytes and early embryos (Kimelman *et al*, 1988). Slack *et al* (1987) reported that the application of bFGF to ectodermal explants of early *Xenopus* embryos induced mesenchymal differentiation. It remains to be determined whether adult tissue can respond to the inductive potential of bFGF and whether it might be the inducer of mesenchymal "reawakening" suggested by McNeal (1984) to be the initiator of the prostatic hyperplastic process.

Despite the requirements for androgen in vivo, the propagation of prostatic fibroblasts and epithelial cells in vitro is not dependent on androgen (McKeehan *et al*, 1984; Peehl and Stamey, 1986; Taketa *et al*, 1990). It may be that the cells that adapt to growth in culture are representative of the androgen independent cells of the prostate. Alternatively, it is possible that prostatic epithelial cells do not require androgen for growth in culture because their requirement for androgen is met by bFGF or another growth factor produced by the stromal cells. Basic FGF production by cultured prostatic fibroblasts appears not to be affected by steroid hormones. Expression of the growth factor was not affected by including androgen, oestrogen or combinations of these hormones in the growth medium (Story *et al*, 1990).

Transcripts for bFGF in the prostate of castrated rats increased dramatically after administration of androgen (Katz *et al*, 1989). Harris *et al* (1989) and Hall *et al* (1990) demonstrated androgen modulation of aFGF mRNA expression in DDT-1 cells. These cells, derived from a hamster ductus deferens smooth muscle tumour, have proved to be a useful model for steroid hormone responsive tumour growth in vitro. The growth of DDT-1 cells in culture was stimulated by testosterone. Fibroblast growth factors could replace testosterone in stimulating cell growth, and the phenomenon was correlated with testosterone's ability to elevate aFGF mRNA. Similarily, the growth of Shionogi carcinoma cells was stimulated by androgen. Growth of a cloned line, SC-3, in serum free medium in the presence of androgen conditioned the medium to support cell growth in the absence of androgen. The androgen induced factor was identified as an FGF like peptide (Nonomura *et al*, 1990) whose action was mediated by binding to the FGF receptor and inhibited by antibody against bFGF (Lu *et al*, 1989). These studies demonstrate that androgen dependent cell growth may be mediated by FGFs.

Angiogenic Properties and Possible Role in Tissue Repair

Acidic and basic FGFs have been studied for their angiogenic activities (reviewed in Folkman and Klagsbrun, 1987; Ingber and Folkman, 1989). The capacity of endothelial cells to undergo proliferation and form blood vessels in response to FGFs has been demonstrated in vitro. However, it is clear that most tissues in which FGFs are found normally show little endothelial proliferation. This might be due to a lack of a signal sequence for secretion, and thus FGFs remain intracellular or complexed with components of the extracellular matrix (ECM). Heparin sulphate containing proteoglycans are major components of the ECM. These structural elements bind and protect FGFs from enzymatic degradation (Schreiber *et al*, 1985; Gospodarowicz *et al*, 1986). The evidence for association of bFGF with heparin sulphate was provided by Baird and Ling (1987) and Vlodavsky *et al* (1987). Their studies showed that bFGF could be released from ECM reservoirs by treatment with heparinase or heparitinase or by brief exposure to high salt solutions or heparin. The storage of the growth factor in the ECM appears to make it inaccessible to its cell surface receptor, thus providing a mechanism to regulate its mitogenic potential. Structure-function studies with synthetic bFGF peptides have identified two sequences that cross react with FGF receptors (Baird *et al*, 1987). Both functional domains share the capacity to bind heparin. This emphasizes the importance of the ECM in modulating the mitogenic activity of the growth factor in vivo.

The formation of new blood vessels occurs during embryonic development and in remodelling of tissues in the adult. It is also a hallmark under pathological conditions such as the development of solid tumours, where capillary development is a prerequisite for expanded tumour growth (Folkman and Klagsbrun, 1987).

Heparin sulphate proteoglycan degradation is a major enzymatic step in the breakdown of the ECM. The degradation of these glycosaminoglycans, produced experimentally by heparinase and heparitinase treatment (Baird and Ling, 1987), results in decreased absorption of newly synthesized bFGF to the ECM and releases the growth factor from the ECM. Thus, one mechanism by which tumours and perhaps some normal cells induce neovascularization and cell proliferation might be the release of heparinase like enzymes (reviewed in Baird and Walicke, 1989). The observation that several tissues, including tumours, are a rich source of heparinase like enzymes (Vlodavsky *et al*, 1983; Matzner *et al*, 1985) supports this hypothesis. It is conceivable that bFGF may be released from ECM reservoirs in prostate in response to injury. The growth factor can be released upon cell lysis or by enhanced enzymatic turnover of the ECM. Heparin like molecules are products of vascular endothelial and smooth muscle cells (Castellot *et al*, 1981). Damage to these cells could release these molecules, which are known to compete with bFGF for binding to the ECM. Infiltrating lymphocytes and macrophages may contribute to the mobilization of bFGF. These cells are also known to release heparin and are a source of enzymes that degrade heparin sulphate containing proteoglycans. Once released, bFGF is free to bind cell surface receptors known to be located on prostatic fibroblasts and epithelial cells. The proliferative response of these cells to bFGF could initiate the fibromatous nodule that is believed to be the earliest pathological feature of BPH (Deming and Neumann, 1939; LeDuc, 1939; Moore, 1943).

Possible Role in Malignant Transformation

The concept of autocrine stimulation of cell proliferation proposes that normal cells acquire the capacity for autonomous growth by acquiring the ability to produce and respond to a growth factor (Todaro *et al*, 1977; Sporn and Todaro, 1980). Uncontrolled production of growth factors has been shown to result in acquisition of the transformed phenotype in vitro and tumorigenicity in vivo (reviewed in Kraus *et al*, 1988; Sinkovics, 1988). Examples include: transfection of rat fibroblasts with the gene coding for transforming growth factor-α (TGF-α) (Rosenthal *et al*, 1986) and expression of either the platelet derived growth factor (PDGF) B gene or its viral counterpart, v-*sis*, in NIH3T3 cells (Gazit *et al*, 1984; Huang *et al*, 1984).

Demonstration that FGFs can transform cells and promote autonomous growth was reported by Neufeld *et al* (1988). These investigators transfected BHK-21 cells, which do not express bFGF, with plasmids carrying the bFGF coding sequence linked to the SV40 enhancer and the metallothionein II promoter. Transformed cells exhibited properties usually associated with transformed cells. Similar studies were done in 3T3 NR-6 cells transfected with plasmids carrying the aFGF gene by Jaye *et al* (1988). Transfected cells grew as transformed cells and formed small tumours when injected in nude mice. Highly tumorigenic transformants were produced by Rogelj *et al* (1988) and Blam *et al* (1988) by fusing the coding sequence for bFGF to signal secretory sequences for the immunoglobulin or growth hormone genes, respectively. These reports suggest that introduction of a secretory peptide sequence for the bFGF coding sequence enhances its oncogenic potential.

Heparin binding growth factor members whose genes code for secretory polypeptides, Int-2, HST, FGF-5 and FGF-6, are expressed in tumours and in cell lines derived from tumours and transform normal cells in vitro (reviewed in Benharroch and Birnbaum, 1990). Prostatic enlargement characterized by epithelial hyperplasia developed in male transgenic mice expressing the *MMTV-Int-2* fusion gene in their prostates (Muller *et al*, 1990). Expression of KGF, also a secreted growth factor, in tumours has not been reported. In addition, expression of secreted HBGF proteins or amplification of their genes in prostate cancer has not been reported. Studies to address these possibilities may prove informative.

TRANSFORMING GROWTH FACTOR-β FAMILY

Structure and Properties

Interest has recently focused on the biology of the transforming growth factor-β (TGF-β) family of polypeptides in the prostate. On the basis of structural and functional similarity, TGF-β family members are divided into two groups: the closely related members, TGF-β1, TGF-β2 and TGF-β3, and those members that are distantly related, Müllerian inhibiting substance, inhibin, activins, the bone morphogenetic proteins and products of the decapentaplegic gene complex in *Drosophila* (reviewed in Roberts and Sporn, 1988; Sporn and Roberts, 1988; Hsuan, 1989). Emphasis will be placed on members of the first group, since the proteins and their receptors have been identified in prostate.

Transforming growth factors β1 and β2 are multifunctional polypeptides first isolated from platelets, human placenta and PC-3 prostatic adenocarcinoma cells (Assoian *et al*, 1983; Derynck *et al*, 1985; Ikeda *et al*, 1987). The polypeptides are widely distributed in many different cells throughout the body and most cells have receptors (Wakefield *et al*, 1987), implying broad physiological significance. Transforming growth factors β1 and β2 are homodimers of 112 aminoacids per chain and exhibit 75% sequence homology; TGF-β3 is a heterodimer with approximately 80% identity with TGF-β2 in the mature region of the peptide (Miller *et al*, 1990). The murine cDNAs for the three closely related members have been cloned. The genes encoding these proteins are located on different chromosomes. The TGF-β gene family is well conserved. Formation of the 25 kDa active polypeptides occur by cleavage from larger precursor forms that first produce a latent peptide that is subsequently cleaved in vivo by proteases to an active form or that can be activated in vitro by treatment with acid.

Transforming growth factor-β1 is the predominant species in almost all tissues, whereas TGF-β2 and TGF-β3 have a more restricted pattern of expression (Derynck *et al*, 1988). Of interest is the finding that all TGF-β mRNAs are expressed more abundantly in the male than in the female submaxillary gland, suggesting that regulation of gene expression or posttranscriptional events may be controlled by steroid hormones.

Transforming growth factors β1 and β2 have been shown to elicit a variety of biological effects, most notably their ability to stimulate growth of some cells while acting as inhibitors of others. In most assays for biological activity, TGF-β1 and TGF-β2 promote growth of fibroblasts in soft agar and inhibit growth of epithelial cells. However, as will be discussed, there are exceptions to this general rule: TGF-β1 and TGF-β2 show similar spectra of biological activity, although restricted specificity of activity is known (reviewed in Sporn and Roberts, 1988). This is in agreement with data indicating that these factors bind with similar affinity to their receptors (Cheifetz *et al*, 1987). However, other investigators have described receptors with preferential binding for TGF-βs, and this may account for conflicting reports concerning the biological activities of these factors.

Aside from the proliferative and antiproliferative properties of TGF-βs, these agents exhibit diverse effects unrelated to proliferation (reviewed in Roberts and Sporn, 1988). In fibroblasts and other connective tissue cells, TGF-β is an important regulator of the synthesis of collagen, fibronectin, proteoglycan and other components of the ECM. Other effects of TGF-β include its ability to induce formation of specific proteins that inhibit plasminogen activator, increase synthesis of protease inhibitors and decrease synthesis of proteases. Thus, these agents affect the composition of the ECM and may be important in modulating the mobilization of HBGFs.

Identification in Prostate and Modulation of bFGF Expression

Our laboratory has found that acid/ethanol extracts of BPH tissue contain a factor(s) that inhibits the proliferation of mink lung CCL64 cells (Story MT, unpublished). These cells are widely used to assess TGF-β activity. The preliminary findings are supported by a recent report by Mori *et al* (1990) showing TGF-β1 and TGF-β2 transcripts in BPH and normal prostate. Transcripts for TGF-β2, but not TGF-β1, were said to be increased in BPH compared with normal prostate. However, to suggest that TGF-β2, but not TGF-β1, is associated with the development of BPH is premature.

Transforming growth factor-β1 transcripts have been identified in rat ventral prostate (Kyprianou and Isaacs, 1989), as have receptors for the factor (Kyprianou and Isaacs, 1988). Cell lines derived from human prostate cancer, PC-82 and PC-3, also express TGF-βs (Wilding *et al*, 1989; Kyprianou *et al*, 1990). Rat prostate cancer cells, AXC/SSh (Shain *et al*, 1990), and the human cell lines, PC-3 and DU-145 (Wilding *et al*, 1989), express TGF-β receptors.

All of the studies that identified TGF-βs in BPH and normal prostate analysed whole tissue. Currently, it is not known whether the factors are synthesized by stromal or epithelial cells, nor has it been determined which cells express TGF-β receptors. This information is needed to understand better the physiological role of TGF-βs in prostate.

The growth of rat prostatic epithelial cells in culture is inhibited by porcine platelet derived TGF-β, predominantly TGF-β1 (McKeehan and Adams, 1988). The inhibition by TGF-β was attenuated by HBGF-1 but not by EGF. We have also found that the growth of human prostate derived fibroblasts was inhibited by TGF-β1 (Story *et al*, 1990). The inhibition by TGF-β1 was overcome by bFGF but not by EGF, PDGF, insulin like growth factor I (IGF-I) or insulin. Furthermore, TGF-β1 enhanced bFGF production and elevated bFGF mRNA levels in these cells (Story MT, Hopp KA, Meier DA, Begun FP and Lawson RK, unpublished). Thus, growth inhibition by TGF-β1 occurs at a time when synthesis of bFGF is increased. It is likely that newly synthesized bFGF is not accessible to its receptor, since levels of the growth factor do not increase in the culture fluid. However, the addition of bFGF to the medium completely overcomes the inhibitory affect of TGF-β1. The inhibition of prostatic fibroblast proliferation by TGF-β1 appears to be an exception to the generalization that stromal cells are growth stimulated by TGF-βs.

Castration dramatically increased the level of TGF-β mRNA in rat ventral prostate (Kyprianou and Isaacs, 1989) while increasing TGF-β receptor binding (Kyprianou and Isaacs, 1988). Androgen administration to rats 4 days after castration lowered TGF-β mRNA levels to levels expressed in intact animals and decreased TGF-β receptor binding. A similar effect of androgen ablation on TGF-β1 mRNA expression in the androgen responsive PC-82, human prostatic adenocarcinoma xenograft was reported by Kyprianou *et al* (1990). These reports suggest that TGF-β and its receptor are negatively regulated by androgen.

The bFGF/TGF-β scenario in the prostate appears to be that androgen withdrawal induces TGF-β gene expression and "programmed cell death" of the epithelium. Elevated tissue TGF-β would be expected to increase bFGF synthesis by the stromal cells while inhibiting their proliferation. Administration of androgen to the androgen depleted prostate further enhances bFGF expression (Katz *et al*, 1989) while decreasing TGF-β expression, overcoming growth inhibition by TGF-β of both the stromal and epithelial cells. Considering the complexity of the stromal and ductal components of prostate, it will be important to utilize in situ hybridization methodology with TGF-β and bFGF specific probes to identify the cellular components within the androgen deprived and reandrogenized prostate in order better to define the physiological role of these growth regulating factors. It would also be of interest to apply the technology to occult and malignant prostatic cancer, since a possible mechanism by which tumour cells could acquire autonomous growth is by failure to respond to inhibition by TGF-β (reviewed in Keski-Oja *et al*, 1987, 1988).

EPIDERMAL GROWTH FACTOR AND TRANSFORMING GROWTH FACTOR-α

Properties

Epidermal growth factor was first isolated from the mouse submaxillary gland (Cohen, 1962), and a similar peptide was isolated from human urine (Cohen and Carpenter, 1975; Gregory, 1975). Both 53 aminoacid peptides exhibit the same biological activities and interact with the same cell surface receptor. The peptide is a mitogen for a variety of cells in vitro and for epithelial cells, in particular, in vivo. A homologous peptide, transforming growth factor-α (TGF-α), was originally observed in the conditioned medium of murine sarcoma virus transformed cells because of its ability to compete with EGF for receptor binding (Sporn and Roberts, 1985). Unlike EGF, which is produced by a variety of normal cells throughout the body, TGF-α is produced by different malignant cells, including those transfected by viruses. The structure, receptor characteristics and biological activities of EGF and TGF-α have been extensively reviewed (Carpenter and Cohen, 1979; Schlessinger *et al*, 1983; Carpenter, 1987; Keski-Oja *et al*, 1987).

Identification in Prostate

The possible role of EGF as a mediator of prostate growth has recently been reviewed by Habib (1990). Harper *et al* (1979) first reported that the guinea pig prostate was a rich source of EGF and nerve growth factor (NGF). Shikata *et al* (1984) localized the growth factor in the cytoplasm of the glandular epithelium with immunohistochemical techniques. Extracts of rat ventral prostate also contain relatively high levels of the 6000 molecular weight peptide, as well as a higher molecular weight form of the growth factor (Jacobs *et al*, 1988). Gregory *et al* (1986) identified EGF in human prostatic secretions.

The EGF content of this fluid exceeded that found in any other biological fluid, with the possible exception of colostrum. This suggests that prostatic EGF is destined for secretion. Its secretion by the rat ventral prostate has been reported to be under α-adrenergic control (Jacobs and Story, 1988).

Immunohistochemical localization of EGF in BPH and prostate cancer specimens was reported by Fowler *et al* (1988). Their studies identified EGF staining in only 6% of BPH specimens, whereas 68% of prostate cancer specimens stained with EGF antiserum. These observations are not consistent with those based on radioimmunoassay quantitation of tissue levels of the growth factor. Habib (1990) reported significantly higher levels of EGF in BPH than in prostate cancer specimens. Similar findings were reported by Shaikh *et al* (1990). No correlation between the amount of EGF detected and clinical stage or Gleason score was observed, nor was there a correlation between EGF and the response to orchidectomy and patient survival.

The level of EGF in the mouse submaxillary gland was increased by androgen (Byyny *et al*, 1972). Castration of adult male mice greatly reduced the amount of EGF in ventral prostate. Testosterone administration to castrates increased EGF to the level found in intact animals (Hiramatsu *et al*, 1988). EGF receptor binding also appears to be modulated by androgen. Castration increased EGF receptor number in rat ventral prostate, and receptor number decreased with subsequent administration of dihydrotestosterone (Traish and Wotiz, 1987).

Studies by Chaproniere and McKeehan (1986) and Peehl and Stamey (1986) demonstrated the importance of EGF, but not androgen, for the growth of prostate epithelial cells in serum free medium. This suggests that the cells that adapt to growth in vitro are not the prostatic cells that produce EGF under androgen control.

Receptors for EGF have been identified in the membrane fraction of prostate tissue from men with BPH (Maddy *et al*, 1987). Lubrano *et al* (1989) observed a negative correlation between EGF receptor binding and nuclear steroid receptor content. Fiorelli *et al* (1989) found that EGF receptor binding was significantly higher in prostate tissue from men treated for 3 months with gonadotrophin releasing hormone agonists, which reduce plasma androgens, than in BPH tissue from untreated men. These studies suggest that androgens negatively affect EGF receptor expression in both rat and human prostate. Since androgens increase EGF levels in prostate, it may be that their effect on receptor binding is a result of receptor downregulation. A different mechanism may function in prostate cancer, since prostate tumours have lower levels of EGF than BPH tissue. BPH exhibits higher EGF binding than do prostate tumours (Habib, 1990). Habib's observations suggest that well differentiated tumours exhibit higher receptor binding than do poorly differentiated tumours. Tumours with Gleason scores of eight to ten did not have detectable EGF receptor binding, nor did they show staining with antiserum to EGF receptor. Additionally, androgens have been found to increase EGF receptor number in human prostate cancer derived cells, LNCaP (Schuurmans *et al*,

1988). Thus, EGF receptor induction by androgen might be a mechanism by which these steroids increase the growth rate of these cells. Transforming growth factor-α transcripts have been identified in LNCaP cells (Schuurmans *et al*, 1988), and the peptide has been identified in the medium conditioned by DU-145 cells (Habib, 1990). Expression of TGF-α and its receptor by human prostate cancer cells could confer on these cells a growth advantage, leading to their autonomous growth. Analysis of EGF/TGF-α expression and expression of its receptor by primary hormone responsive prostate cancer tumours and androgen insensitive prostate cancer cells may be a fruitful area for investigation.

OSTEOBLASTIC FACTORS

Human prostatic cancer is unique in that it is the only cancer that consistently produces osteoblastic metastases to bone. More than 90% of bone lesions due to prostatic cancer are osteoblastic rather than osteolytic. The malignant prostatic cells spread to the red marrow spaces of cancellous bone. New bone formation then follows, surrounding the nests of malignant prostatic cells. Osteoblasts become more numerous on the trabecular surfaces. New bone is laid down by the osteoblasts in the vicinity of the malignant prostatic cells (Jacobs and Story, 1987). Using histomorphometric analysis of bone metastases, Charhon *et al* (1983) concluded that a local trophic factor (paracrine factor) released by the cancer cells could account for the histological picture.

Extracts of normal prostate, BPH and prostate cancer were reported to be mitogenic for fetal rat calvarial derived osteoblasts (Jacobs *et al*, 1979). As previously indicated, prostatic extracts are a rich source of bFGF. Demonstration that recombinant bFGF can elicit events leading to the formation of new bone in implants of demineralized bone matrix in vivo has been provided by Aspenberg and Lohmander (1989). It is not clear from this report, however, whether bFGF directly controls mineralization of the matrix or whether it facilitates ossification through its properties as a stimulator of capillary formation.

Other investigators have provided evidence that osteoblast specific factors, whose properties are distinct from any of the characterized growth factors, may be present in the prostate. None of the putative osteoblast specific factors have yet been purified to permit structural analysis. Additionally, osteoblast specificity was often based on enhanced mitogenic potential for cultured cells derived from bone. Yet it is known that fetal rat calvaria derived cells are stimulated to divide by EGF, FGFs, PDGF and IGF-I.

Nishi *et al* (1988) reported that prostate cancer tissue, but not normal prostate or BPH, contained a mitogen with specificity for MC3T3-E1 mouse osteoblasts. The factor has not been characterized, nor has this observation been confirmed by others. Koutsilieris *et al* (1986, 1987a,b) described the chromatographic properties of a factor(s) from extracts of BPH and prostatic adenocarcinoma tissue with enhanced activity for freshly isolated rat osteoblasts and osteoblast derived osteosarcoma cells. The properties of the 10 000 molecular weight factor appear to be different from those of known growth factors. It remains to be determined whether the factor is specifically expressed by prostate. A mitogen with specificity for human osteoblasts over fibroblasts was identified in the medium conditioned by PC-3 cells (Perkel *et al*, 1990). The properties of the factor appear to be different from those of the mitogen described by Koutsilieris *et al* (1987a) and distinct from those of other known growth factors. PC-3 mRNA microinjected into *Xenopus* oocytes has been reported to direct the synthesis of substances mitogenic for osteoblastic cells (Simpson *et al*, 1985).

Bone is also a rich source of endogenously produced factors with possible autocrine or paracrine action. Transforming growth factors β are present in high concentration in bone (Seyedin *et al*, 1986), as are PDGFs, HBGFs (Hauschka *et al*, 1986) and haematopoietic growth factors. The medium conditioned by bone marrow derived stromal cells has been reported to stimulate growth of PC-3 cells (Chackal-Roy *et al*, 1989). Therefore, it is conceivable that the osteoblastic response to metastatic prostate cancer may involve not only extrinsic factors of prostate cancer cell origin but also bone derived factors. The recognition of the basis for the osteoblastic response to metastatic prostate cancer would be a major accomplishment towards understanding the control of skeletal metabolism by prostate cancer cells.

CONCLUSION

The prostate has proved to be a fascinating but formidable organ for the investigation of growth control mechanisms. The human prostate undergoes both normal and abnormal developmental stages. These include: (a) embryonic development, (b) pubertal growth and adult secretory activity, (c) development of BPH and (d) development of prostate cancer (including androgen dependent and androgen insensitive growth).

An understanding of how steroid hormones and autocrine or paracrine growth stimulating and inhibiting factors are involved in prostatic development is in its infancy. Tenniswood (1986) presented a hypothesis to explain the effects of stromal-epithelial interactions on the mechanism of action of androgens in regulating growth of the prostate. The hypothesis proposed the existence of three factors—two growth stimulating factors referred to as "stromally derived growth factor" (SDGF) and "epithelially derived growth factor" (EDGF), and one inhibiting factor, "epithelially derived inhibiting factor" (EDIF)—that modulate the replication and transcriptional processes of the prostate. It was proposed that during embryonic development, androgen binds to its stromal cell receptor, inducing the gene for SDGF; SDGF induces replication of the embryonic epithelium, and EDGF induces stromal cell replication.

The nature of these putative regulatory agents is not known. On the basis of current information about the biology of the growth factors identified in the prostate, it may be that the role of SDGF is played by EGF, whereas bFGF may function as the EDGF. This speculation is supported by the following: (a) EGF production is under androgen control, (b) EGF is required for epithelial cell proliferation in vitro, (c) embryonic mesenchymal cells, but not epithelial cells, have androgen receptors and (d) stromal cell proliferation in vitro is stimulated by bFGF but not by EGF. It remains to be determined whether the urogenital sinus mesenchyme synthesizes EGF under androgen control and whether embryonic epithelial cells express EGF receptors. The answers to these questions are amenable to study with embryonic tissue recombinant technology.

As embryonic development of the prostate comes to completion, there is a need to check the induction loop of SDGF/EDGF to prevent uncontrolled growth. Tenniswood proposed that this may be accomplished by the acquisition of androgen receptors by the epithelial cells. Accompanying androgen control of the epithelium is the secretion of the EDIF, which serves to inhibit SDGF gene expression and ultimately EDGF expression by the epithelial cells. Tenniswood proposed that, in the adult prostate, epithelial cells constitutively express EDIF, suppressing SDGF expression by the stroma and preventing replication of both cell types.

It is tempting to suggest that TGF-β may function as the EDIF, since it is known to inhibit proliferation of both cell populations in prostate. However, the negative regulation of TGF-β by androgen in the prostate and the finding that TGF-β increases stromal cell synthesis of bFGF argue against this role. Stimulation of bFGF production by TGF-β would seem to lead to uncontrolled growth of the stroma and perhaps the epithelium. However, in cultured cells, increased bFGF levels are not accompanied by stromal cell proliferation; instead, TGF-β inhibits division of these cells. Tenniswood's model also proposed that EDIF inhibits SDGF synthesis. It remains to be determined whether TGF-β regulates EGF production. However, it is clear that EGF is produced in the adult prostate. If EGF fulfills the proposed role for SDGF, its continued synthesis in the adult gland would suggest that epithelial cell proliferation would be uncontrolled. However, it is likely that in the adult prostate, the epithelial cells control EGF synthesis. This would be possible if the epithelial cells, like the stromal cells, lack receptors for the growth factor on their apical surfaces and are therefore unable to respond to the growth factor.

Castration preferentially decreases the epithelial to stromal ratio in the prostate. According to Tenniswood's hypothesis, this would be expected to reduce EDIF levels in the gland. Androgen replacement would activate the SDGF/EDGF loop until once again EDIF was increased to a level that inhibits SDGF gene expression. There may be important differences between developmental process and events that follow androgen replacement. Nevertheless, it should be possible to use animal models and the techniques of molecular biology to identify regulatory factors with properties required of an EGIF.

Tenniswood also suggested ways in which failure in control mechanisms could lead to prostate disease. Loss of EDIF expression by the epithelial cells or insensitivity of the stroma to EDIF would be expected to result in continued synthesis of SDGF and uncontrolled replication. If regulation of SDGF and EDGF production were not coordinated, overproduction of one or the other would be expected to lead to prostate growth that is either predominantly epithelial or stromal, as is evident in BPH. Prostate cancer could result from failure to respond to an inhibitor factor or by the acquisition of receptors for a growth factor produced by the cell to complete an autocrine loop. In the absence of adequate models for human BPH and prostate cancer, studies to determine the role of prostatic growth factors in these developmental events that are unique to the human gland will have to be conducted with tissue available at surgery and with isolated prostatic cells in culture.

SUMMARY

Normal and abnormal developmental events in the prostate are strongly influenced by androgens. There is abundant evidence, however, that androgens are not the only substances present that have the capacity to influence prostatic growth. A number of polypeptides that either stimulate or inhibit growth have now been identified in the prostate. These include members of the HBGF family, TGF-β family, EGF and TGF-α, PDGF, NGF, and the less well characterized osteoblast growth factors. In some cases, the prostatic cell population, stromal or epithelial, that synthesizes the growth factor and its receptor is known. This information and the properties of the growth factors suggest ways in which these polypeptides may be involved in regulating growth of the prostate, including benign prostatic hyperplasia and prostate cancer.

Acknowledgements

I thank my colleagues Dr Russell K Lawson, Dr Frank P Begun, Dr Herbert Lepor of the Department of Urology, Medical College of Wisconsin, and Dr Stephen C Jacobs of the Department of Urology, University of Maryland, for valuable discussion. The author's original work presented in this article was supported by National Institutes of Health grant DK31063.

References

Aspenberg P and Lohmander SL (1989) Fibroblast growth factor stimulates bone formation. *Acta Orthopaedica Scandinavica* **60** 473–476

Assoian RK, Komoriya A, Meyers CA, Miller DM and Sporn MB (1983) Transforming growth factor-beta in human platelets. *Journal of Biological Chemistry* **258** 7155–7160

Baird A and Ling N (1987) Fibroblast growth factors are present in the extracellular matrix produced by endothelial cells in vitro: implications for a role of heparinase-like enzymes in the neovascular response. *Biochemical and Biophysical Research Communications* **142** 429–435

Baird A and Walicke PA (1989) Fibroblast growth factors. *British Medical Bulletin* **45** 438–452

Baird A, Ueno N, Esch F and Ling N (1987) Distribution of fibroblast growth factor (FGFs) in tissue and structure function studies with synthetic fragments of basic FGF. *Journal of Cellular Physiology* **5** 101–106

Benharroch D and Birnbaum D (1990) Biology of the fibroblast growth factor gene family. *Israel Journal of Medical Sciences* **26** 212–219

Blam S, Mitchell R, Tischer E *et al* (1988) Addition of growth hormone secretion signal to bFGF results in cell transformation and secretion of aberrant forms of the protein. *Oncogene* **3** 129–136

Bottaro DP, Rubin JS, Ron D, Finch PW, Florio C and Aaronson SA (1990) Characterization of the receptor for keratinocyte growth factor. *Journal of Biological Chemistry* **265** 12767–12770

Burrus LW and Olwin BB (1989) Isolation of a receptor for acidic and basic fibroblast growth factor from embryonic chick. *Journal of Biological Chemistry* **264** 18647–18653

Byyny RL, Orth DN and Cohen S (1972) Radioimmunoassay of epidermal growth factor. *Endocrinology* **90** 1261–1266

Carpenter G (1987) Receptors for epidermal growth factor and other polypeptide mitogens. *Annual Review of Biochemistry* **56** 881–914

Carpenter G and Cohen J (1979) Epidermal growth factor. *Annual Review of Biochemistry* **48** 193–216

Castellot JJ, Addonizio ML, Rosenberg R and Karnovsky MJ (1981) Cultured endothelial cells produce a heparin-like inhibitor of smooth muscle cell growth. *Journal of Cellular Biology* **90** 372–379

Chackal-Roy M, Niemeyer C, Moore M and Zetter BR (1989) Stimulation of human prostatic carcinoma cell growth by factors present in human bone marrow. *Journal of Clinical Investigation* **84** 43–50

Chaproniere DM and McKeehan WL (1986) Serial culture of single adult human prostatic epithelial cells in serum-free medium containing low calcium and a nerve growth factor from bovine brain. *Cancer* **46** 819–824

Charhon SA, Chapuy MC, Delvin EE, Valentin-Opran A, Edouard CM and Meunier PJ (1983) Histomorphometric analysis of sclerotic bone metastases from prostatic carcinoma with special reference to osteomalacia. *Cancer* **51** 918–924

Cheifetz S, Weatherbee JA, Tsang MLS *et al* (1987) The transforming growth factor beta system, a complex pattern of cross-reactive ligands and receptors. *Cell* **48** 409–415

Coffey DS (1986) The biochemistry and physiology of the prostate and seminal vesicles, In: Walsh PC, Gittes RF and Stamey TA (eds). *Campbell's Urology*, 5th edition, pp 233–274, WB Saunders Company, Philadelphia

Cohen S (1962) Isolation of a mouse submaxillary gland protein accelerating incisor eruption and eyelid opening in the newborn animal. *Journal of Biological Chemistry* **237** 1555–1562

Cohen S and Carpenter G (1975) Human epidermal growth factor: isolation of chemical and biological properties. *Proceedings of the National Academy of Sciences of the USA* **72** 1317–1321

Connolly JM and Rose DP (1989) Secretion of epidermal growth factor and related polypeptides by the DU 145 human prostate cancer cell line. *Prostate* **15** 177–186

Cunha GR (1984) Androgenic effects upon prostatic epithelium via trophic influences from stroma, In: Kimball FA, Buhl AF and Carter DB (eds). *New Approaches to the Study of Benign Prostatic Hyperplasia*, pp 81–102, Alan R Liss, Inc, New York

Deming CL and Neumann C (1939) Early phases of prostatic hyperplasia. *Surgery, Gynecology and Obstetrics* **68** 155–160

Derynck R, Jarrett JA, Chen EY *et al* (1985) Human transforming growth factor-beta complementary DNA sequence and expression in normal and transformed cells. *Nature* **316** 701–705

Derynck R, Lindquist PB, Lee A *et al* (1988) A new type of transforming growth factor-beta, TGF-beta 3. *EMBO Journal* **7** 3737–3743

Dionne C, Crumley G, Bellot F *et al* (1990) Cloning and expression of two distinct high-affinity receptors cross-reacting with acidic and basic fibroblast growth factors. *EMBO Journal* **9** 2685–2692

Esch F, Baird A, Ling N *et al* (1985) Primary structure of bovine pituitary basic fibroblast growth factor (FGF) and comparison with the amino-terminal sequence of bovine brain acidic FGF. *Proceedings of the National Academy of Sciences of the USA* **82** 6507–6511

Finch PW, Rubin JS, Miki T, Ron D and Aaronson SA (1989) Human KGF is FGF-related with properties of a paracrine effector of epithelial cell growth. *Science* **245** 752–755

Fiorelli G, De Bellis A, Longo A, Natali A, Costantini A, and Serio M (1989) Epidermal growth factor receptors in human hyperplastic prostate tissue and their modulation by chronic treatment with a gonadotropin-releasing hormone analog. *Journal of Clinical Endocrinology and Metabolism* **68** 740–743

Folkman J and Klagsbrun M (1987) Angiogenic factors. *Science* **235** 442–447

Fowler Jr JE, Lau JLT, Ghosh L, Mills SE and Mounzer A (1988) Epidermal growth factor and prostatic carcinoma: an immunohistochemical study. *Journal of Urology* **139** 857–861

Gazit AH, Igarashi IM, Chiu A *et al* (1984) Expression of the normal human sis/PDGF-2 coding sequence induces cellular transformation. *Cell* **39** 89–97

Gospodarowicz D (1990) Fibroblast growth factor and its involvement in developmental processes. *Current Topics in Developmental Biology* **24** 57–93

Gospodarowicz D, Baird A, Cheng J, Lui GM, Esch F and Bohlen P (1986) Isolation of fibroblast growth factor from bovine adrenal gland: physiochemical and biological characterization. *Endocrinology* **118** 82–90

Gregory H (1975) Isolation and structure of urogastrone and its relationship to epidermal growth factor. *Nature* **257** 325–327

Gregory H, Willshire IR, Kavanagh JP, Blacklock NJ, Chowdury S and Richards RC (1986) Urogastrone-epidermal growth factor concentrations in prostatic fluid of normal individuals and patients with benign prostatic hypertrophy. *Clinical Science* **70** 359–363

Habib FK (1990) Peptide growth factors: a new frontier in prostate cancer. *Progress in Clinical and Biological Research* **357** 107–115

Hall JA, Harris MA, Malark M, Mansson P-E, Zhou H and Harris SE (1990) Characterization of the hamster DDT-1 cell aFGF/HGBF-I gene and cDNA and its modulation by steroids. *Journal of Cellular Biochemistry* **43** 17–26

Harper GP, Barde YA, Burnstock G *et al* (1979) Guinea pig prostate is a rich source of nerve growth factor. *Nature* **279** 160–162

Harris SE, Smith RG, Zhou H, Mansson P-E and Malark M (1989) Androgens and glucocorticoids modulate heparin-binding growth factor-I mRNA accumulation in DDT1 cells as analyzed by in situ hybridization. *Molecular Endocrinology* **3** 1839–1844

Hauschka PV, Mavrakos AE, Iafrati MD, Doleman SE and Klagsbrun M (1986) Growth factors in bone matrix. *Journal of Biological Chemistry* **261** 12665–12674

Hiramatsu M, Kashimata M, Minami N, Sato A, Murayama M and Minami N (1988) Androgenic regulation of epidermal growth factor in the mouse ventral prostate. *Biochemistry International* **17** 311–317

Hsuan JJ (1989) Transforming growth factor beta. *British Medical Bulletin* **45** 425–437

Huang JS, Huang SS and Deuel TF (1984) Transforming protein on simian sarcoma virus stimulates autocrine growth of SSV-transformed cells throgh PDGF cell-surface receptors. *Cell* **39** 79–87

Ikeda T, Lioubin MN and Marquardt H (1987) Human transforming growth factor type beta 2: production by a prostatic adenocarcinoma cell line, purification and initial characterization. *Biochemistry* **26** 2406–2410

Ingber DE and Folkman J (1989) Mechanochemical switching between growth and differentiation during fibroblast growth factor-stimulated angiogenesis in vitro: role of extracellular matrix. *Journal of Cell Biology* **109** 317–330

Jacobs SC and Story MT (1987) Growth factors in urology, In: Ratliff TL and Catalona WJ (eds). *Genitourinary Cancer*, pp 43–70, Martinus Nijhoff Publishers, Boston

Jacobs SC and Story MT (1988) Exocrine secretion of epidermal growth factor by the rat prostate: effect of adrenergic agents, cholinergic agents and vasoactive intestinal peptide. *Prostate* **13** 79–87

Jacobs SC, Pikna D and Lawson RK (1979) Prostatic osteoblastic factor. *Investigative Urology* **17** 195–198

Jacobs SC, Story MT, Sasse J and Lawson RK (1988) Characterization of growth factors derived from the rat ventral prostate. *Journal of Urology* **139** 1106–1110

Jaye M, Howk R, Burgess W *et al* (1986) Human endothelial cell growth factor: cloning, nucleotide sequence and chromosome localization. *Science* **233** 541–545

Jaye M, Lyall RM, Mudd R, Schlessinger J and Sarver N (1988) Expression of aFGF cDNA confers growth advantage and tumorigenesis to Swiss 3T3 cells. *EMBO Journal* **7** 963–969

Kabalin JN, Peehl DM and Stamey TA (1989) Clonal growth of human prostatic epithelial cells is stimulated by fibroblasts. *Prostate* **14** 251–263

Kan M, DiSorbo D, Jinzhao H, Hoshi H, Mansson P-E and McKeehan WL (1988) High and low affinity binding of heparin-binding growth factor to a 130-kDa receptor correlates with stimulation and inhibition of growth of a differentiated human hepatoma cell. *The Journal of Biological Chemistry* **263** 11306–11313

Katz, AE, Benson MC, Wise GW *et al* (1989) Gene activity during the early phase of androgen-stimulated rat prostate regrowth. *Cancer Research* **49** 5889–5894

Keski-Oja J, Leof EB, Lyons RM, Coffey Jr RJ and Moses HL (1987) Transforming growth factors and control of neoplastic cell growth. *Journal of Cellular Biochemistry* **33** 95–107

Keski-Oja J, Postlethwaite AE and Moses HL (1988) Transforming growth factors in the regulation of malignant cell growth and invasion. *Cancer Investigation* **6** 705–724

Kimelman D, Abraham JA, Haaparanta T, Palisi TM and Kirschner MW (1988) The presence of fibroblast growth factor in the frog egg: its role as a natural mesoderm inducer. *Science* **242** 1053–1056

Kishi H, Ishibe T, Usui T and Miyachi Y (1988) Epidermal growth factor (EGF) in seminal plasma and prostatic gland: a radioreceptor assay. *Archives of Andrology* **20** 243–249

Koutsilieris M, Rabbani SA and Goltzman D (1986) Selective osteoblast mitogens can be extracted from prostatic tissue. *The Prostate* **9** 109–115

Koutsilieris M, Rabbani SA, Bennett HPJ and Goltzman D (1987a) Characteristics of prostate-derived growth factors for cells of the osteoblast phenotype. *Journal of Clinical Investigation* **80** 941–946

Koutsilieris M, Rabbani SA and Goltzman D (1987b) Effects of human prostatic mitogens on rat bone cells and fibroblasts. *Journal of Endocrinology* **115** 447–454

Kozlowski JM, McEwan R, Keer H *et al* (1988) Prostate cancer and the invasive phenotype: application of new in vivo and in vitro approaches, In: Nicolson GL (ed). *Tumor Progression and Metastasis*, pp 189-231, Alan R Liss, Inc, New York

Kraus MH, Pierce JH, Fleming TP, Robbins KC, DiFiore PP and Aaronson SA (1988) Mechanisms by which genes encoding growth factors and growth factor receptors contribute to malignant transformation. Annals of the New York Academy of Sciences **551** 320–336

Kurokawa T, Sasada R, Iwan M and Igarashi K (1987) Cloning and expression of cDNA encoding human basic fibroblast growth factor. *FEBS Letters* **213** 189–194

Kyprianou N and Isaacs JT (1988) Identification of a cellular receptor for transforming growth factor beta in rat ventral prostate and its negative regulation by androgens. *Endocrinology* **123** 2124–2131

Kyprianou N and Isaacs JT (1989) Expression of transforming growth factor beta in the rat ventral prostate during castration-induced programmed cell death. *Molecular Endocrinol-*

ogy **3** 1515–1522

Kyprianou N, English HF and Isaacs JT (1990) Programmed cell death during regression of PC-82 human prostate cancer following androgen ablation. *Cancer Research* **50** 3748–3753

LeDuc IE (1939) The anatomy of the prostate and the pathology of early benign hypertrophy. *Journal of Urology* **42** 1217–1241

Lee C (1981) Physiology of castration-induced regression in rat prostate, In: Murphy GP, Sandberg AA and Karr JP (eds). *The Prostatic Cell: Structure and Function*, pp 145–159, Alan R Liss, Inc, New York

Lu J, Nishizawa Y, Tanaka A *et al* (1989) Inhibitory effect of antibody against basic fibroblast growth factor on androgen- or glucocorticoid-induced growth of Shionogi carcinoma 115 cells in serum-free culture. *Cancer Research* **49** 4963–4967

Lubrano C, Petrangeli E, Catizone A *et al* (1989) Epidermal growth factor binding and steroid receptor content in human benign prostatic hyperplasia. *Journal of Steroid Biochemistry* **34** 499–504

McKeehan WL and Adams PS (1988) Heparin-binding growth factor/prostatropin attenuates inhibition of rat prostate tumor epithelial cell growth by transforming growth factor type beta. *In Vitro Cellular and Developmental Biology* **24** 243–246

McKeehan WL, Adams PS and Rosser MP (1984) Direct mitogenic effects of insulin, epidermal growth factor, glucocorticoid, cholera toxin, unknown pituitary factors and possibly prolactin, but not androgen on normal rat prostate epithelial cells in serum-free, primary cell culture. *Cancer Research* **44** 1998–2010

McKeehan WL, Adams PS and Fast D (1987) Different hormonal requirements for androgen-independent growth of normal and tumor epithelial cells from rat prostate. *In Vitro Cellular and Developmental Biology* **23** 147–152

McNeal JE (1984) Anatomy of the prostate and morphogenesis of BPH, In: Kimball FA, Buhl AE and Carter DB (eds). *New Approaches to the Study of Benign Prostatic Hyperplasia*, pp 27–53, Alan R Liss, Inc, New York

Maddy SQ, Chisholm GD, Hawkins RA and Habib FK (1987) Localization of epidermal growth factor receptors in the human prostate by biochemical and immunocytochemical methods. *Journal of Endocrinology* **113** 147–153

Mannson P-E, Adams P, Kan M and McKeehan WL (1989) Heparin-binding growth factor gene expression and receptor characteristics in normal rat prostate and two transplantable rat prostate tumors. *Cancer Research* **49** 2485–2494

Matuo Y, Nishi N, Matsui S, Sandberg AA, Isaacs JT and Wada F (1987) Heparin binding affinity of rat prostatic growth factor in normal and cancerous prostates: partial purification and characterization of rat prostatic growth factor in the Dunning tumor. *Cancer Research* **47** 188–192

Matzner Y, Bar-Ner M, Yahalom J, Ishai-Michaelis R, Fuks Z and Vlodavsky I (1985) Degradation of heparin sulfate in the subendothelial extracellular matrix by a readily released heparanase from human neutrophile. *Journal of Clinical Investigation* **76** 1306–1313

Miki T, Fleming TP, Bottaro DP, Rubin JS, Ron D and Aaronson SA (1991) Expression cDNA cloning of the KGF receptor by creation of a transforming autocrine loop. *Science* **251** 72–75

Miller DA, Pelton RW, Derynck R and Moses HL (1990) Transforming growth factor beta. *Annals of the New York Academy of Sciences* **593** 208–217

Moore RA (1943) Benign hypertrophy of the prostate: a morphological study. *Journal of Urology* **50** 680–710

Mori H, Maki M, Oishi K *et al* (1990) Increased expression of genes for basic fibroblast growth factor and transforming growth factor type 2 in human benign prostatic hyperplasia. *Prostate* **16** 71–80

Muller WJ, Lee FS, Dickson C, Peters G, Pattengale P and Leder P (1990) The int-2 gene product acts as an epithelial growth factor in transgenic mice. *EMBO Journal* **9** 907–913

Mydlo JH, Bulbul MA, Richon VM, Heston WDW and Fair WR (1988) Heparin-binding growth factor isolated from human prostatic extracts. *Prostate* **12** 343–355

Neufeld G, Mitchell R, Ponte P and Gospodarowicz D (1988) Expression of human basic fibroblast growth factor cDNA in baby hamster kidney-derived cells results in autonomous cell growth. *Journal of Cell Biology* **106** 1385–1394

Nishi N, Matuo Y, Kunitomi K *et al* (1988) Comparative analysis of growth factors in normal and pathologic human prostates. *Prostate* **13** 39–48

Nonomura N, Lu J, Tanaka A *et al* (1990) Interaction of androgen-induced autocrine heparin-binding growth factor with fibroblast growth factor receptor on androgen-dependent Shionogi carcinoma 115 cells. *Cancer Research* **50** 2316–2321

Peehl DM and Stamey TA (1986) Serum-free growth of adult human prostatic epithelial cells. *In Vitro Cellular and Developmental Biology* **22** 82–90

Perkel VS, Mohan S, Herring SJ, Baylink DJ and Linkhart TA (1990) Human prostatic cancer cells, PC3, elaborate mitogenic activity which selectively stimulated human bone cells. *Cancer Research* **50** 6902–6907

Roberts AB and Sporn MB (1988) Transforming growth factor beta. *Advances In Cancer Research* **51** 107–145

Rogelj S, Weinberg RA, Fanning P and Klagsbrun M (1988) Basic fibroblast growth factor fused to a signal peptide transforms cells. *Nature* **331** 173–175

Rosenthal A, Lindquist PB, Bringman TS, Goeddel DV and Derynck R (1986) Expression in rat fibroblasts of a human transforming growth factor cDNA results in transformation. *Cell* **46** 301–309

Schlessinger J, Schreiber AB, Levi A, Lax I, Libermann T, and Yarden Y (1983) Regulation of cell proliferation by epidermal growth factor. *Critical Reviews in Biochemistry* **14** 93–111

Schreiber AB, Kenney J, Kowlaski WJ, Friesek R, Mehlman T and Maciag T (1985) Interaction of endothelial cell growth factor with heparin: characterization by receptor and antibody recognition. *Proceedings of the National Academy of Sciences of the USA* **82** 6138–6142

Schuurmans ALG, Bolt J and Mulder E (1988) Androgens stimulate both growth rate and epidermal growth factor receptor activity of the human prostate tumor cell LNCaP. *Prostate* **12** 55–63

Seyedin SM, Thompson AY, Bentz H *et al* (1986) Cartilage-inducing factor-A: apparent identity to transforming growth factor beta. *Journal of Biological Chemistry* **261** 5693–5695

Shaikh N, Lai L, McLoughlin J, Clark D and Williams G (1990) Quantitative analysis of epidermal growth factor in human benign prostatic hyperplasia and prostatic carcinoma and its prognostic significance. *Anticancer Research* **10** 873–874

Shain SA, Lin AL, Koger JD and Karaganis AG (1990) Rat prostate cancer cells contain functional receptors for transforming growth factor beta. *Endocrinology* **126** 818–825

Shikata H, Utsumi N, Hiramatsu M, Minami N, Nemoto N and Shikata T (1984) Immunohistochemical localization of nerve growth factor and epidermal growth factor in guinea pig prostate gland. *Histochemistry* **80** 411–413

Sinkovics JG (1988) Oncogenes and growth factors. *CRC Critical Reviews in Immunology* **8** 217–297

Sitaras NM, Sariban E, Bravo M, Pantazis P and Antoniades HN (1988) Constitutive production of platelet-derived growth factor-like proteins by human prostate carcinoma cell lines. *Cancer Research* **48** 1930–1935

Simpson E, Harrod J, Eilon G, Jacobs JW and Mundy GR (1985) Identification of a messenger ribonucleic acid fraction in human prostatic cancer cells coding for a novel osteoblast-stimulating factor. *Endocrinology* **117** 1615–1620

Slack JM, Darlington BG, Heath JK and Godsave SF (1987) Mesoderm induction in early Xenopus embryos by heparin-binding growth factors. *Nature* **326** 197–200

Sporn MB and Roberts AB (1985) Autocrine growth factors and cancer. *Nature* **313** 747–749

Sporn MB and Roberts AB (1988) Transforming growth factor-beta: new chemical forms and new biological roles. *Biofactors* **1** 89–93

Sporn MB and Todaro G (1980) Autocrine secretion and malignant transformation of cells. *New*

England Journal of Medicine **303** 878–880

Story MT, Sasse J, Jacobs SC and Lawson RK (1987a) Prostatic growth factor: purification and structural relationship to basic fibroblast growth factor. *Biochemistry* **26** 3843–3849

Story MT, Esch F, Shimasaki S, Sasse J, Jacobs SC and Lawson RK (1987b) Amino-terminal sequence of a large form of basic fibroblast growth factor isolated from human benign prostatic hyperplastic tissue. *Biochemical and Biophysical Research Communications* **142** 702–709

Story MT, Livingston B, Baeten L *et al* (1989) Cultured human prostate-derived fibroblasts produce a factor that stimulates their growth with properties indistinguishable from basic fibroblast growth factor. *Prostate* **15** 355–365

Story MT, Baeten LA, Molter MA and Lawson RK (1990) Influence of androgen and transforming growth factor beta on basic fibroblast growth factor levels in human prostate-derived fibroblast cell cultures. *Journal of Urology* **143** 241A

Taketa S, Nishi N, Takasuga H, Okutani T, Takenaka I and Wada F (1990) Differences in growth requirements between epithelial and stromal cells derived from rat ventral prostate in serum-free primary culture. *Prostate* **17** 207–218

Tenniswood M (1986) Role of epithelial-stromal interactions in the control of gene expression in the prostate: an hypothesis. *Prostate* **9** 375–385

Todaro GJ, De Larco JE, Nissley SP and Rechler MM (1977) MSA and EGF receptors on sarcoma virus-transformed cells and human fibrosarcoma cells in culture. *Nature* **267** 526–528

Traish AM and Wotiz HH (1987) Prostatic epidermal growth factor receptors and their regulation by androgens. *Endocrinology* **121** 1461–1467

Vlodavsky I, Folkman J, Sullivan R *et al* (1987) Endothelial cell-derived basic fibroblast growth factor: synthesis and deposition into subendothelial extra-cellular matrix. *Proceedings of the National Academy of Sciences of the USA* **84** 2292–2296

Vlodavsky I, Fuks Z, Bar-Ner M, Ariav Y and Schirrmacher V (1983) Lymphoma cells mediated degradation of sulfated proteoglycans in the subendothelial extracellular matrix: relationship to tumor cell metastasis. *Cancer Research* **43** 2704–2711

Wakefield LM, Smith DM, Masui T, Harris CC and Sporn MB (1987) Distribution and modulation of the cellular receptor for transforming growth factor-beta. *Journal of Cell Biology* **105** 965–975

Wilding G, Zugneier G, Knabbe C, Flanders K and Gelmann E (1989) Differential effects of transforming growth factor beta on human prostate cancer cells in vitro. *Molecular and Cellular Endocrinology* **62** 79–87

The author is responsible for the accuracy of the references.

Response of Prostate Cancer Cells to Peptide Growth Factors: Transforming Growth Factor-β

G WILDING

University of Wisconsin Clinical Cancer Center, Madison, Wisconsin 53792

INTRODUCTION: THE ROLE OF PEPTIDE GROWTH FACTORS IN CANCER GROWTH, DIFFERENTIATION AND METABOLISM

Peptide Growth Factors

Understanding the control of epithelial cell growth, differentiation and metabolism is crucial to understanding why many of these cellular functions are controlled differently in transformed cancer cells and non-transformed cells. For example, transformed cells, unlike their normal counterparts, are often immortal, can grow without anchorage, are less apt to perform differentiated functions and commonly have a higher level of expression of a broad variety of metabolic enzymes. Non-transformed epithelial cells exist in a tightly controlled state maintained, seemingly, by a balance between the effects of stimulatory factors and inhibitory factors. Holley (1975) proposed that transformed cells escape this control and require fewer exogenous growth factors in culture than their normal counterparts. In fact, transformed cells very frequently require less serum to grow in culture than non-transformed cells. These observations formed the basis of the autocrine growth control hypothesis, whereby transformed cells produce and respond to their own growth factors (DeLarco and Todaro, 1978; Sporn and Todaro, 1980).

Growth Factors and Cancer

The role of growth factors in the growth control and carcinogenesis of prostate cancer, as in many other cancer types, appears to be vital (Thompson 1990). Members of many of the known families of peptide growth factors have been found in prostatic tissue, both malignant and normal. The prostate gland and cancer cells derived from the prostate gland contain growth factors from the fibroblast growth factor (FGF) (Crabb *et al*, 1986a,b), insulin like growth factor (Matuo *et al*, 1988), transforming growth factor-β (TGF-β) (Wilding *et al*, 1989b) and transforming growth factor-α/epidermal growth factor (TGF-α/EGF) (Wilding *et al*, 1989a) families. In addition, platelet derived growth factor (PDGF) production has been documented in human prostate cancer cell lines (Sitaras *et al*, 1988). Other factors have been purified from prostatic tissue and represent either distinct factors or family members of the above mentioned groups (Maehama *et al*, 1986; Matuo *et al*, 1987). In some instances, prostate cancer cells have been shown to transcribe, produce, secrete and respond to growth factors such as TGF-α and TGF-β in autocrine fashion (Wilding *et al*, 1989a,b). The aetiological role of these factors in prostate carcinogenesis has not been established.

Paracrine versus Autocrine Influences

The effects of peptide growth factors are not limited to growth. Stromal-epithelial interactions are important in the normal development of the prostate gland (Cunha *et al*, 1980; Lasnitzki and Mizano 1980) and in prostate cancer (Tenniswood, 1986). Because most growth factors are secreted and therefore can influence the cells surrounding their cell of origin in a paracrine fashion, it is possible that growth factors mediate stromal-epithelial interactions and account for many of the metastatic and invasive characteristics of cancer cells (Keski-Oja *et al*, 1988).

Positive versus Negative Growth Factors

Not all growth factor effects are mitogenic. Growth factors can exert both stimulatory and inhibitory effects depending on the target cell, and, as noted above, even if there is no effect on the growth of cells, many important characteristics of transformed cells can be mediated via growth factors (Keski-Oja *et al*, 1988; Thompson, 1990; Goldstein and Wilding in press). Growth factor production and growth factor receptors are covered by Story and McKeehan, respectively, elsewhere in this issue. This chapter will concentrate on the response of prostate cancer cells to growth factors. In particular, TGF-β, because of its pluripotent actions on cell growth and cell-cell interactions, will be the primary focus.

TRANSFORMING GROWTH FACTOR-β FAMILY

TGF-β Subtypes

Transforming growth factors that have the ability to support anchorage independent growth of indicator cells include TGF-α and TGF-β families of growth factors. Transforming growth factor-α generally supports growth in a wide variety of cell types (Goustin *et al*, 1986). The TGF-βs, on the other hand, exhibit both stimulatory and inhibitory properties, depending on the cell type examined (Massague, 1987). For example, normal rat kidney cells require both TGF-α and a member of the TGF-β family for optimum colony formation in soft agar medium, whereas mouse embryo AKR 2B cells require only TGF-β to grow under anchorage independent conditions. Overall, the effects of TGF-β on epithelial cells are complex and are probably a manifestation of growth regulatory factors and their receptors that are present in and around the cell at a given time (Roberts *et al*, 1985).

The initial observation that density arrested BSC-1 cells secrete a growth inhibitor identical to or closely related to TGF-β raised the possibility that autocrine inhibitory factors may be contributory factors in growth control (Tucker *et al*, 1984a). However, just as important may be the effects these factors have on neighbouring cells and surrounding tissue. For example, TGF-β seems to promote chemotaxis and pericellular proteolysis, as well as to stimulate stromal development (Keski-Oja *et al*, 1988). The net effect of these factors on tumour development thus appears to represent the summation of these disparate influences.

Transforming growth factor-β was initially discovered as one of the components of conditioned medium of murine sarcoma virus transformed fibroblasts, which supported anchorage independent growth of non-transformed fibroblasts (Anzano *et al*, 1983). In addition, TGF-β was discovered as a stimulatory factor for AKR 2B mouse embryo cells and NRK 49F cells (Moses *et al*, 1981; Roberts *et al*, 1985). Thus, from the very beginning, it was apparent that TGF-β was a pluripotent molecule with multifunctional effects on a wide variety of cells.

Transforming growth factor-β1 is ubiquitous (Assoian *et al*, 1983). The active growth factor has a molecular weight of 23 000 and is a homodimer of two 12 500 molecular weight subunits with 112 aminoacids each. The dissociated subunits are inactive (Assoian *et al*, 1983). Transforming growth factor-β1 is derived from a larger precursor and is secreted from the cell in a latent form (Derynck *et al*, 1985). In addition to acid activation, the latent form of the molecule undergoes proteolytic activation (Lyons *et al*, 1988). It binds to a cell surface receptor that is a dimeric glycoprotein of 560 000 molecular weight, with lower molecular weight forms also described (Massague and Like 1985; Cheifetz *et al*, 1986; Fanger *et al*, 1986). No enzymatic activity has been associated with the receptor, although receptor binding activity can be found in most cells (Tucker *et al*, 1984b; Wakefield *et al*, 1987).

The widespread distribution of TGF-β1 receptors and the release of latent forms of TGF-β1 by most cells seem to indicate that the influence of TGF-β1 on cells may be controlled by the activation process or via postreceptor mechanisms. This allows one to postulate that other growth factors may exert control or at least modulate the activation process of TGF-β1 and therefore its biological effects. This is consistent with the hypothesis that normal growth control reflects a balance between positive and negative factors. The very tight homology between TGF-β1 of human and murine origin showing only one aminoacid difference (Derynck *et al*, 1985) emphasizes the importance of this molecule in normal growth and development.

The members of the TGF-β family share many characteristics. The prototypical form, TGF-β1, was the first member of this family identified; its gene is located on chromosome 19q subbands q13.1-q13.3 (Fujii *et al*, 1986). Northern analysis shows a 2.5 kb transcript. Transforming growth factor-β2 was initially isolated from a tamoxifen treated human prostatic carcinoma cell line (PC-3) (Ikeda *et al*, 1987; Madisen *et al*, 1988). The cDNA sequence indicates that TGF-β2 is synthesized as a 442 aminoacid polypeptide precursor from which the mature 112 aminoacid TGF-β2 subunit is derived by proteolytic cleavage. The proteins coded for by the human TGF-β1 and TGF-β2 cDNAs show an overall homology of 71%. Heterodimers can form and are designated TGF-β1.2. Similar to types one and two, the TGF-β3 gene codes for a protein that includes a signal peptide of 20–30 aminoacids and a precursor protein of 412 aminoacids, which is processed to form a final subunit of 112 aminoacids (Derynck *et al*, 1988; Jakowlew *et al*, 1988a; TenDijke *et al*, 1988). At the aminoacid level, TGF-β3 shows 76% identity with TGF-β1 and 79% with TGF-β2. Transforming growth factor-β3 mRNA is mainly expressed in cell lines from mesenchymal origin, suggesting a biological role different from the other species of TGF-β. Transforming growth factor-β4, which lacks a signal peptide (Jakowlew *et al*, 1988b), and TGF-β5, which is expressed in *Xenopus laevis* (Kondaian *et al*, 1990), are recent additions to the TGF-β family. Other factors, such as the inhibins (de Kretser 1990), the Mullerian inhibitory substance (Cate *et al*, 1986) and the decapentaplegic gene complex of *Drosophila* (Padgett *et al*, 1987), constitute an array of more distant relatives to the TGF-β family.

Biological Effects of TGF-β

The role of TGF-β in cancer biology is not limited to negative growth regulation. Its paracrine effects on stromal cells, the immune system and bone metabolism may be even more important. One of the primary targets for TGF-β is fibroblasts. Transforming growth factor-β has been shown to enhance the proliferative effect of epidermal growth factor on fibroblasts and is mitogenic alone towards many cells of mesenchymal origin (Fine and Goldstein 1987). It also enhances the production of collagen (Roberts *et al*, 1986; Fine and Goldstein, 1987) and fibronectin (Ignotz and Massague, 1986) by fibroblasts. Increased production of these proteins by fibroblasts exposed to TGF-β suggests that TGF-β may have an important regulatory role in the synthesis and deposition of extracellular matrices during wound healing and tumour formation (Sporn *et al*, 1983; Masui *et al*, 1986; Roberts *et al*, 1986; Sporn and Roberts, 1986; Twardzik *et al*, 1989). In addition, TGF-β appears to modulate the action of other growth factors such as basic fibroblast growth factor (bFGF), as well as the expression of collagenase and protease genes (Edwards *et al*, 1989). Induction of the proteases by TGF-β may, in turn, foster increased activation of latent forms of TGF-β.

Immune surveillance may also be altered by TGF-β. In its activated form, TGF-β suppresses activation/differentiation of T and B lymphocytes, as well as natural killer cells (Kerhl *et al*, 1986; Rook *et al*, 1986; Wrann *et al*, 1987). However, TGF-β has little effect on lymphocyte proliferation once an immune response has been initiated, and it does not suppress functions of activated lymphocytes, such as cytolysis. Torre-Amione and coworkers (1990) demonstrated the ability of TGF-β to promote the escape of tumour cells from immune surveillance. In addition, TGF-β has been shown to induce monocyte chemotaxis and the production of growth factors such as interleukin-1 (IL-1) (Assoian *et al*, 1987; Wahl *et al*, 1987). As a modulator of inflammation and tissue repair, TGF-β1 increases the secretion of positive acute phase proteins such as α-1-protease inhibitor and α-1-antichymotrypsin, whereas it decreases secretion of the negative acute phase protein albumin. When TGF-β1 and IL-6 are combined, additive induction of the above two positive acute phase proteins is observed, along with a decrease in albumin and α-fetoprotein secretion.

Transforming growth factor-β inhibits the induction of fibrinogen caused by IL-6 (Mackiewicz *et al*, 1990). Thus, TGF-β not only mediates, in part, the inflammatory response but can also modulate the actions of other factors involved in inflammation and tissue repair.

Although endothelial cell proliferation and motility are inhibited by TGF-β (Muller *et al*, 1987; Takehara *et al*, 1987), osteoblasts are mitogenically and metabolically stimulated by TGF-β (Centrella *et al*, 1987; Pfeilschifter and Mundy, 1987), an indication that TGF-β may be important in the regulation of bone remodelling. In fact, demineralized bone is a very rich source of TGF-β. In cancers such as prostate cancer, which commonly metastasize to bone, production of and secretion by tumour cells may play an important part in the establishment of metastases in the bone. One could hypothesize that the blastic characteristics of prostate cancer bone metastases are the result of TGF-β production by the prostate cancer cells.

TGF-β IN PROSTATE CANCER

Growth Response

The simplest assessment of the effect of a growth factor on cancer cells is the measurement of the effect of a factor on an established cancer cell line's growth in tissue culture. As mentioned above, TGF-β in general exerts inhibitory growth effects on cancer cells derived from epithelial tissue. Wilding *et al* (1989b) examined the effects of TGF-β on the human prostate cancer cell lines DU-145, PC-3 and LNCaP for possible inhibitory activity. Growth in monolayer was initially inhibited in a dose response fashion in the two androgen independent cell lines, PC-3 and DU-145, but not in the androgen dependent LNCaP cells. However, the rate of growth of the PC-3 and DU-145 cells treated with TGF-β eventually returned to control levels despite retreatment with TGF-β. Anchorage independent growth was inhibited to 55% and 16% of control levels in PC-3 and DU-145, respectively. Scatchard analysis showed 1500 and 2900 TGF-β binding sites per cell on DU-145 and PC-3 cells. Whereas these high affinity binding sites could be found on the PC-3 and DU-145 cells, high affinity binding has not been demonstrated on the LNCaP cells. Similarly, Fernandez-Pol *et al* (1986) have shown PC-3 and DU-145 anchorage independent growth to be inhibited by TGF-β, and Shain *et al* (1990) have demonstrated the presence of functional TGF-β receptors on rat prostate cancer cells. Zugmaier *et al* (1989) have demonstrated that TGF-β1 and TGF-β2 are equipotent growth inhibitors of human breast cancer cells, but no similar data on prostate cancer cells are available.

The possibility that TGF-β is produced and secreted by prostate cancer cells was also explored by Wilding *et al* (1989b). Analysis of conditioned media by immunoprecipitation and a radioreceptor assay showed secretion of TGF-β into the media by DU-145 and PC-3 but not by LNCaP. Northern analysis showed the presence of TGF-β mRNA in DU-145 and PC-3, but not LNCaP. These data indicate that TGF-β might serve as an autoinhibitory factor in prostate cancer.

Mitchen *et al* (1990) and Wilding G (unpublished) examined the effects of TGF-β1 on epithelial cells derived from normal, benign hyperplastic and cancerous human prostate tissue. All of the primary cultures were inhibited by TGF-β1 with a 50% inhibitory concentration of approximately 10 pM. No differential response was observed for epithelial cells derived from normal versus benign hyperplastic versus cancerous tissue. Doses of TGF-β1 more than tenfold higher than those required for the primary cultures were required to achieve 50% inhibition of the established cell lines PC-3 and DU-145. Similarly, immortalized but non-tumorigenic neonatal prostate epithelial cells were not inhibited by TGF-β1 (Kaighn *et al*, 1989). The inhibition of primary epithelial cultures by TGF-β1 observed by Mitchen *et al* (1990) was not reversed by the addition of bovine pituitary extract, EGF or acidic fibroblast growth factor (aFGF). Inhibition as characterized by flow cytometry showed an increase in the fraction of cells in G_0/G_1 with a decrease of the fraction of cells in S phase after TGF-β1 treatment. Hosobuchi and Stampfer (1989) have observed similar effects of TGF-β on the growth of primary human mammary epithelial cells in culture. Thus, it appears that primary epithelial cultures of human prostate tissue are very sensitive to the inhibitory effects of TGF-β1, and in the human cultures, this might not be reversed by mitogenic factors such as EGF, aFGF and bovine pituitary extract. As in other cell systems, response to the inhibitory effects of TGF-β1 is attenuated by transformation when compared to non-transformed epithelial cells of the same tissue origin.

The control of TGF-β expression in prostate tissue is poorly understood. Elevated levels of mRNA encoding TGF-β2 have been demonstrated in benign hyperplastic prostate tissue compared to normal controls (Mori *et al*, 1990). Thompson (1990) has recently shown that TGF-β1 mRNA levels are markedly elevated in poorly differentiated mouse prostate adenocarcinomas induced by the overexpression of the *ras* and *myc* oncogenes. Although changes in growth factor expression have been associated with the expression of mutated *ras* oncogenes in breast cancer cells, it is not known what the effect of *ras* expression is on the expression of growth factors in human prostate cancer cells. It is, however, of interest that the overexpression of mutated *ras* in the human prostate cancer cell line LNCaP results in an increase in androgen independent growth of these cells in vitro (Voeller *et al*, in press), and Viola *et al* (1986), using immunohistochemistry to determine the expression of *ras* p21, noted increased expression of the *ras* p21 protein on the surface of less differentiated prostate cancer cells compared with normal prostate epithelial of well differentiated prostate cancer cells.

Does TGF-β interact with other growth factors and alter their effects on prostate cancer cells? McKeehan and Adams (1988) showed that normal rat prostate epithelial cell growth requires both EGF and heparin binding growth factor I (HBGF)/aFGF. In contrast, epithelial cells derived from the transplantable Dunning R-3327H rat tumour required either EGF or aFGF. TGF-β inhibited normal epithelial cell growth, whereas TGF-β inhibited EGF dependent growth of tumour epithelial cells, independent of EGF concentrations. TGF-β increased the effectiveness of aFGF to support tumour epithelial cell growth tenfold, but saturating levels of aFGF completely attenuated the inhibitory effect of TGF-β. Although Schuurmans *et al* (1988) reported that TGF-β decreased the growth response of LNCaP cells to EGF, TGF-β receptors were not found on these cells when examined by Wilding *et al* (1989b), and TGF-α did not reverse the inhibitory effects of TGF-β on human prostate cancer cell lines (Wilding *et al*, 1989a,b). Overall, these results suggested that rat prostate cancer cells may escape the inhibitory effect of TGF-β as a consequence of alteration of the concurrent requirement for both EGF and aFGF.

Non-growth Responses

As stated in the introduction, Sitaras *et al* (1988) reported the production of PDGF by DU-145 human prostate cancer cells. Although prostate epithelial cells have not been reported to respond to PDGF, many cell types of mesenchymal origin have been shown to be stimulated by PDGF. Bronzert *et al* (1990) reported that normal mammary epithelial cells are induced to increase the transcription of the PDGF mRNA by TGF-β, even though the TGF-β inhibits the growth of the same mammary epithelial cells. The mechanism by which TGF-β can influence the transcription of PDGF was explored further by Battegay *et al* (1990), who described modulation of the autocrine production of PDGF in cultured smooth muscle cells by TGF-β. These data serve as reminders that TGF-β may not directly influence the growth of cancer cells or the stroma that surrounds them, but it may modulate tumour growth by altering the production of other growth factors by the tumour cells or the stroma.

A body of information in the literature indicates that tissue of mesenchymal origin can influence the embryologic development of prostate epithelial tissue (Cunha *et al*, 1980; Lasnitzki and Mizano, 1980), and it can be postulated that stromal tissue may be involved in the pathological processes of cancer and benign prostatic hypertrophy. The frequently seen complication of bone marrow metastasis in prostate cancer may involve a favourable microenvironment for growth in bone. This hypothesis is supported by the recent report of growth stimulation of the human prostate cancer cell lines DU-145 and PC-3 by human bone marrow and bone stromal conditioned media, but not by conditioned media derived from other organs (Chackel-Roy *et al*, 1989). Co-culture of prostate fibroblasts has been shown to stimulate primary human prostate epithelial cultures (Kabalin *et al*, 1989). Growth inhibition of the established prostate cancer cell lines has also been demonstrated. It has been shown that normal human fetal lung fibroblasts can either inhibit or stimulate the growth of PC-3 cells in soft agar, depending on whether the fibroblasts were grown under anchorage dependent or anchorage independent conditions (Kirk *et al*, 1981). Confluent prostate fibroblast monolayers have been shown to produce an activity that inhibits the growth of PC-3 and LNCaP cells (Konig *et al*, 1987). Finally, Rago and Wilding (unpublished) have shown that an inhibitory activity distinct from TGF-β and the interferons is secreted by bone marrow stroma. These experiments show that it is possible to modulate the growth of prostate cancer cells with paracrine factors released by stromal cells and that the nature of these factors can be influenced by the growth state of the stromal cells.

Osteoblasts are mitogenically and metabolically stimulated by TGF-β (Centrella *et al*, 1987; Pfeilschifter and Mundy, 1987), an indication that TGF-β may be important in the regulation of bone remodeling. Prostate cancer cells, as described above, secrete TGF-β. Koutsilieris *et al* (1987) have demonstrated the presence of potent osteoblast stimulating activity in hyperplastic and cancerous prostatic tissue. Gelb *et al* (1990) have shown that growth plate chondrocytes produce TGF-β and that TGF-β might serve as an important autocrine or paracrine regulator of endochondral calcification. Similarly, Bassols and Massague (1988) have demonstrated that TGF-β regulates the expression and structure of extracellular matrix chondroitin/dermatan sulphate proteoglycans. The secretion of TGF-β by prostate cancer cells can therefore disrupt the regulation of bone remodelling and extracellular matrix structure. Although it is not known whether TGF-β can alter the metastatic potential of prostate cancer cells, Welch *et al* (1990) have shown that TGF-β stimulates mammary adenocarcinoma cell invasion and metastatic potential.

As noted previously, growth factors, including TGF-β, can mediate and modulate the interactions of prostate cancer cells with stromal cells and may also influence androgenic responses (Chang and Chung, 1989). Can TGF-β also modulate metabolic pathways and through such mechanisms alter the response of prostate cancer cells to chemotherapeutic agents? Chapekar and coworkers (1990) isolated rat liver hepatocyte cell lines according to their resistance to the antiproliferative effects of TGF-β. Cells showing stable resistance to TGF-β exhibited a five- to tenfold resistance to chemotherapy agents such as adriamycin and vinblastine. This drug resistance was accompanied by an increase in the steady state mRNA levels of the multiple drug resistance gene and glutathione S-transferase P, two proteins involved in the detoxification and metabolism of chemotherapeutic agents. This study raises the possibility of an association between resistance to the growth inhibitory effects of TGF-β and drug resistance. Equally pertinent to the treatment of human prostate cancer is control of steroidogenesis and the response of prostate cancer cells to androgens. Insight into the role of TGF-β in steroidogenesis has been supplied by Rainey and coworkers (1990), who demonstrated that TGF-β is a potent inhibitor of steroid production in ovine adrenocortical cells. Specifically, TGF-β inhibited the expression of 17α-hydroxylase cytochrome P-450. This is a key enzyme controlling the formation of cortisol and androgens.

In Vivo Effects

Because of the plethora of effects induced by members of the TGF-β family, the question arises as to whether these peptide growth factors can be used in a therapeutic sense in the treatment of prostate cancer. A limited number of in vivo studies have been performed using exogenously administered TGF-β. Two of the first reports of the effects of TGF-β administration were by Sporn *et al* (1983) and Roberts *et al* (1986), who demonstrated the rapid induction of fibrosis and angiogenesis when the factor was administered subcutaneously by injection. Coffey and coworkers (1987) studied the hepatic processing of radioactively labelled, biologically active TGF-β in the rat. After injection into the tail vein, radioactively labelled TGF-β disappeared from the plasma with a half life of 2.2 minutes. Partial hepatectomy prolonged the plasma half life of the injected TGF-β. The first pass hepatic extraction efficiency of labelled TGF-β was approximately 36%, and nearly all of the radioactivity found in the bile was not precipitable with trichloroacetic acid. These data thus suggested that the liver is a major target tissue or site of metabolism for biologically active TGF-β. Silberstein and Daniel (1987) examined the effect of TGF-β on developing epithelial tissue in situ by using slow release plastic pellets containing TGF-β to treat developing mouse mammary gland. They observed powerful but reversible inhibition of mammary growth and morphogenesis.

One of the first descriptions of the effects of TGF-β on tumour cells in vivo was made by Twardzik and coworkers (1989). This group described the effects of natural and recombinant TGF-βs on the growth and differentiation of a xenograft of human lung adenocarcinoma A549 in male athymic Balb/c mice. In these studies, subcutaneous, peritumoural injection of both forms of TGF-β inhibited, in a dose dependent manner, the growth of established human lung tumours. Tumours exposed to TGF-β appeared to be more differentiated, as determined by a lower mitotic activity and a predominance of highly specialized mucous secreting goblet like cell types.

Kyprianou and Isaacs (1988, 1989) demonstrated that both the receptor and the mRNA for TGF-β1 increase rapidly in the ventral prostate after castration. More recently, Martikainen and Issacs (1990) and Martikainen *et al* (1990) reported that TGF-β1 can induce the death of androgen dependent prostatic glandular cells even when physiological levels of androgen are present. These results suggest that TGF-β1 may be a physiological intermediate in the programmed cell death of rat prostatic glandular cells activated after androgen ablation. Information on the effects of TGF-β on prostatic cancer cells in vivo is very limited. Zugmaier *et al* (in press) have administered TGF-β by intraperitoneal injection and measured the effects on xenografts, intraperitoneal and subcutaneous, of human breast cancer cells in athymic nude mice. Although the growth of the breast cancers was not inhibited, the administration of TGF-β intraperitoneally on a daily basis for 10 days proved to be very toxic, many mice becoming cachectic. Similarly, subcutaneous injection of TGF-β in athymic nude mice carrying DU-145 human prostate cancer xenografts did not inhibit the growth of the prostate cancer (Wilding G and Zugmaier G, unpublished). It is entirely possible that despite the inhibitory effects of TGF-β on prostate cancer cells in vitro, TGF-β secretion by the prostate cancer cells or their stromal neighbors may render an advantage to the cancer cells in the process of tumour development.

TGF-β Mechanism of Action

Recent studies have greatly elucidated our understanding of the mechanisms by which TGF-β can inhibit or stimulate cell proliferation (Moses *et al*, 1990). Thus far, TGF-β appears to function through or modulate the expression of the retinoblastoma gene (*RB*) (Laiho *et al*, 1990; Pietenpol *et al*, 1990a) and the early response genes such as c-*fos*, c-*myc* and c-*jun* (Li *et al*, 1990; Moses *et al*, 1990; Pietenpol *et al*, 1990b). Pientenpol and coworkers (1990a,b) recently proposed that the mechanism of TGF-β1 growth inhibition involves the synthesis or modification of a protein that may interact with a specific element in the 5′ regulatory region of the c-*myc* gene and that this results in inhibition of transcriptional initiation. They subsequently showed that the RB protein may mediate TGF-β1 regulation of c-*myc* gene expression and growth inhibition. In these studies, binding of the RB protein with gene products of several of DNA viruses such as the large T antigen of the SV40 (Ludlow *et al*, 1989, 1990) abrogated the TGF-β1 inhibition of c-*myc* and growth in keratinocytes (Pietenpol, 1990a). In addition, Laiho *et al* (1990) showed that TGF-β1 and RB protein appear to function in a common growth inhibitory pathway in which TGF-β1 acts to retain RB protein in its underphosphorylated, growth suppressive state. Other studies have shown that other early response genes and their mRNA expression are also effected by TGF-β (Li, 1990; Moses *et al*, 1990). For example, three members of the Jun family exhibit distinct responses to TGF-β (Li, 1990).

Although the relationship of TGF-β inhibition and the RB protein has not yet been determined in prostate cancer cells, the possible role of the RB protein in prostate tumour formation has been explored by Bookstein *et al* (1990). These investigators examined *RB* expression in three human prostate carcinoma cell lines. One of the lines, DU-145, contained an abnormally small protein translated from an *RB* mRNA transcript that lacked 105 nucleotides. When DU-145 cells had a normal *RB* gene introduced by retrovirus mediated gene transfer, cells that maintained stable exogenous *RB* gene expression lost their ability to form tumors in athymic nude mice. However, their growth rate in vitro was unchanged compared with controls. Thus, tumour suppressor gene products, such as *RB* or *RB* like proteins, may function in the cellular response to growth factors (Hollingsworth and Lee, 1991), since addition of TGF-β prevents the phosphorylation of the RB protein in late G_1 (Laiho, 1990) and since the *RB* binding domains of viral transforming proteins appear to antagonize the growth inhibitory effects of TGF-β (Pientenpol, 1990a). These data suggest that alterations in the *RB* gene may play a part in prostate carcinogenesis.

SUMMARY

The growth of human prostate cancer and its relationship to the surrounding stroma are controlled by complex mechanisms that are incompletely understood. Clearly, peptide growth factors appear to have crucial roles in these processes. One of these factors, TGF-β, and its family members are notable for their wide spectrum of biological effects. In terms of growth, TGF-β inhibits the growth of prostate cancer cells in a cytostatic fashion while stimulating the growth of critical stromal cells, such as fibroblasts. Since the inhibitory effects of TGF-β on prostate cancer cells appear to diminish as the process of transformation progresses towards less differentiated states, the net effect on prostate tumour growth may be positive. Recent evidence suggests that the inhibitory effects of TGF-β on growth, at least, might be mediated through the *RB* tumour suppressor gene product and the proto-oncogene c-*myc*. Beyond its direct growth effects, TGF-β also alters the response of prostate cancer cells to positive mitogenic factors, such as members of the EGF and FGF families, suggesting that growth control is a delicate balance between positive and negative influences. Non-mitogenic responses to TGF-β by prostate cancer cells, the immune system, the stroma and the vascular system provide evidence that TGF-β might also be important in the processes of carcinogenesis, tumour establishment and metastases. In addition, TGF-β appears to influence metabolic pathways important to drug metabolism and steroidogenesis. In vivo, limited evidence suggests that TGF-β can alter the growth and differentiation of some tumour types but appears to be very toxic when administered in high doses. A better understanding of the response of prostate cancer cells to members of the TGF-β family may open new avenues of treating and controlling this disease.

References

Anzano MA, Roberts AB, Smith JM *et al* (1983) Sarcoma growth factors from conditioned medium of virally transformed cells is composed of both type a and b transforming growth factors. *Proceedings of the National Academy of Sciences of the of the USA* **80** 6264–6268

Assoian RK, Komoriya A, Meyers CA *et al* (1983) Transforming growth factor β in human platelets: Identification of a major storage site, purification and characterization. *Journal of Biological Chemistry* **258** 7155–7160

Assoian RK, Fleurdelys BS, Stevenson HD, Miller PD, Madtes DK, Raines EW, Ross R and Sporn MB (1987) Expression and secretion of type beta transforming growth factors by activated human macrophages. *Proceedings of the National Academy of Sciences of the USA* **84** 6020–6024

Bassols A and Massague J (1988) Transforming growth factor β regulates the expression and structure of extracellular matrix chondroitin/dermatan sulfate proteoglycans. *Journal of Biological Chemistry* **263** 3039–3045

Battegay EJ, Raines EW, Seifert RA, Bowen-Pope DF and Ross R (1990) TGF-β induces bimodal proliferation of connective tissue cells via complex control of an autocrine PDGF loop. *Cell* **63** 515–524

Bookstein R, Shew JY, Chen PL, Scully P and Lee WH (1990) Suppression of tumorigenicity of human prostate carcinoma cells by replacing a mutated *RB* gene. *Science* **247** 712–715

Bronzert DA, Bates SE, Sheridan JP *et al* (1990) Transforming growth factor-β induces platelet-derived growth factor (PDGF) messenger RNA and PDGF secretion while inhibiting growth in normal human mammary epithelial cells. *Molecular Endocrinology* **4** 981–

Cate RL, Mattaliano RJ, Hession C *et al* (1986) Isolation of the bovine and human genes for Mullerian inhibiting substance and expression of the human gene in animals. *Cell* **45** 685–698

Centrella M, McCarthy TL and Canalis E (1987) Transforming growth factor beta is a bifunctional regulator of replication and collagen synthesis in osteoblast-enriched cell cultures from fetal rat bone. *Journal of Biological Chemistry* **262** 2869–2874

Chackel-Roy M, Niemeyer C, Moore M and Zetter BR (1989) Stimulation of human prostatic carcinoma cell growth by factors present in human bone marrow. *Journal of Clinical Investigation* **84** 43–50

Chang SM and Chung LWK (1989) Interaction between prostatic fibroblast and epithelial cells in culture: role of androgen. *Endocrinology* **125** 2719–2727

Chapekar MS, Huggett AC, Cheng CC, Hampton LL, Lin KH and Thorgeirsson SS (1990) Isolation and characterization of a rat liver epithelial cell line resistant to the antiproliferative effects of transforming growth factor β (type I). *Cancer Research* **50** 3600–3604

Cheifetz S, Like B and Massague J (1986) Cellular distribution of types I and II receptors for transforming growth factor β. *Journal of Biological Chemistry* **261** 9972–9978

Coffey RJ Jr, Kost LJ, Lyons RM, Moses HL and LaRusso NF (1987) Hepatic processing of transforming growth factor β in the rat. *Journal of Clinical Investigation* **80** 750–757

Crabb JW, Armes LG, Johnson CM and McKeehan WL (1986a) Characterization of multiple forms of prostatropin (prostate epithelial cell growth factor) from bovine brain. *Biochemical and Biophysical Research Communications* **136** 1155–1161

Crabb JW, Armes LG, Carr SA *et al* (1986b) Complete primary structure of prostatropin, a prostate epithelial cell growth factor. *Biochemistry* **25** 4988–4993

Cunha GR, Chung LWK, Shannon JM and Reese BA (1980) Stromal-epithelial interactions in sex differentiation. *Biology of Reproduction* **22** 19–42

de Kretser DM (1990) Inhibin. *Molecular and Cellular Endocrinology* **69** C17–C20

Delarco JE and Todaro GJ (1978) Growth factors from murine sarcoma virus transformed cells. *Proceedings of the National Academy of Sciences of the USA* **75** 4001–4005

Derynck R, Jarrett JA, Chen EY *et al* (1985) Human transforming growth factor β complementary DNA sequence and expression in normal and transformed cells. *Nature* **316** 701–705

Derynck R, Lindquist PB, Lee A *et al* (1988) A new type of transforming growth factor β, TGFβ3. *EMBO Journal* **7** 3737–3743

Edwards DR, Murphy G, Reynolds JJ *et al* (1989) Transforming growth factor beta modulates the expression of collagenase and metalloproteinase inhibitor. *EMBO Journal* **6** 1899–1904

Fanger BO, Wakefield LM and Sporn MB (1986) Structure and properties of the cellular receptor for transforming growth factor type β. *Biochemistry* **25** 3083

Fernandez-Pol JA, Klos DJ and Grant GA (1986) Purification and biologic properties of type β transforming growth factor from mouse transformed cells. *Cancer Research* **46** 5153–5161

Fine A and Goldstein RH (1987) The effect of transforming growth factor beta on cell proliferation and collagen formation by lung fibroblasts. *Journal of Biological Chemistry* **262** 3897–3902

Fujii D, Brissenden JE, Derynck R *et al* (1986) Transforming growth factor β gene maps to human chromosome 19 long arm and to mouse chromosome 7. *Somatic Cell and Molecular Genetics* **12** 281–288

Gelb DE, Rosier RN and Puzas JE (1990) The production of transforming growth factor β by chick growth plate chondrocytes in short term monolayer culture. *Endocrinology* **127** 1941–1946

Golstein D and Wilding G The effects of inhibitory growth factors and cytokines on cell proliferation, In: Foa PP (ed). *Endocrinology and Metabolism*, Springer-Verlag, New York (in press)

Goustin AS, Leof EB, Shipley GD and Moses HL (1986) Growth factors and cancer. *Cancer Research* **46** 1015–1029

Hollingsworth RE and Lee WH (1991) Tumor suppressor genes: new prospects for cancer research. *Journal of the National Cancer Institute* **83** 91–96

Holley RW (1975) Control of growth of mammalian cells in culture. *Nature* **258** 487–

Hosobuchi M and Stampfer MR (1989) Effects of transforming growth factor β on growth of human mammary epithelial cells in culture. *In Vitro Cellular & Developmental Biology* **25** 705–713

Ignotz RA and Massague J (1986) Transforming growth factor beta stimulates the expression of fibronectin and collagen and their incorporation into the extracellular matrix. *Journal of Biological Chemistry* **261** 4337–4345

Ikeda T, Lioubin MN and Marquardt H (1987) Human transforming growth factor type β2: production by a prostatic adenocarcinoma cell line, purification and initial characterization. *Biochemistry* **26** 2406–2410

Jakowlew SB, Dillard PJ, Kondaian P *et al* (1988a) Complementary deoxyribonucleic acid cloning of a novel transforming growth factor β messenger ribonucleic acid from chick embryo chondrocytes. *Molecular Endocrinology* **2** 747–755

Jakowlew SB, Dillard PJ, Sporn MB and Roberts AB (1988b) Complementary deoxyribonucleic acid encoding transforming growth factor β4 from chick embryo chondrocytes. *Molecular Endocrinology* **2** 1186–1195

Kabalin JN, Peehl DM and Stamey TA (1989) Clonal growth of human prostatic epithelial cells is stimulated by fibroblasts. *Prostate* **14** 251–263

Kaighn ME, Reddel RR, Lechner JF *et al* (1989) Transformation of human neonatal prostate epithelial cells by strontium phosphate transfection with a plasmid containing SV40 early region genes. *Cancer Research* **49** 3050–3056

Kerhl JH, Roberts AB, Wakefield LM, Jakowlew S, Sporn MB and Fauci AS (1986) Transforming growth factor beta is an important immunomodulatory protein for human B-lymphocytes. *Journal of Immunology* **137** 3855–3860

Keski-Oja J, Postlethwaite AE and Moses HL (1988) Transforming growth factors in the regulation of malignant cell growth and invasion. *Cancer Investigation* **6** 705–

Kirk D, Szalay MF and Kaighn ME (1981) Modulation of growth of a human prostatic cancer line (PC3) in agar culture by normal human lung fibroblasts. *Cancer Research* **41** 1100–1103

Kondaian P, Sands MJ, Smith JM *et al* (1990) Identification of a novel transforming growth factor-β (TGFβ5) mRNA in *Xenopus laevis*. *Journal of Biological Chemistry* **265** 1089–1093

Konig JJ, Romijn JC and Schroder FH (1987) Prostate epithelium inhibiting factor (PEIF): organ specificity and production by prostatic fibroblasts. *Urologic Research* **15** 145–149

Koutsilieris M, Rabbani SA and Goltzman D (1987) Effects of human prostatic mitogens on rat bone cells and fibroblasts. *Journal of Endocrinology* **115** 447–454

Kyprianou N and Isaacs JT (1988) Identification of a cellular receptor for transforming growth factor beta in rat ventral prostate and its negative regulation by androgens. *Endocrinology* **123** 2124–2131

Kyprianou N and Isaacs JT (1989) Expression of transforming growth factor beta in the rat ventral prostate during castration induced programmed cell death. *Molecular Endocrinology* **3** 1515–1522

Laiho M, DeCaprio JA, Ludlow JW, Livingston DM and Massague J (1990) Growth inhibition by TGF-β linked to suppression of retinoblastoma protein phosphorylation. *Cell* **62** 175–185

Lasnitzki I and Mizano T (1980) Prostatic induction: interaction of epithelium and mesenchyme from normal wild-type mice and androgen-insensitive mice with testicular feminization. *Journal of Endocrinology* **85** 423–428

Li L, Hu JS and Olsen EN (1990) Different members of the jun proto-oncogene family exhibit distinct patterns of expression in response to type β transforming growth factor. *Journal of Biological Chemistry* **265** 1556–1562

Ludlow JW, DeCaprio JA, Huang CM, Lee WH, Paucha E and Livingston DM (1989) SV40 large T antigen binds preferentially to an underphosphorylated member of the retinoblastoma susceptibility gene product family. *Cell* **56** 57–65

Ludlow JW, Shon J, Pipas JM, Livingston DM and DeCaprio JA (1990) The retinoblastoma susceptibility gene product undergoes cell cycle-dependent dephosphorylation and binding to and release from SV40 large T. *Cell* **60** 387–396

Lyons RM, Keski-Oja J and Moses HL (1988) Proteolytic activation of latent transforming growth factor β from fibroblast conditioned medium. *Journal of Cellular Biology* **106** 1597–1605

McKeehan WL and Adams PS (1988) Heparin-binding growth factor/prostatropin attenuates inhibition of rat prostate tumor epithelial cell growth by transforming growth factor type beta. *In Vitro Cellular & Developmental Biology* **24** 243–246

Mackiewicz A, Ganapathi MK, Schultz D *et al* (1990) Transforming growth factor β1 regulates production of acute phase proteins. *Proceedings of the National Academy of Sciences of the*

USA **87** 1491–1495

Madisen L, Webb NR, Rose TM *et al* (1988) Transforming growth factor β2: cDNA cloning and sequence analysis. *DNA* **7** 1–8

Maehama S, Li D, Nanri H, Leykam JF and Deuel TF (1986) Purification and partial characterization of prostate derived growth factor. *Proceedings of the National Academy of Sciences of the USA* **83** 8162–8166

Martikainen P and Isaacs JT (1990) An organ culture system for the study of programmed cell death in the rat ventral prostate. *Endocrinology* **127** 1268–1277

Martikainen P, Kyprianou N and Isaacs JT (1990) Effect of transforming growth factor-β1 on proliferation and death of rat prostatic cells. *Endocrinology* **127** 2963–2968

Massague J (1987) The TGFβ family of growth and differentiation factors. *Cell* **49** 437–438

Massague J and Like B (1985) Cellular receptors for type β transforming growth factor: Ligand binding and affinity labelling in human and rodent cell lines. *Journal of Biological Chemistry* **260** 2636–2645

Masui T, Wakefield LM, Lechner JF *et al* (1986) Type beta transforming growth factor is the primary differentiation inducing serum factor for normal human bronchial epithelial cells. *Proceedings of the National Academy of Sciences of the USA* **83** 2438–2442

Matuo Y, Nishi N, Matusi S, Sandberg AA, Isaacs JT and Wada F (1987) Heparin binding affinity of rat prostatic growth factor in normal and cancerous prostates: partial purification and characterization of rat prostatic growth factor in the Dunning tumor. *Cancer Research* **47** 188–192

Matuo Y, Nishi N, Tanaka H, Sasaki I, Isaacs JT and Wada F (1988) Production of IGF-II-related peptide by an anaplastic cell line (AT3) established from the Dunning prostatic carcinoma of rats. *In Vitro Cellular & Developmental Biology* **24** 1053–1056

Mitchen JL, Rago R and Wilding G (1990) Effects of suramin and TGFβ on the proliferation of primary epithelial cultures from normal, benign hyperplastic and cancerous human prostates. *American Association of Cancer Research* **31** 1289

Mori HM, Maki K, Oishi M, Jaye K, Igarashi O and Hatanaka M (1990) Increased expression of genes for basic fibroblast growth factor and transforming growth factor type β2 in human benign prostatic hyperplasia. *Prostate* **16** 71–80

Moses HL, Branum EB, Proper JA *et al* (1981) Transforming growth factor production by chemically transformed cells. *Cancer Research* **41** 2842–2848

Moses HL, Yang EY and Pietenpol JA (1990) TGF-β stimulation and inhibition of cell proliferation: new mechanistic insights. *Cell* **63** 245–247

Muller G, Behrens J, Nussbaumer U, Bohlen P and Birchmeier W (1987) Inhibitory action of transforming growth factor β on endothelial cells. *Proceedings of the National Academy of Sciences of the USA* **84** 5600–5604

Padgett RW, St Johnston RD and Gelbart WM (1987) A transcript from a Drosophila pattern gene predicts a protein homologous to the transforming growth factor β family. *Nature* **325** 81–84

Pfeilschifter J and Mundy GR (1987) Modulation of type beta transforming growth factor activity in bone cultures by osteotropic hormones. *Proceedings of the National Academy of Sciences of the USA* **84** 2024–2028

Pietenpol JA, Holt JT, Stein RW and Moses HL (1990a) Transforming growth factor β1 suppression of c-*myc* gene transcription: role in inhibition of keratinocyte proliferation. *Proceedings of the National Academy of Sciences of the USA* **87** 3758–3762

Pietenpol JA, Stein RW, Moran E *et al* (1990b) TGF-β1 inhibition of c-*myc* transcription and growth in keratinocytes is abbrogated by viral transforming proteins with *pRB* binding domains. *Cell* **61** 777–785

Rainey WE, Naville D, Saez JM *et al* (1990) Transforming growth factor-β inhibits steroid 17α-hydroxylase cytochrome P-450 expression in ovine adrenocortical cells. *Endocrinology* **127** 1910–1915

Roberts AB, Anzano MA, Wakefield LM, Roche NS, Stern DF and Sporn MB (1985) Type β transforming growth factor: a bifunctional regulator of cell growth. *Proceedings of the National Academy of Sciences of the USA* **82** 119–123

Roberts AB, Sporn MB, Assoian RK *et al* (1986) Transforming growth factor beta: rapid induction of fibrosis and angiogenesis in vivo and stimulation of collagen formation in vitro. *Proceedings of The National Academy of Sciences of the USA* **83** 4167–4174

Rook AH, Kerhl JH, Wakefield LM *et al* (1986) Effects of transforming growth factor beta on the functions of normal killer cells: depressed cytolytic activity and blunting of interferon responsiveness. *Journal of Immunology* **136** 3916–3920

Schuurmans ALG, Bolt J and Mulder E (1988) Androgens and transforming growth factor β modulate the growth response to epidermal growth factor in human prostate tumor cells (LNCaP). *Molecular and Cellular Endocrinology* **60** 101–104

Shain SA, Lin AL, Koger JD and Karaganis AC (1990) Rat prostate cancer cells contain functional receptors for transforming growth factor-β. *Endocrinology* **126** 818–825

Silberstein GB and Daniel CW (1987) Reversible inhibition of mammary gland growth by transforming growth factor β. *Science* **237** 291–293

Sitaras NM, Sariban E, Bravo M, Pantazis P and Antoniades HN (1988) Constitutive production of platelet derived growth factor-like proteins by human prostate carcinoma cell lines. *Cancer Research* **48** 1930–1935

Sporn MD and Todaro GJ (1980) Autocrine secretion and malignant transformation of cells. *New England Journal of Medicine* **303** 878–880

Sporn MB and Roberts AB (1986) Peptide growth factors and inflammation, tissue repair and cancer. *Journal of Clinical Investigation* **78** 329–332

Sporn MB, Roberts AB, Shull JH *et al* (1983) Polypeptide transforming growth factors isolated from bovine sources and used for wound healing in vivo. *Science* **219** 1329–1331

Takehara K, Leroy EC and Grotendorst GR (1987) TGFβ inhibition of endothelial cell proliferation: alteration of EGF binding and EGF induced growth regulatory gene expression. *Cell* **49** 415–422

TenDijke PT, Hanson P, Iwata KK, Piela C and Foulkes JG (1988) Identification of another member of the transforming growth factor type β gene family. *Proceedings of the National Academy of Sciences of the USA* **85** 4715–4719

Tenniswood M (1986) Role of epithelial-stromal interactions in the control of gene expression in the prostate: an hypothesis. *Prostate* **9** 375–385

Thompson TC (1990) Growth factors and oncogenes in prostate cancer. *Cancer Cells* **2** 345–354

Torre-Amione G, Beauchamp RD, Koeppen H *et al* (1990) A highly immunogenic tumor transfected with a murine transforming growth factor β1 cDNA escapes immune surveillance. *Proceedings of the National Academy of Sciences of the USA* **87** 1486–1490

Tucker RF, Shipley GD, Moses HL and Holley RW (1984a) Growth inhibitor from BSC-1 cells closely related to type beta transforming growth factor. *Science* **226** 705–709

Tucker RF, Barnum EL, Shipley GD *et al* (1984b) Specific binding to cultured cells of 125I-labelled transforming growth factor β from human platelets. *Proceedings of the National Academy of Science* **81** 6757–6761

Twardzik DR, Ranchalis JE, McPherson JM *et al* (1989) Inhibition and promotion of differentiated-like phenotype of a human lung carcinoma in athymic mice by natural and recombinant forms of transforming growth factor β. *Journal of the National Cancer Institute* **81** 1182

Viola MV, Fromowitz F, Oravez S *et al* (1986) Expression of ras oncogene p21 in prostate cancer. *New England Journal of Medicine* **314** 133–137

Voeller HJ, Wilding G and Gelmann EP (1991) v-H-ras expression confers hormone independent in vitro growth to LNCaP prostate carcinoma cells. *Molecular Endocrinology* **5** 209–216

Wahl SM, Hunt DA, Wakefield LM *et al* (1987) Transforming growth factor beta induces monocyte chemotaxis and growth factor production. *Proceedings of the National Academy of Sciences of the USA* **84** 5788–5792

Wakefield LM, Smith DM, Masui T, Harris CC and Sporn MB (1987) Distribution and modulation of the cellular receptor for transforming growth factor beta. *Journal of Cell Biology* **105** 965–975

Welch DR, Fabra A and Nakajima M (1990) Transforming growth factor β stimulates mammary adenocarcinoma cell invasion and metastatic potential. *Proceedings of the National Academy of Sciences of the USA* **87** 7678–7682

Wilding G, Valvarius E, Knabbe C and Gelmann EP (1989a) The role of transforming growth factor alpha in human prostate cancer cell growth. *Prostate* **15** 1–12

Wilding G, Knabbe C, Zugmaier G, Flanders K and Gelmann EP (1989b) Differential effects of TGFβ on human prostate cancer cells in vitro. *Molecular and Cellular Endocrinology* **62** 79–87

Wrann M, Bodmer S, deMartin A, Siepl C, Hofer-Warbinek R, Frei K, Hofer E and Fontant A (1987) T cell suppressor factor from human glioblastoma cells is a 25 KD protein closely related to transforming growth factor beta. *EMBO Journal* **6** 1633–1636

Zugmaier G, Ennis B, Deschauer B *et al* (1989) Transforming growth factors type β1 and β2 are equipotent growth inhibitors of human breast cancer cell lines. *Journal of Cellular Physiology* **141** 353–361

Zugmaier G, Paik S, Wilding G *et al* Transforming growth factor beta-1 induces cachexia and systemic fibrosis without an antitumor effect in nude mice. *Cancer Research* (in press)

The author is responsible for the accuracy of the references.

Growth Factor Receptors and Prostate Cell Growth

WALLACE L McKEEHAN

W Alton Jones Cell Science Center, Inc, Lake Placid, New York 12946

Introduction: Growth factor families acting on the prostate
Growth factor receptors in the prostate
    Insulin like growth factors
    Platelet derived growth factors
    The epidermal growth factor family
    Transforming growth factor-β
    Heparin binding (fibroblast) growth factors
Summary

INTRODUCTION: GROWTH FACTOR FAMILIES ACTING ON THE PROSTATE

Analysis of effect on isolated prostate cells and prostate tissues reveals that a minimum of five major growth factor families are probably active in prostate tissues (Table 1). The failure to implicate androgen directly in regulation of prostate growth at the cellular or molecular levels has stimulated tests of the hypothesis that polypeptide growth factors or their receptors may be the mediators of the dramatic control of blood borne androgens on prostate cell growth in vivo. In contrast to classical endocrine hormones, growth factors are generally of local origin and have effects within local tissues, although some factors, such as platelet derived growth factors (PDGF) and transforming growth factor-β (TGF-β), may originate from cellular elements of the circulatory system. Locally acting growth factors have been classified as paracrine and autocrine to describe their origin and target cells in the local tissue (Sporn and Todaro, 1980). Paracrine factors are those that originate in one cell type and affect another cell type, whereas an autocrine factor both originates in and affects the same cell type. Polypeptide growth factors are categorized as families of polypeptides primarily according to their structural homology, despite the name assigned to individual factors, which usually refers to a tissue or cell of origin, a biological activity or a property of the factor. Although growth factors differ from circulating hormones in that they originate and act in the local tissue environment, they are thought to act predominantly at the external cell surface by binding and activating specific transmembrane glycoprotein receptors (Ullrich and Schlessinger, 1990). Growth factor transmembrane receptors are characterized by an aminoterminal extracellular do-

Cancer Surveys Volume 11: *Prostate Cancer*
© 1991 Imperial Cancer Research Fund. 0-87969-368-1/91. $3.00 + .00

TABLE 1. Major growth factor families acting on the prostate

Family	Cloned members	Reference
Insulin like growth factor (IGF)	insulin (pancreatic); IGF-I, II	Czech (1989)
Platelet derived growth factors (PDGF)	PDGF-AA, BB,AB	Ross *et al* (1986)
Epidermal growth factor (EGF)	EGF; TGF-α; pox virus GF; amphiregulin	Carpenter and Cohen (1989)
Transforming growth factor-β (TGF-β)	TGF-β1,2,3,5,1.2; inhibin A,B; activin A,B; Mullerin inhibiting substance (MIS)	Massague (1990)
Heparin binding (fibroblast) growth factors (HBGF/FGF)	HBGF-1 (acidic FGF) HBGF-2 (basic FGF) HBGF-3 (Int-2) HBGF-4 (hst/KFGF) HBGF-5 (FGF-5) HBGF-6 (FGF-6) HBGF-7 (KGF)	Burgess and Maciag (1989)

main, which constitutes the growth factor binding site, a 16–22 aminoacid hydrophobic transmembrane domain, an intracellular juxtamembrane domain and an additional carboxyterminal intracellular catalytic domain. The intracellular catalytic domains of characterized receptors for three of the five growth factor families (insulin, epidermal growth factor [EGF] and PDGF) at play in the prostate consist of structural domains containing the ATP binding and catalytic sites characteristic of tyrosine kinases. An additional carboxyterminal subdomain consists of multiple tyrosine phosphorylation sites, which are autophosphorylated upon binding of the growth factor to the receptor. The receptor for one member of the insulin like growth factor (IGF) family (IGF-II) does not exhibit tyrosine kinase structural domains in the intracellular sequence (Czech, 1989). Receptors for the heparin binding (fibroblast) growth factor family (HBGF) consist of both tyrosine kinase and non-kinase intracellular domains fused with the same extracellular ligand binding domains (Hou *et al*, 1991). The structures of receptors for the TGF-β family remain to be characterized.

GROWTH FACTOR RECEPTORS IN THE PROSTATE

Insulin Like Growth Factors

The IGF family currently consists of three members, pancreatic insulin, IGF-I and IGF-II (Table 1). Specific high affinity receptors for each have been cloned and fully characterized (Czech, 1989). Insulin, IGF-I and IGF-II bind with low affinity to the high affinity insulin and IGF-I receptors, whereas insulin and IGF-I do not bind significantly to the specific IGF-II receptor (Czech, 1989). There has been little study of the molecular structure of the three receptors in prostate tissues. The importance of the specific IGF-I receptor in the growth of prostate cells has been inferred from analysis of the comparative dose response of cultured prostate cells to insulin, IGF-I and IGF-II. Low levels of IGF-I, which are near the apparent dissociation constant (K_d) of the IGF-I receptor, are sufficient to support proliferation of both normal and tumour derived cultured prostate epithelial and mesenchymal cell proliferation, whereas much higher doses of insulin and IGF-II are required to elicit the same response (McKeehan *et al*, 1984, 1991, in press and unpublished). Elevated levels of IGF-I gene expression are seen in regenerating normal prostate after androgen treatment of castrated rats and appear to be constitutive in slow growing, androgen responsive and highly malignant variants of the Dunning R-3327 model transplantable tumours (McKeehan *et al*, 1991, in press). IGF-I gene expression appears to occur predominantly in the mesenchymal cells of both regenerating normal prostate and slow growing tumours (Wang F and McKeehan WL, unpublished). Expression of the IGF family of receptors (IGF-I in particular) deserves careful study in epithelial and mesenchymal cells of both normal prostate and prostatic tumours.

Platelet Derived Growth Factors

The PDGF receptor family has not been characterized at the molecular level in prostate tissues. As with most tissues, isolated prostate epithelial cells exhibit neither a response to nor specific receptors for the PDGF polypeptides (McKeehan WL, unpublished). Growth of isolated prostate mesenchymal cells, like the growth of mesenchymal cells from other tissues, is stimulated by PDGF (McKeehan WL, unpublished).

The Epidermal Growth Factor Family

The EGF family of receptors currently consists of products of three distinct genes (Schlessinger, 1986; Kraus *et al*, 1989; Carpenter and Cohen, 1990; Ullrich and Schlessinger, 1990). Products of the *EGFr* gene (also called *ERB-B* and *HER-1*) appear to exhibit equal affinity for homologues EGF and TGF-α, whereas products of the *neu* gene (also called *ERB-B2*, *HER-2* and *NGL*) do not bind EGF and TGF-α with high affinity. A potentially specific ligand for the *neu* receptor has been identified recently that also binds to the *EGFr* gene product (Lupu *et al*, 1990). Both *EGFr* and *neu* genes exhibit structural variants that are ligand independent and oncogenic. The EGF receptor family has not been extensively characterized at the molecular level in prostate tissues.

Ligand binding and immunochemical analysis suggest that the EGF receptor family is a candidate for regulation by androgen, but whether the family is a mediator of androgen regulation of prostate cell growth and a factor in unregulated growth of prostate tumour cells remains to be established. Castration of normal male rats resulted in a two- to sixfold increase in EGF binding in membranes and whole homogenates, whereas subsequent androgen treatment decreased the binding (Traish and Wotiz, 1987; St-Arnaud *et al*, 1988). Unfractionated benign prostatic hyperplastic (BPH) tissue exhibited lower EGF binding than normal and cancerous human prostate tissues (Maddy *et al*, 1987; Eaton *et al*, 1988; Davies and Eaton, 1989), but fractionated epithelial cells exhibited equal levels of binding in the three tissues (Davies and Eaton, 1989). No clear correlation between EGF receptor levels and tumour grade could be established. An immunohistochemical analysis suggested that BPH stroma was deficient in the EGF receptor content relative to epithelium (Maddy *et al*, 1987). The level of nuclear steroid hormone receptors, including androgen receptors, inversely correlated with the level of EGF receptor in membranes from BPH tissues (Lubrano *et al*, 1989). In contrast to its effect in prostate tissues, androgen increased EGF receptor number in an androgen responsive cell line (LNCaP) derived from a lymph node metastasis of human prostate (Schuurmans *et al*, 1988b; Mulder *et al*, 1989). Recent studies indicate that the LNCaP cell line expresses an altered steroid hormone and agonist/antagonist receptor phenotype, which may underlie its unusual androgen responsiveness relative to the great majority of isolated normal and tumour derived prostate epithelial cells (Wilding *et al*, 1989a; Harris *et al*, 1990).

Although there is a paucity of molecular study of the EGF receptor and tyrosine kinases in the prostate, the studies of Lin and Clinton (1988) are noteworthy. These authors have suggested that the phosphorylated species of the EGF receptor is a substrate for human prostatic acid phosphatase (PrPYP). An inverse correlation between PrPYP and tyrosine kinase activities has been observed in prostate carcinoma cells. Recently, specific protein tyrosine phosphatases have been implicated as important controllers of tyrosine kinase signal cascades (Hunter, 1989).

Transforming Growth Factor-β

Binding sites for the various members of the TGF-β family of polypeptides are heterogeneous and have so far been resistant to molecular characterization (Massague, 1990). Three size classes of binding sites have been characterized from various cells and tissues by covalent labelled ligand affinity cross linking (Massague, 1990). Type I binding sites of 60–70 kDa are the most common and have high affinity for TGF-β1 and lower affinity for TGF-β2. Type II sites of 85–110 kDa vary between species and cell types. Type III binding sites with an apparent mass of 250–350 kDa have high affinity for at least three members of the family, TGF-β1, TGF-β2 and TGF-β1.2 (Massague, 1990). Occupancy of type I and II binding sites correlates with biological effects of TGF-β (Massague, 1990). Type III binding sites, which are membrane bound proteogly-cans (betaglycans), have not been directly implicated in signal transduction and may have a passive role as a reservoir of the factors in the local tissue environment (Massague, 1990).

Specific TGF-β binding sites with an apparent kDa of 140 pM have been characterized in membranes of rat prostate (Kyprianou and Isaacs, 1988). Covalent affinity cross linking revealed a dominant species of 260 kDa, a size that correlates with the type III binding site (Kyprianou and Isaacs, 1988). Receptor levels increased in the prostate after castration and were restored to normal by androgen therapy. The expression pattern correlated with that of TGF-β1 mRNA (Kyprianou and Isaacs, 1989). Transforming growth factor-β binding sites have been detected in two of three human prostate carcinoma derived cell lines concurrently with expression of TGF-β antigen (Wilding *et al*, 1989b). Neither TGF-β binding sites nor the factor could be detected in the androgen responsive LNCaP cell line (Wilding *et al*, 1989b). The absence of binding sites in the LNCaP line contradicts an earlier report that showed that TGF-β inhibits the response of the same line to EGF (Schuurmans *et al*, 1988b).

Although TGF-β receptors have not been analysed, epithelial cells derived from both normal rat prostate and androgen responsive Dunning R-3327PAP tumours exhibit active TGF-β receptors, which presumably mediate growth inhibitory effects of the factor (McKeehan and Adams, 1988). Transforming growth factor-β expression is very low in normal rat prostate tissue but is constitutively expressed in R-3327PAP ("slow tumour") and the androgen independent, highly malignant variant, R-3327AT3 ("fast tumour") (Wang F and McKeehan WL, unpublished). Transforming growth factor-β completely abrogates the mitogenic effect of EGF/TGF-α on epithelial cells from the slow tumour, but inhibition of HBGF stimulated proliferation of the slow tumour derived epithelial cells depends on the ratio of HBGF to TGF-β (McKeehan and Adams, 1988). Conceivably, this dose dependent interaction reflects the variable affinity of both HBGF and TGF-β receptor phenotypes for ligand. This contrasts with the low dose inhibitory effects of TGF-β1 on normal prostate epithelial cells, which require both EGF and HBGF for proliferation (McKeehan *et al*, 1984; McKeehan and Adams, 1988).

Heparin Binding (Fibroblast) Growth Factors

The HBGF receptor family (HBGF-R) has only recently been characterized at the molecular level. Currently, the family consists of the products of at least three distinct genes termed *Flg* (*F*ms *l*ike *g*ene) (Dionne *et al*, 1990; Hou *et al*, 1991), *Bek* (*B*acterially *e*xpressed *k*inase) (Dionne *et al*, 1990) and *Cek-2* (*C*hicken *e*mbryo *k*inase) (Pasquale, 1990). The *Flg* and *Bek* gene products exhibit extensive structural variation as a consequence of alternate splicing during transcription. Structural variants in the aminoterminal domains consist of three (HBGF-Rα) and two (HBGF-Rβ) immunoglobulin like disulphide loop structures, the presence and absence of a characteristic sequence of acidic residues ("the acidic box") (Miki *et al*, 1991) and a two aminoacid variation just downstream from the acidic box (Hou *et al*, 1991). Two additional amino-terminal variants consist of an alternate splice of a nucleotide sequence in place of the coding sequence for the outermost IgG like loop and a deletion of the first five base pairs of the coding sequence for the loop (Hou *et al*, 1991; McKeehan WL, Hou J and Wang F, unpublished). Both mRNA variants cause appearance of stop codons in-frame with the common translational initiation site and transmembrane signal coding sequence. Both variants predict an alternate product initiated at a favourable downstream translational initiation site that does not contain a favourable membrane translocation sequence. The existence of these mRNAs has raised the possibility of intracellular structural variants of HBGF-R that are not translocated to the cell surface. The *Bek* gene also exhibits an additional variant in the second IgG like loop of the two loop HBGF-β extracellular domain, which has also been called *K-Sam* (*K*ato-III cell derived *s*tomach cancer *am*plified gene) (Hattori *et al*, 1990) and *KGF-R* (*K*eratinocyte *G*rowth *F*actor *R*eceptor) (Miki *et al*, 1991). *HBGF-R* genes exhibit splice variants in the juxtamembrane sequence, which vary in the presence and absence of a threonine residue that may constitute a serine-threonine kinase phosphorylation site (Hou *et al*, 1991). The most common intracellular (carboxyterminal) domain of HBGF-R species consists of consensus sequences typical of the ATP binding and catalytic domains of tyrosine kinases followed by a carboxyterminus exhibiting multiple candidate tyrosine phosphorylation sites (Dionne *et al*, 1990; Hattori *et al*, 1990; Pasquale, 1990; Hou *et al*, 1991; Miki *et al*, 1991). Alternate splicing in the *HBGF-R* (*Flg*) gene results in a truncated translational product beginning at the 5′ end of the catalytic domain sequence (Hou *et al*, 1991). This structural variant has no tyrosine kinase activity (McKeehan WL, Hou J and Shi E, unpublished) and is devoid of the carboxyterminal tyrosine phosphorylation sites (Hou *et al*, 1991; McKeehan WL, unpublished). The role and regulation of each of these structural variants on ligand binding, receptor oligomerization, metabolism and signal transduction in cells and tissues are unclear and will require extensive quantitative analysis.

The HBGF family of polypeptides currently consist of seven cloned gene products (Burgess and Maciag, 1989). The two most widely studied members of the family, HBGF-1 (acidic fibroblast growth factor, aFGF) and HBGF-2 (basic [b]FGF) have been extensively implicated in prostate cell growth (Mansson *et al*, 1989; Gelmann, 1991; McKeehan *et al*, 1991, in press). The other five members of the family need extensive analysis in prostate. Only the *Int-2* gene (*HBGF-3*) has been additionally implicated (Muller *et al*, 1990). The gene caused the development of prostatic hypertrophy in male mice carrying the *Int-2* transgene. Epithelial and mesenchymal cells from normal prostate and various grades of model rat prostate tumours exhibit specific membrane receptor sites for HBGF-1 and HBGF-2 (Mansson *et al*, 1989). Both epithelial and mesenchymal cells derived from normal prostate exhibit biphasic Scatchard binding plots, indicating heterogeneity of binding sites in respect to ligand affinity (Mansson *et al*, 1989). In contrast, both cell types from slow growing, hormone responsive tumours ("slow tumours") and cells from highly malignant variants ("fast tumours") exhibit simple linear plots. The hallmark of the slow tumour epithelial cells is a dramatic reduction in amount of HBGF-1 required to elicit maximal proliferative response relative to normal cells (McKeehan *et al*, 1987; Mansson *et al*, 1989). Cells derived from fast tumours are completely independent of exogenous HBGF. The lower requirement in slow tumour epithelial cells correlates with ligand occupancy of the high affinity binding site predicted by the biphasic Scatchard plot of normal epithelial cells, whereas the dose required for normal epithelial cell proliferation correlates with complete occupancy of both high and low affinity sites (Mansson *et al*, 1989). In sum, the data suggest that an alteration in receptor phenotype in epithelial cells may underlie a progressively relaxed requirement for HBGF in both slow and fast tumours.

In view of the extensive heterogeneity of the emergent HBGF receptor family at the genetic and structural level, analysis of expression of isoforms in prostate tissues is in early stages. Normal and tumour prostate tissues express a 4.2–4.5 kb *HBGF-R* (*Flg*) mRNA (McKeehan *et al*, 1991, in press). Expression of *HBGF-R* (*Bek*) mRNA at about 4.2–4.5 kb is about 10% of *HBGF-R* (*Flg*) expression (Yan G and McKeehan WL, unpublished). *HBGF-R* (*Flg*) expression appears limited to both normal and slow tumour derived stromal cells and is undetectable in the epithelial cells (McKeehan *et al*, 1991). Fast tumour cells express elevated levels of *HBGF-R* (*Flg*), whereas expression of *HBGF-R* (*Bek*) is about equal in normal and slow tumour epithelial cells (Yan G and McKeehan WL, unpublished). Castration causes a significant increase in *Flg* gene expression in normal and slow tumours (McKeehan *et al*, 1991). Administration of testosterone causes a more dramatic increase in *Flg* gene expression in normal prostate and a transient increase in the slow tumour (McKeehan *et al*, 1991). Cloning and analysis of *HBGF-R* (*Flg*) cDNAs from the fast AT-3 tumour tissue predict the presence of isoforms of the HBGF-R α, β and γ aminoterminal, the a and b juxtamembrane and the type I carboxyterminus (McKeehan *et al*, 1991; Hou J, Wang F and McKeehan WL, unpublished). A cDNA predicting the exact type 2 truncated isoform reported from human hepatoma cells (Hou *et al*, 1991) has not been detected. However, cDNAs cloned from normal and tumour prostate tissue predict carboxyterminal truncations upstream of the kinase consensus sequence that may have a similar consequence, an isoform of HBGF-R (Flg) that does not have kinase activity (Kan M, Hou J and McKeehan WL, unpublished). The isoforms of HBGF-R (Bek) present in prostate cells and tissues have not been analysed. The HBGF-R (Flg) family appears to be associated with the mesenchymal cells and the HBGF-R (Bek) family with the epithelial cells from normal prostate and the slow growing, hormone responsive tumours (McKeehan *et al*, 1991; Yan G and McKeehan WL, unpublished). Aaronson and colleagues have suggested that a variant in the second IgG like loop of HBGF-R (Bek) and devoid of the acidic box constitutes the predominant HBGF-R in epithelial cells and has higher affinity for HBGF-1 and the homologue keratinocyte growth factor (KGF/HBGF-7) than HBGF-2 (Miki *et al*, 1991). Keratinocyte growth factor has been proposed as an HBGF that originates in mesenchymal cells and acts on epithelial cells by a paracrine mechanism (Finch *et al*, 1989), a profile similar to HBGF-1 expression in the slow R-3327PAP prostate (slow) tumour (Mansson *et al*, 1989). The fast AT-3 tumour variant expresses KGF mRNA, and the complete coding sequence for the rat factor has been deduced from a cloned cDNA from the tumour (Yan *et al*, 1991).

In contrast to KGF and other members of the HBGF family (HBGF-3 to 7), HBGF-1 and HBGF-2 differ in that no apparent hydrophobic signal for conventional secretion is encoded in their mRNAs (Burgess and Maciag, 1989). This has led to speculation about the participation of the two factors at an intracellular, possibly nuclear, site, rather than binding to the extracellular domain of transmembrane receptors (Acland *et al*, 1990; Imamura *et al*, 1990). A cDNA of the *HBGF-R* (*Flg*) gene present in normal tissue but elevated in rat tumours predicts a variant of the two-loop β form of the receptor, which is probably not transported to the cell surface (McKeehan *et al*, 1991; Wang F and McKeehan WL, unpublished). This raises the possibility that a complete intracellular autocrine circuit consisting of both intracellular HBGF and receptor isoforms may be operative in some prostate cells.

Distinct structural domains of polypeptide receptors have distinct roles in various activities of the receptor (Ross *et al*, 1986; Schlessinger, 1986; Burgess and Maciag, 1989; Czech, 1989; Carpenter and Cohen, 1990; Ullrich and Schlessinger, 1990). Ligand affinity is generally determined by the amino-terminal domain, although modifications in other domains, eg phosphorylation sites, may alter affinity. The juxtamembrane intracellular domain exhibits serine/threonine phosphorylation sites, which can alter both ligand affinity and metabolism by internalization. The structural motifs between the two kinase consensus regions and the carboxyterminal tail, which usually contain tyrosine phosphorylation sites, have been implicated in substrate binding specificity. Receptors are thought to act at the molecular level through formation of clusters of oligomers, predominantly dimeric structures, upon ligand binding. The structural requirements for active dimer formation are unclear. The HBGF-R family consists of structural variants that may differ in all of the above activities. A major challenge lies ahead to analyse and understand the contribution of this extremely diverse family of effectors and their receptors to normal prostate physiology and progression of prostate tumours.

SUMMARY

Five major growth factor families and their receptors have been implicated in prostate cell growth. The regulation of expression of individual members of individual families and their aberrant expression are candidates for causal factors underlying normal prostate development, androgen regulated compensatory growth of prostate and prostate pathologies (BPH and cancer). Despite the fact that prostate cancer is the most common male malignancy in Western countries and second only to lung cancer in black American males, the cellular and molecular biology of growth factor and receptor action in prostate is a relatively neglected area of study. The characterization of individual growth factors and receptors is progressing rapidly and provides the molecular basis to establish which factors by what mechanism underlie progressive prostate malignancies.

NOTE ADDED IN PROOF

While this review was in press, a fourth distinct gene coding for an HBGF-R was reported, FGFR-4, a novel acidic fibroblast growth factor receptor with a distinct expression pattern (Partenen *et al*, 1991). The first receptor for a member of the TGF-β family (activin) which exhibits an intracellular domain that has sequence homology with serine kinases was also described (Mathews and Vale, 1991).

References

Acland D, Dixon M, Peters G and Dickson C (1990) Subcellular fate of the Int-2 oncoprotein is determined by choice of initiation codon. *Nature* **343** 662–665

Burgess WH and Maciag T (1989) The heparin-binding (fibroblast) growth factor family of proteins. *Annual Review of Biochemistry* **58** 575–606

Carpenter G and Cohen S (1990) Epidermal growth factor. *Journal of Biological Chemistry* **265** 7709–7712

Czech M (1989) Signal transmission by the insulin-like growth factors. *Cell* **59** 235–238

Davies P and Eaton CL (1989) Binding of epidermal growth factor by human normal, hypertropic, and carcinomatous prostate. *Prostate* **14** 123–132

Dionne CA, Crumley G, Bellot F *et al* (1990) Cloning and expression of distinct high-affinity receptors cross-reacting with acidic and basic fibroblast growth factors. *EMBO Journal* **9** 2685–2692

Eaton CL, Davies P and Phillips MEA (1988) Growth factor involvement and oncogene expression in prostatic tumors. *Journal of Steroid Biochemistry* **30** 341–345

Finch DW, Rubin JS, Miki T, Ron D and Aaronson SA (1989) Human KGF is FGF-related with properties of a paracrine effector of epithelial cell growth. *Science* **245** 752–755

Gelmann EP (1991) Oncogenes and growth factors in prostate cancer. *Journal of NIH Research* **3** 62–64

Harris SE, Rong Z, Harris MA and LuBahn DB (1990) Androgen receptor in human prostate carcinoma LNCaP/ADEP cells contains a mutation which alters the specificity of the steroid-dependent transcriptional activation region. *The Endocrine Society 72nd Annual Meeting* **272** 93 [Abstract]

Hattori Y, Odagiri H, Nakatani H *et al* (1990) K-*sam*, an amplified gene in stomach cancer, is a member of the heparin-binding growth factor receptor genes. *Proceedings of the National Academy of Sciences of the USA* **87** 5983–5987

Hou J, Kan M, McKeehan K, McBride G, Adams P and McKeehan WL (1991) Fibroblast growth factor receptors from liver vary in three structural domains. *Science* **251** 665–668

Hunter T (1989) Protein-tyrosine phosphatases: the other side of the coin. *Cell* **58** 1013–1016

Imamura T, Engleka K, Zhan X *et al* (1990) Recovery of mitogenic activity of a growth factor mutant with a nuclear translocation sequence. *Science* **249** 1567–1574

Kraus MH, Issing W, Miki T, Popescu NC and Aaronson SA (1989) Isolation and characterization of ERBB3, a third member of the ERBB/epidermal growth factor receptor family: evidence for overexpression in a subset of human mammary tumors. *Proceedings of the National Academy of Sciences of the USA* **86** 9193–9197

Kyprianou N and Isaacs JT (1988) Identification of a cellular receptor for transforming growth factor-b in rat ventral prostate and its negative regulation by androgens. *Endocrinology* **123** 2124–2131

Kyprianou N and Isaacs JT (1989) Expression of transforming growth factor-b in the rat ventral prostate during castration-induced programmed cell death. *Molecular Endocrinology* **3** 1515–1522

Lin MF and Clinton GM (1988) The epidermal growth factor receptor from prostate cells is dephosphorylated by a prostate-specific phosphotyrosyl phosphatase. *Molecular and Cellular Biology* **8** 5477–5485

Lubrano C, Petrangeli E, Catizone A *et al* (1989) Epidermal growth factor binding and steroid receptor content in human benign prostatic hyperplasia. *Journal of Steroid Biochemistry* **34** 499–504

Lupu R, Colomer R, Zugmaier G *et al* (1990) Direct interaction of a ligand for the erbB2 oncogene product with the EGF receptor and p185erbB2. *Science* **249** 1552–1555

Mathews LS and Vale WW (1991) Expression cloning of an activin receptor, a predicted transmembrane serine kinase. *Cell* **65** 973–982

McKeehan WL and Adams PS (1988) Heparin-binding growth factor/prostatropin attenuates inhibition of rat prostate tumor epithelial cell growth by transforming growth factor type beta. *In Vitro Cellular and Developmental Biology* **24** 243–246

McKeehan WL, Adams PS and Rosser MP (1984) Direct mitogenic effects of insulin, epidermal growth factor, glucocorticoid, cholera toxin, unknown pituitary factors and possibly prolactin, but not androgen, on normal rat prostate epithelial cells in serum-free, primary cell culture. *Cancer Research* **44** 1998–2010

McKeehan WL, Adams PS and Fast D (1987) Different hormonal requirements for androgen-independent growth of normal and tumor epithelial cells from rat prostate. *In Vitro Cellular and Developmental Biology* **23** 147–152

McKeehan WL, Kan M, Hou J, Wang F, Adams P and Mansson PE (1991) Heparin-binding (fibroblast) growth factor/receptor gene expression in the prostate, In: Karr J, Coffey DS, Smith RG and Tindall DJ (eds). *Molecular and Cell Biology of Prostate Cancer*, pp 115–126, Plenum Press, New York

McKeehan WL, Hou J, Adams P, Wang F, Yan G and Kan M Heparin-binding fibroblast growth factors and prostate cancer, In: Stringer-Wang S (ed). *Underlying Molecular, Cellular and Immunological Factors in Age-related Cancers*, Plenum Press, New York (in press)

Maddy SQ, Chisholm GD, Hawkins RA and Habib FK (1987) Localization of epidermal growth factor receptor in the human prostate by biochemical and immunochemical methods. *Journal of Endocrinology* **113** 147–153

Mansson PE, Adams P, Kan M and McKeehan WL (1989) Heparin-binding growth factor gene expression and receptor characteristics in normal rat prostate and two transplantable rat prostate tumors. *Cancer Research* **49** 2485–2494

Massague J (1990) The transforming growth factor-b family. *Annual Review of Cell Biology* **6** 597–641

Miki T, Fleming TP, Bottaro DP, Rubin JS, Ron D and Aaronson SA (1991) Expression cDNA cloning of the KGF receptor by creation of a transforming autocrine loop. *Science* **251** 72–74

Mulder E, vanLoon D, DeBoer W *et al* (1989) Mechanisms of androgen action: recent observations on the domain structure of androgen receptors and the induction of EGF receptors by androgens in prostate tumor cells. *Journal of Steroid Biochemistry* **32** 151–156

Muller WJ, Lee FS, Dickson C, Peters G, Pattengale P and Leder P (1990) The INT-2 gene product acts as an epithelial growth factor in transgenic mice. *EMBO Journal* 9 907–910

Partenen J, Makela TP, Eerola E *et al* (1991) FGFR-4, a novel acidic fibroblast growth factor receptor with a distinct expression pattern. *The EMBO Journal* 10 1347–1354

Pasquale EB (1990) A distinctive family of embryonic protein-tyrosine kinase receptors. *Proceedings of the National Academy of Sciences of the USA* 87 5812–5816

Ross R, Raines EW and Bowen-Pope DF (1986) The biology of platelet-derived growth factor. *Cell* 46 155–169

Schlessinger J (1986) Allosteric regulation of the epidermal growth factor receptor kinase. *Journal of Cell Biology* 103 2067–2072

Schuurmans ALG, Bolt J and Mulder E (1988a) Androgens stimulate both growth rate and epidermal growth factor receptor activity of the human prostate tumor cell LNCaP. *Prostate* 12 55–63

Schuurmans ALG, Bolt J and Mulder E (1988b) Androgens and transforming growth factor β modulate the growth response to epidermal growth factor in human prostatic tumor cells (LNCaP). *Molecular and Cellular Endocrinology* 60 101–104

Sporn MB and Todaro GJ (1980) Autocrine secretion and malignant transformation of cells. *New England Journal of Medicine* 303 878–880

St-Arnaud R, Poyet P, Walker P and Labrie F (1988) Androgens modulate epidermal growth factor receptor levels in the rat ventral prostate. *Molecular and Cellular Endocrinology* 56 21–27

Traish AM and Wotiz HH (1987) Prostatic epidermal growth factor receptors and their regulation by androgens. *Endocrinology* 121 1461–1467

Ullrich A and Schlessinger J (1990) Signal transduction by receptors with tyrosine kinase activity. *Cell* 61 203–212

Wilding G, Chen M and Gelmann EP (1989a) Aberrant response in vitro of hormone-responsive prostate cancer cells to antiandrogens. *Prostate* 14 103–115

Wilding G, Zugmeier G, Knabbe C, Flanders K and Gelmann E (1989b) Differential effects of transforming growth factor β on human prostate cancer cells in vitro. *Molecular and Cellular Endocrinology* 62 79–87

Yan G, Nikolaropoulos S, Wang F and McKeehan WL (1991) Sequence of keratinocyte growth factor (heparin-binding growth factor type 7) from a rat prostate tumor. *In Vitro Cellular and Developmental Biology* 27A 437–438

The author is responsible for the accuracy of the references.

Endocrine Therapy: Where Do We Stand and Where Are We Going?

FRITZ H SCHRÖDER

Department of Urology, Academic Hospital and Erasmus University, 3000 DR Rotterdam, The Netherlands

INTRODUCTION

Endocrine management, initially consisting exclusively of castration, was introduced into the treatment of human prostate cancer by Huggins and his associates (1941). This was done after careful and extensive studies of the endocrine dependence of the dog prostate and after exploration of the effect of castration in a selected group of patients with benign prostatic hyperplasia (BPH) (Huggins and Stevens, 1940). The impressive palliative effects in patients with symptoms were clearly evident early on, and it was assumed that this excellent palliation was also associated with increased survival. This was firmly believed until in 1967 the results of a large placebo controlled study of the Veterans Administration Cooperative Urological Research Group (VACURG) were published. In the first VACURG study, placebo was compared with standard endocrine treatment, such as orchidectomy, diethylstilboestrol (DES), 5 mg/day, and orchidectomy plus DES 5 mg/day. The policy of this study allowed that treatment could be changed if patients progressed. For this reason, 44% of patients in the placebo arm were switched to endocrine treatment. Patients with stages III and IV (non-metastatic and metastatic) disease were included. These studies confirmed the excellent palliative effect of endocrine treatment that, compared with placebo, was associated with a statistically significant benefit in terms of pain reduction, decrease of their performance status, urethral obstruction and neurological symptoms. Prostatic size, pretreatment elevation of acid phosphatase and the time until metastases occur in the non-metastatic group were also favourably influenced in a statistically significant fashion, as reported by Blackard *et al* (1971). Later, randomized studies added little to this description of the palliation achievable by endocrine management. A complete summary of the VACURG studies has recently been published by Byar and Corle (1988). Many problems still remain (Schröder, 1990).

Endocrine management of prostate cancer is associated with significant side effects. Up to very recently, these consisted of minimally the side effects of castration such as loss of potency and libido. Treatment with oestrogenic hormones, which utilize pituitary testicular feedback mechanisms to suppress plasma testosterone, is, especially in the case of DES, associated with cardiovascular thromboembolic side effects, which have significantly increased the death rate from such diseases in the VACURG studies. A detailed account is given by Byar and Corle (1988). The side effects of DES have also been confirmed by other studies, especially those of the European Organization for Research on Treatment of Cancer (EORTC), as reported by de Voogt *et al* (1986).

Because of the weak evidence that endocrine treatment prolongs survival and because of the evident side effects, endocrine treatment has in general been limited to patients with metastatic disease, usually associated with symptoms.

In spite of an increasing number of prospective randomized studies in the field of endocrine management of prostate cancer, very few studies have described significant differences in overall survival. Significantly poorer results were seen for medroxyprogesterone acetate than with DES and cyproterone acetate in EORTC Genitourinary Group protocol 30761, as reported by Pavone-Macaluso *et al* (1986). In protocol 0036 of the National Cancer Institute Southwest Oncology Group, reported by Crawford *et al* (1989), overall survival was significantly better when total androgen suppression was achieved with flutamide and the luteinizing hormone releasing hormone (LHRH) agonist leuprolide than with leuprolide alone. Controversy about whether daily injections of leuprolide represent a standard treatment persists. Comparison of total androgen suppression applied as flutamide plus castration versus castration alone did not confirm these differences in the meta-analysis of two large European studies reported by Iversen *et al* (1990a,b). In spite of descriptions of long term survival under endocrine treatment, reports of apparent cure of prostate cancer by endocrine management based on necropsy findings are rare in the urological literature. Johansson and Ljunggren (1981) reported on two patients, of whom one had no evidence of disease within his prostate and the other showed reduction of the primary tumour to minimal focal disease. In spite of the fact that, due to the age group involved, many patients with prostate cancer will die of unrelated, concomitant disease, virtually all those under endocrine management will eventually have a relapse of prostate cancer. This relapse is due to tumour progression that can no longer be influenced by means of endocrine manipulations. In spite of extensive research, the mechanisms of autonomous progression are still ill understood. The key to improvement of the prognosis of prostate cancer that is not amenable to local curative measures lies either in the prevention of transition to the autonomous state or in the combination of effective treatment of the endocrine independent tumour cell populations in addition to effective endocrine management. Unfortunately, reported improvements resulting from non-endocrine treatment in patients with hormone insensitive prostate cancer were marginal and do not warrant hope for a major short term improvement of the prognosis of this disease.

Methods of endocrine treatment will be discussed later in this chapter. Although their effectiveness has not improved in terms of prolongation of survival, the higher selectivity of anti-androgens and of 5α-reductase inhibitors seems to be combined with a significant reduction of side effects. This may in the future allow the very early application or maybe even the preventive application of such treatment principles. This will undoubtedly be an area of future clinical research.

The purpose of this chapter is to outline the achievements of endocrine therapy, including the recent developments around treatment methods. This will be followed by a summary of possible future developments, which for a large part are still limited to laboratory investigations.

METHODS OF TREATMENT

All types of endocrine management of prostate cancer make use of mechanisms that are related either to hypothalamic, pituitary, testicular feedback mechanisms or to the capability of anti-androgens to counteract the effect of androgens at target cells. Very recently, a new group of drugs with as yet unknown potential in the field of prostate cancer has been added, the 5α-reductase inhibitors. The hormonal interconnections between endocrine organs and the prostate as a target are depicted in Fig. 1; 90% of the circulating androgenic activity comes from the testes and 10% from the adrenal gland. Oesterling and coworkers (1986) have convincingly shown that adrenal androgens alone are not capable of supporting growth and function of the normal human prostate.

Castration

Castration can probably be considered standard treatment of prostate cancer at this time. In their original report, Huggins and Hodges (1941) showed that 15 (71%) of 21 patients with metastatic prostate cancer had at least subjective improvement in pain. They also showed that those patients who had an ele-

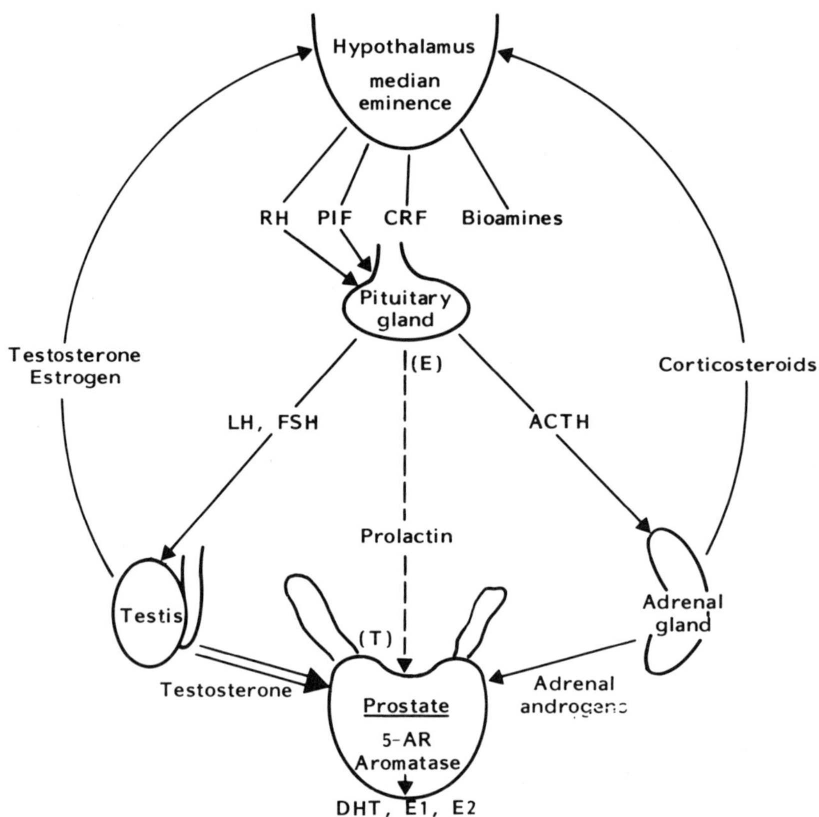

Fig. 1. Endocrine factors regulating prostatic growth and function. (RH) Releasing hormones; (PIF) pituitary factor for prolactin; (E) oestrogen; (LH) luteinizing hormone; (FSH) follicle stimulating hormone; (ACTH) corticotraphin; (T) testosterone; (DHT) 5-α-dihydrotestosterone; (5-AR) 5-α-reductase; (CRF) corticotrophic releasing factor

vated serum acid phosphatase showed a decrease of enzyme activity after castration. Castration reduces circulating testosterone levels from 20 fmol/l to 2 fmol/l. This reduction occurs within 24 hours and is followed in virtually all patients by a reduction of prostatic size and also of the palpable prostatic tumour mass within 3 months (Carpentier *et al*, 1986). Median times to progression of metastatic prostatic cancer patients after castration are 12 to 18 months and median survival 24 to 30 months. This has been shown by many different prospective studies and was recently confirmed by the data resulting from EORTC protocol 30853, which compared complete androgen blockade with castration, as reported by Denis *et al* (1990). Castration obviously has the disadvantages of some psychological impact and the necessity to undergo an operation, which, however, is small and can be carried out under local anaesthesia. Castration has the advantage of not being associated with any adverse effects except for loss of libido and potency. The treatment is definitive, and plasma testosterone remains low once castration levels are reached (Robinson and Thomas, 1971).

Adrenalectomy

It has long been speculated that removal of the adrenal androgenic stimulus may enhance the palliation seen with castration alone. Adrenalectomy can obviously be achieved by removal of both adrenal glands, an operation that is associated with significant side effects and requires substitution treatment with glucocorticoids and mineralocorticoids at least. Adrenal androgen production can also be excluded medically with the use of glucocorticoids, aminoglutethimide and spironolactone or by suppression of corticotrophin production. In the past, surgical and medical adrenalectomy was widely used as a second line endocrine treatment. With the use of various types of response criteria, an average of 44% of objective responses with a mean duration of 2.5 months was seen in 116 patients reported by various authors. These data were recently summarized by Schröder and Roehrborn (in press). Results of medical adrenalectomy are similar. However, considering the less involving nature of this treatment as well as the non-tumour related favourable effects of glucocorticoids on general well-being, this treatment still has a place in the management of prostate cancer showing progression after primary endocrine treatment. In a study by Tannock *et al* (1989), 38% of 37 patients with endocrine independent, progressive prostate cancer showed a subjective response, which could be maintained for 3 to 30 months.

Interference with Pituitary Feedback Mechanisms

Hypophysectomy will obviously lead to the elimination of luteinizing hormone (LH) and corticotrophin (ACTH), the hormones that stimulate testicular and adrenal androgen production. Luteinizing hormone releasing hormone secretion is dependent on a negative feedback with androgens and oestrogenic hormones. As with corticotrophin, which can be suppressed with hydrocortisone, the commonest and oldest way of suppressing LHRH is with exogenous oestrogens. More recently, after the description of the structure and the synthesis of LHRH agonists and antagonists by Schally *et al* (1971), it has become possible to suppress LH production more selectively with virtually no oestrogenic side effects. There is some evidence (Grayhack *et al*, 1955) of a synergism between testosterone and prolactin in their stimulation of the growth and function of the rat ventral prostate. This mechanism has been exploited for the treatment of prostate cancer by the use of prolactin inhibitors. The treatment, however, has not reached clinical importance.

Oestrogens were first used successfully in the treatment of prostate cancer by Herbst (1942). Oestrogens were probably the most widely used endocrine treatment of prostate cancer until their cardiovascular side effects were described in the VACURG studies. Besides LH suppression, oestrogens exert a number of effects in the human. They lead to an increase of the production of sex hormone binding globulin (SHBG) and thereby decrease the amount of free testosterone available for stimulating target cells. Oestrogens also lead to an increase of prolactin production through interference with the prolactin inhibiting factor (PIF). They cause gynaecomastia in men. Oestrogens at high dose may have a direct effect at prostate cancer cells and they have been described to interfere with the receptor binding of 5α-dihydrotestosterone and testosterone.

Most commonly used are synthetic oestrogen preparations such as the stilbenes and oestradiolesters. Diethylstilboestrol reliably suppresses plasma testosterone to castration levels at a dose of 3 mg and probably also of 2 mg, and 1 mg has been reported to exert an incomplete effect by Shearer *et al* (1973) and by Beck *et al* (1978). A dose of 1 mg of DES is associated with significantly fewer cardiovascular side effects than higher dosages. Although it does not lower plasma testosterone to castration levels, this dose has been shown to be as effective as castration and even as effective as total androgen suppression castration with cyproterone acetate (Robinson and Hetherington 1986).

The most extensive exploration of the effect of oestrogens has been done by VACURG. Results have recently been summarized by Byar and Corle (1988). The main conclusions from these studies, involving more than 4000 patients, are that 5 mg of DES is associated with significant cardiovascular side effects and cardiovascular death rates, these side effects are less common with 1 mg DES, orchidectomy plus DES is no better than DES alone and the delay in progression and cancer death seems to be similar whether 1 mg or 5 mg DES is given. Older patients are more likely to suffer serious cardiovascular side effects. Delaying endocrine treatment until symptomatic metastases occur did not lead to a reduction of overall survival. In the VACURG studies, DES was more effective than orchidectomy in preventing cancer death. However, this finding was not confirmed by others, especially not by the EORTC Genitourinary Group protocol 30805, as reported by Robertson and Hetherington (1986).

Other substances that have been used to decrease LH and testosterone production are chlorotrianisene (TACE), a stilbene derivate, diethylstilboestroldiphosphate (stilphostrol), polyestradiolphosphate and the gestagens megestrol acetate (MGA) and medroxyprogesterone acetate (MPA). These substances and their effect in clinical studies will not be reviewed in detail. They are not considered standard treatment of prostate cancer at present. Estramustine phosphate is a molecule that combines oestradiol with nitrogen mustard. It is claimed that this substance has oestrogenic as well as cytostatic properties. In primary treatment, it was shown not to be superior to standard endocrine regimens by Andersson (1988) and by Smith *et al* (1986). Since estramustine phosphate is most commonly used as a cytostatic agent in the treatment of hormone independent prostate cancer, it will not be further reviewed in this context.

Palliative effectiveness in terms of pain relief and improvement of performance status, serum markers and micturition complaints are identical if castration and effective forms of LH suppression are compared. Response rates, if objective criteria are used and if stability is not considered, amount to

30% to 40%, as was clearly shown by the EORTC Genitourinary Group. Roughly 40% show stabilization of their disease process. Also, progression and survival rates are similar within groups of metastatic prostatic cancer patients randomized between castration and oestrogen treatment.

A similar response is seen with the use of LHRH agonists. Paradoxically, after an initial rise due to stimulation of the Leydig cells, plasma testosterone can be reliably brought down to castration levels, especially with slow release depot formulations of LHRH agonists. The initial rise of plasma testosterone, which occurs during the first week of LHRH treatment, is associated with objective and subjective signs of a syndrome that has been called "flare phenomenon". Evidence from the literature has recently been reviewed by Boccon-Gibod (1990). Anti-androgens can counteract the increase of pain, rise in plasma testosterone and other signs of exacerbation of prostate cancer that are usually seen in patients with a heavy tumour load. The same author has also reviewed the effect of anti-androgens in this situation and recommended a treatment scheme.

Several randomized prospective studies have compared LHRH therapy alone with other standard forms of treatment. No differences in time to progression and survival were found by the leuprolide study group in comparison with 3 mg DES or by Parmar and coworkers (1985) in comparison with castration. The same was also confirmed by Peeling (1989), who used a depot preparation of goserelin in comparison to DES.

Anti-androgens

Anti-androgens are substances that counteract hormones at their target cells. One side effect is the simultaneous inhibition of the hypothalamic feedback mechanism, which results in a subsequent increase of LH and testosterone production. So called "pure anti-androgens" of the flutamide (FL) type are associated with a rise of plasma testosterone and LH that may need to be counteracted by other means. Steroidal anti-androgens of the cyproterone acetate type partially counteract the rise of LH because of their gestagenic properties. The effects of cyproterone acetate and of flutamide in monotherapy have been reviewed by Schröder (1990). In brief, cyproterone acetate has been shown in prospective randomized studies to be as effective as 3 mg DES and, indirectly, as castration. Cyproterone acetate is therefore considered standard endocrine treatment. Cardiovascular side effects are significantly less common with cyproterone acetate than with DES or MPA. Gynaecomastia, breast tenderness and leg oedema are rarely seen with cyproterone acetate. These data refer to EORTC protocol 30761, which compares 3 mg DES with 250 mg cyproterone acetate, and to a regimen of low dose MPA, as reported by Pavone-Macaluso *et al* (1986). Patients treated with cyproterone acetate usually become impotent. Flutamide as monotherapy is not recognized as standard treatment and has been shown in a valid prospective randomized study to be equivalent to castration or other forms of standard management of prostate cancer. The rise of plasma testosterone, described by Knuth *et al* (1984) among others, and the fact that most patients remain potent (which could be a sign of persistent androgenic stimulation) have discouraged many clinicians from using flutamide or other pure anti-androgens as monotherapy. Sogani *et al* (1984) has clearly shown short term effectiveness in a phase II study that was limited to an observation period of 1 year. Side effects of flutamide are gynaecomastia, diarrhoea and other intestinal disturbances. The short half life of the drug necessitates treatment three times a day.

Non-steroidal anti-androgens are most commonly used in combination with castration or LHRH agonists to achieve what is called "total androgen blockade".

Total Androgen Blockade

The term "total androgen blockade" indicates the simultaneous exclusion or blockade of testicular and adrenal androgens as initial forms of endocrine management of prostate cancer. This approach was propagated in the medical literature by Labrie *et al* (1983) and also in the lay press. Labrie and his associates used the combination of an LHRH analogue with a pure anti-androgen. The treatment was designed to exclude testicular androgen production and to counteract with the anti-androgen the remaining circulating androgens at the target cell level. In a series of 29 patients with very short follow up and very limited response parameters available, an objective response rate of 96% was reported. Before the first publication from Labrie's group, total androgen suppression was used by the EORTC Genitourinary Group in a prospective randomized study conducted from 1980 to 1985. In this study, castration was compared with castration plus cyproterone acetate and with 1 mg DES per day as a third arm. Preliminary results were reported by Robinson and Hetherington (1986). The final analysis of this study has confirmed that neither progression nor survival rates show any significant difference. In 1983, the combination of a treatment strategy, eliminating testicular androgens in combination with a pure anti-androgen, had not been studied. This uncertainty and the widespread publicity given to the data emerging from Labrie's group contributed to a major research effort into both basic scientific and clinical approaches in subsequent years. Labrie *et al* (1988) and Schröder and van Steenbrugge (1988) summarized the arguments for and against total androgen suppression. The hope that the initial very favourable impression might be confirmed was based mainly on the assumption that cancer cells might be hypersensitive to the androgenic stimulus and that primary exclusion of adrenal androgen might lead to prolonged survival and a reduction in cancer deaths in time. As mentioned above, adrenal androgens amount to about 10% of the normally circulating androgens. However, these lower plasma concentrations are capable of maintaining a higher level of dihydrotestosterone within prostatic tissues (Geller *et al*, 1984; Belanger *et al*, 1989). However, classical animal models such as the ventral prostate of the rat and the transplantable human cancer line PC-82 cannot be stimulated by very low amounts of androgens. There seems to be a threshold for stimulation, which is higher than castration tissue levels. These data are summarized by Kyprianou and Isaacs (1987), van Weerden *et al* (1991a) and van Weerden *et al* (1991b). It should soon be possible to argue on clinical grounds rather than on the basis of speculations arising from experimental observations. Large clinical studies will undergo their final analysis soon.

During the past year, a large volume of clinical data has emerged from studies utilizing regimens of total androgen blockade. The information comes from two types of trials—those that use LHRH in the control arm and those that use castration in the control arm. Luteinizing hormone releasing hormone control studies on which information on the outcome is available have recruited 2465 patients and castration control studies have recruited 2049 patients. The anti-androgens used in these studies are flutamide, nilutamide and cyproterone acetate. In many of the clinical studies, follow up is not yet long enough for final analysis, and the median times to progression and survival have not been reached. So far, within the group of LHRH controlled studies, only protocol 0036 of the NCI Southwest Oncology Group/National Prostatic Cancer Project has shown significant differences in progression and survival rates. This study was reported by Crawford *et al* (1989); 603 evaluable patients were randomized between leuprolide daily injections plus placebo (300 patients) and leuprolide daily injections plus flutamide (303 patients). Time to progression and overall survival showed significant differences (p = 0.039 and 0.035 in favour of the total androgen blockade regimen). Median time to progression was 13.9 months in the leuprolide plus placebo group and 16.5 months in the total androgen blockade group. Similarly, median survival showed a difference of 7.3 months between the treatment groups (28.3 months in the leuprolide only and 35.6 months in the combination treatment group). This important study gives strong arguments for the use of total androgen suppression regimens in routine treatment of prostate cancer patients. However, a number of important questions remain. Does the 7 months difference in median survival justify the routine use of a very expensive treatment? Are there groups of patients who might benefit more or less from this regimen? Why have other studies up to now not confirmed the results of this protocol? Can the LHRH agonist leuprolide applied in daily injections really be considered standard treatment? The study of the Leuprolide Study Group, which compared leuprolide applied according to the same scheme with 3 mg DES daily, showed no significant differences (Leuprolide Study Group, 1984). However, in this trial, unequal numbers of patients suffered early progression. This might have been due to flare in the LHRH only group. Flare may lead to early progression and perhaps even to early death in patients with a critical tumour load, as reported by Boccon-Gibod (1990) and Schröder *et al* (1987).

Arguments are unlikely to solve the remaining questions. Fortunately, a large volume of clinical information has become available from studies of total

TABLE 1. Prospective randomized studies comparing castration with total androgen blockade in previously untreated patients with M0-M1 prostate cancer

Author	Design	No. of patients	Preliminary results
Robinson and Hetherington (1986) EORTC 30805	castration v. + CPA v. DES 1 mg	112 115 108	mature study, no difference in time progression and survival
Janknegt *et al* (1990)	castration + placebo v. castration nilutamide	232 225	follow up 26 months time to progression p = 0.034, survival NS
Kueppens *et al* (1990) EORTC 30853	castration v. gosereline + FL	163 164	follow up 18 months, time to progression p = 0.01, survival NS
Iversen *et al* (1990) (DAPROCA)	castration v. gosereline + FL	133 129	follow up 30 months, time to progression and survival NS
de Voogt *et al* (1990) EORTC 30843	castration v. busereline v. busereline + CPA		follow up too short, time to progression and survival NS
Namer M (personal (communication)	castration + placebo v. castration + nilutamide	125	mature, time to progression and survival NS
Béland *et al* (in press)	castration + placebo v. castration + nilutamide	96 98	mature, time to progression NS, survival p = 0.048[a]
Total		2049	

CPA = cyproterone acetate; DES = diethylstilboeshol; FL = flutamide; NS = not significant
[a]No significant differences found in more recent analysis

androgen blockade utilizing castration as a control arm. These are summarized in Table 1, which reports on a total of 2049 patients. Significant differences concerning either time to progression or survival are reported in three studies. In the study by Janknegt *et al* (1990), time to progression in the total androgen blockade arm is significantly longer (p = 0.034). This is also reflected in a delay of the time to cancer death. Overall survival shows no significant difference. EORTC protocol 30853 reported by Keuppens *et al* (1990) has also revealed a difference in time to progression. The average follow up in this study is 18 months and is still too short for final analysis. This study, because of the identical protocol, was analysed in a meta-analysis together with the DAPROCA study (Iversen, 1990). In this meta-analysis, which included 589 patients, the significant difference in time to progression persisted, but there was no difference in survival. A Canadian study reported by Béland *et al* (in press) is a mature study that does not show a difference in time to progression. A difference in survival is reported (p = 0.048). Median survival time was 18 months for castration plus nilutamide, compared with 24 months for castration alone. Unfortunately, in a later analysis of this study reported by Trachtenberg at the European Urological Association congress in Amsterdam (1990), the significance of this difference in survival had disappeared. A trend, however, remained.

WHERE DO WE STAND?

What, then, can be considered standard endocrine treatment of prostate cancer in 1991? The answer still does not seem to be entirely clear. However, unless clear-cut advantages are shown for a new regimen, especially for total androgen suppression, new treatments should not be considered standard treatment, especially if they are much more expensive than previous routines. Clear-cut advantages of any regimen over castration or other methods that counteract testicular testosterone production have not been shown to satisfaction. However, the possibility that there is some use for total androgen blockade cannot be excluded. In the study by Crawford *et al* (1989), patients with favourable prognostic factors had significantly more benefit than those with unfavourable prognostic factors. However, the groups of patients were too small for subgroup analysis to be valid. Studies by Brisset *et al* (1987), Schröder *et al* (1987) and other authors have shown that the rate of first responses was higher in groups of patients treated with total androgen blockade. This may be a valid observation, which may indicate that patients with a very heavy tumour load and metastases in critical locations may benefit from an initial, very rapid and complete withdrawal of androgens. There is no doubt that with increasing maturity of the existing trials subgroup, analyses will be possible and the indications for total androgen blockade will be clearly defined.

Castration, in spite of being less effective in preventing cancer death in the VACURG studies, has subsequently been shown in several studies to be equivalent to other forms of standard treatment. Castration is efficient, producing a fall in plasma testosterone levels to castration levels within 24 hours, it is definite, it can be carried out with more favourable cosmetic results as intracapsular orchidectomy and it lacks the side effects of some of the other compounds. Probably, at this time, castration comes closest to what may be called standard treatment of prostate cancer.

In situations where castration for whatever reason is not desirable, the anti-androgen cyproterone acetate is probably a next choice. Because of its gestagenic effects, it partially excludes the rise of plasma testosterone that results from the blockade of the diencephalic feedback mechanism of testosterone. The role of pure anti-androgens as monotherapy needs to be determined further. Long term observations are lacking, and side effects are significant, but the prospect of preserving potency and still counteracting prostate cancer is very attractive.

Long acting depot LHRH preparations provide a new, viable but expensive alternative for situations where castration is not desired. Oestrogen, if used at all, should be applied with great caution, considering all the lessons the VACURG studies have taught. Oestrogens should not be used in patients with a previous history of cardiovascular disease or in older, frail patients. If DES is used, probably a dose of 1 mg or 2 mg per day should be applied. It must, however, be seriously doubted whether DES still has a place in the treatment of prostate cancer. The only valid argument for its use may lie in the fact that it is very cheap.

WHERE ARE WE GOING?

Considering the strong efforts that have been made to show the superiority of total androgen blockade, it is very unlikely that much progress can be made by considering further a very radical withdrawal of androgens. It seems that endocrine independent tumour growth is and remains the limiting factor of endocrine management of whatever type. Loss of endocrine dependence, on a cell kinetic basis, is very well explained by clonal selection and clonal overgrowth. These mechanisms, however, do not explain the origin of endocrine independent cells. Whatever causes genetic instability and chromosomal alteration probably also causes endocrine independence. However, there are a number of observations that may contribute more directly and more concretely to our understanding of endocrine independence.

It was thought for some time that endocrine independence would be associated with the loss of the nuclear androgen receptor. Recently, with the availability of antibodies against various parts of the androgen receptor (AR), molecule localization studies have become possible. Preliminary results coming from several groups, including a publication by Ruizeveld de Winter (1990), show that androgen receptor is present in the nuclei of hormone dependent as well as hormone independent prostate cancer cells. Prostatic cancer nuclei not containing AR seemed to be an exception. Obviously, the possibility that alterations of the androgen receptor molecule not involving its immunologically active part may explain the loss of androgenic response of these cells. This finding will have to be followed up with molecular biological techniques.

Kyprianou and Isaacs (1988, 1989 and this issue) have clearly shown that the apoptotic cell death occurring in hormone dependent cell populations of the ventral rat prostate is an active process which is associated with a cascade of events that are normally repressed by androgen. These events include the expression of the transforming growth factor-β (TGF-β) gene, the c-*myc* proto-oncogene, the c-*fos* proto-oncogene, the 70 000 molecular weight heat shock gene, the *TRPM-2* gene and the glutathione S-transferase *Xb1* gene. The same authors have shown, by using the transplantable human prostate carcinoma line PC-82 in nude mice, that identical mechanisms are involved in cell death occurring in human prostate cancer (Kyprianou *et al*, 1990). They have also shown that the same mechanism still exists in androgen independent prostate cancer cells. In this situation, there seems to be a cellular defect present that causes failure of the programmed cell death pathway to be activated by androgen removal. Obviously, these mechanisms offer a new possibility for a better understanding of the transition to androgen independence. Research will concentrate on the possibility of triggering the programmed cell death mechanisms even where androgen independence has occurred.

Further progress could be made by better utilization of the available therapies. The question of whether pure anti-androgens, which allow the persistence of potency in most patients, are compatible with standard treatment of prostate cancer needs to be explored. Lund and Rasmussen (1988) have compared 3 mg of DES with 750 mg of flutamide in 40 previously untreated patients with metastatic prostate cancer. Their study included the evaluation of plasma testosterone over a period of 1 year. The predicted rise of plasma testosterone occurs but reaches a maximum after 6 months. After 1 year, plasma testosterone values fall to the normal range. The mechanisms of preservation of potency and the reason for gynaecomastia, which occurs frequently with this treatment, are unknown. It is likely that comparative studies, such as the one undertaken by the EORTC Genitourinary Group at this time and long term studies of prostatic volume in conjunction with proliferation markers, will produce the answer to the question of the usefulness of pure anti-androgens as monotherapy.

A new approach to the treatment of prostatic disease has emerged with the development of 5α-reductase inhibitors. 5α-Dihydrotestosterone (DHT) is synthesized by this enzyme from its main precursor, testosterone; it has the highest affinity to the androgen receptor and is the most powerful androgen in men. It is probably for these reasons that DHT is the main androgen in stimulating growth and function of the prostate. It is known from observations by Imperato-McGinley *et al* (1974) in men with inherited 5α-reductase deficiency that these males with ambiguous genitalia have a normal male libido. Libido and potency seem to be maintained by normal testosterone levels. This discrepant action of testosterone and DHT opens the possibility of utilizing 5α-reductase inhibitors in the treatment of benign prostatic hyperplasia as well as prostate cancer, provided their effectiveness can be shown. Brooks *et al* (1982, 1986) have studied a series of newly synthesized 5α-reductase inhibitors and described their effects on the rat and canine prostate. Eventually, the compound MK-906 was singled out as the most potent and most suitable drug for further exploration in human use. The effect of MK-906 on serum androgens and androgen conjugates in normal men was subsequently reported by Rittmaster *et al* (1989). MK-906 and other 5α-reductase inhibitors are now under experimental and clinical investigation. The potential of these substances lies in their very specific mechanism of action, the lack of side effects in preliminary studies and the possibility of maintaining libido and potency with the potential of arresting the growth of prostatic cancer. Clinical studies, which are on their way, will have to show whether 5α-reductase inhibitors have a role in treating prostate cancer.

It is unknown at present at what stage of the morphogenesis of prostate cancer the transition from hormone dependence to hormone independence occurs. There is a distinct impression that small cancers are more endocrine dependent than very large tumour masses. Also, the primary tumour seems to react longer and more frequently to androgen withdrawal. On the other hand, the VACURG studies have shown that considering locally advanced but not metastasized prostate cancer together with metastatic disease, early and delayed endocrine treatments do not differ in their effect on overall survival. From a clinical view, it is mainly because of the pronounced side effects of endocrine management, especially the loss of potency, that early endocrine treatment is not frequently applied. Whether early endocrine treatment of locally confined prostate cancer or of very limited metastatic disease has advantages over delayed endocrine treatment is at present unknown. Clinical studies of patients with limited lymph node metastases (reviewed in van Aubel *et al*, 1985) but otherwise locally confined disease, comparing early and delayed endocrine treatment in a historic fashion, have shown clearly that time to progression is prolonged about two to three times by early castration. A treatment that maintains potency and libido and at the same time controls growth of endocrine dependent prostate cancer would undoubtedly be used early on in the disease process, perhaps even for prevention. Considerable progress may be expected from such an approach. An obvious patient group to be treated are those in whom focal disease is identified at the time of surgery for benign disease. These studies would also show whether early endocrine manipulations can prevent the transition to endocrine independence of prostate cancer.

SUMMARY

Endocrine management is the best palliative management available for patients with carcinoma of the prostate. It is based on androgen withdrawal by castration or other means. Endocrine management was introduced into clinical medicine by Huggins and his associates in the early 1940s on the basis of careful clinical and experimental research establishing the biological effects of androgen withdrawal in animal systems and in humans.

It was believed for a long time that endocrine treatment would prolong life. This, however, in spite of extensive clinical research, remains unproven. The possibility that the life span of prostate cancer patients is determined by the hormone independent cell populations within virtually all prostate cancers still remains a possibility. Endocrine treatment has, however, been shown to have a significant impact on symptoms related to prostate cancer, especially on bone pain, urethral and ureteral obstruction. It has also been shown to prolong time to progression and to death from prostate cancer.

Although castration and the application of exogenous oestrogens with the purpose of interfering with pituitary testicular feedback have been standard treatment of prostate cancer for more than 30 years, new treatment methods have recently become available. Luteinizing hormone releasing hormone agonists allow suppression of plasma testosterone to castration levels without exerting the side effects associated with oestrogens (eg cardiovascular incidents, gynaecomastia). Also, the application of pure or steroidal anti-androgens allows direct counteraction of circulating androgens at the target cell. The possibility that initial suppression of adrenal androgen production, which contributes about 10% of circulating androgens in males, may be more beneficial than suppression of testicular androgens alone has been subject to intense clinical research recently. Simultaneous suppression of testicular and adrenal androgens in primary management of prostate cancer is called total androgen blockade or total androgen suppression. Up to now, however, no convincing advantages of total androgen suppression regimens above castration have been shown. Total androgen suppression seems to produce significantly better survival when compared with daily injections of LHRH alone.

The use of pure anti-androgens or of 5α-reductase inhibitors could potentially prevent the most significant side effect of all androgen withdrawal regimens, loss of libido and impotence. However, neither the use of pure anti-androgens as monotherapy nor the use of 5α-reductase inhibitors as monotherapy has been shown to produce clinical results that are equal to castration.

Where do we stand? At this moment, castration probably must still be considered standard treatment of prostate cancer. However, there are a number of important questions in this field that await answers through clinical and experimental research. Are there subgroups of patients who may profit from total androgen suppression? Is pure anti-androgen therapy equivalent to standard treatment? Is endocrine treatment associated with an increased overall survival? Is pure anti-androgen monotherapy or treatment with 5α-reductase inhibitors equivalent to castration? Is early or delayed endocrine treatment more beneficial? Can prognostic groups be identified that are better treated by other means? Can the processes that regulate cell death in the prostate be utilized in the treatment of prostate cancer? Can the loss of endocrine dependence in prostate cancer in some way be manipulated?

With the answers to at least some of these questions, major progress in the field of prostate cancer can still be made.

References

Andersson L (1988) Estrogens and Estramustine phosphate, In: Denis L (ed). *The Medical Management of Prostate Cancer*, pp 37–42, Springer-Verlag, Heidelberg
Beck PH, McAnich JW, Goebel JL and Stutman RE (1978) Plasma testosterone in patients

receiving DES. *Urology* **11** 157–160

Béland G, Elhilali M, Fradet Y *et al* A controlled trial of castration with and without nilutamide in metastatic prostatic carcinoma. *Cancer* **66** (in press)

Belanger B, Belanger A, Labrie F, Dupont A, Cusan L and Monfette G (1989) Comparison of residual C-19 steroids in plasma and prostatic tissue of human, rat and guinea pig after castration: unique importance of extratesticular androgens in men. *Journal of Steroid Biochemistry* **32** 695–698

Blackard CE, Mellinger GT and Gleason DF (1971) Treatment of stage 1 carcinoma of the prostate a preliminary report. *Journal of Urology* **106** 729–733

Boccon-Gibod L (1990) The prevention of LHRH induced disease flares in patients with metastatic carcinoma of the prostate, In: Schröder FH (ed). *EORTC Genitourinary Group Monograph 8: Treatment Prostatic Cancer Facts and Controversies*, pp 125–129, Wiley-Liss, New York

Brisset JM, Boccon-Gibod L and Botto H *et al* (1987) Anandron (RU 23908) associated to surgical castration in previously untreated stage D prostate cancer a multicenter comparative study of two doses of the drug and of a placebo, In: Khoury S, Murphy GP (eds). *Prostate Cancer*, pp 411–422, Alan Liss, New York

Brooks JR, Berman D, Glitzer MS *et al* (1982) Effect of a new 5α-reductase inhibitor on size, histologic characteristics, and androgen concentrations of the canine prostate. *Prostate* **3** 35–44

Brooks JR, Berman C, Primka RL, Reynolds GF and Rasmusson GH (1986) 5α-reductase inhibitory and antiandrogenetic activities of some 4-azasteroids in the rat. *Steroids* **47/1** 1–19

Byar DP and Corle DK (1988) Hormone therapy for prostate cancer results of the Veterans Administration Cooperative Urological Research Group Studies. *NCI Monograph* **7** 165–170

Carpentier PJ, Schröder FH and Schmitz PIM (1986) Transrectal ultrasonometry of the prostate the prognostic relevance of volume changes under endocrine management. *World Journal of Urology* **4** 159–162

Crawford ED, Eisenberger MA, McLeod DG *et al* (1989) A controlled trial of leuprolide with and without flutamide in prostatic carcinoma. *New England Journal of Medicine* **321** 419–424

Denis L, Keuppens F, Robinson M *et al* (1990) Complete androgen blockade data from an EORTC 30853 trial *Seminars in Urology* Vol VIII, No 3 (August) 166–174

Geller J, de la Vega DJ, Albert JD and Nachtsheim DA (1984) Tissue dihydrotestosterone levels and clinical response to hormonal therapy in patients with advanced prostate cancer. *Journal of Clinical Endocrinology & Metabolism* **58** 36–40

Grayhack JT, Bunce PL, Kearns JW and Scott WW (1955) Influence of the pituitary on prostatic response to androgen in the rat. *Bulletin of the Johns Hopkins Hospital* **96** 154–163

Herbst WP (1942) Biochemical therapeusis in carcinoma of the prostate gland. *Journal of the American Medical Association* **120** 1116–1122

Huggins C and Stevens RA (1940) The effect of castration on benign hypertrophy of the prostate in man. *Journal of Urology* **43** 705–714

Huggins C and Hodges CV (1941) Studies on prostate cancer I The effect of estrogen and of androgen injection on serum phosphatases in metastatic carcinoma of the prostate. *Cancer Research* **1** 293–297

Huggins C, Stevens RE and Hodges CV (1941) Studies in prostatic cancer II: The effects of castration on advanced carcinoma of the prostate gland. *Archives of Surgery* **43** 209

Imperato-McGinley J, Guerrero L, Gautier T and Peterson RE (1974) 5α-reductase deficiency in man: an inherited form of male pseudohermaphroditism. *Science* **186** 1213–1215

Iversen P (1990) Is there a case for total androgen blockade? In: Schröder FH (ed). *EORTC Genitourinary Group Monograph 8: Treatment Prostatic Cancer, Facts and Controversies*, pp 109–111, Wiley-Liss, New York

Iversen P, Suciu S, Sylvester R, Christensen I and Denis L (1990a) Zoladex and flutamide versus orchiectomy in the treatment of advanced prostatic cancer: a combined analysis of two European studies-EORTC 30853 and DAPROCA 86 *Cancer* **66** 61–67

Iversen P, Christen MG, Friis E *et al* (1990b) A phase III trial of zoladex and flutamide versus orchiectomy in the treatment of patients with advanced carcinoma of the prostate. *Cancer* **66** 52–60

Janknegt RA and the International Anandron Study Group (1990) Results of a double-blind study comparing orchiectomy and anandron to orchiectomy and placebo in metastatic prostate cancer. *European Urology* **18** (**Supplement 1**) [Abstract 191]

Johansson S and Ljunggren X (1981) Prostatic carcinoma cured with hormonal treatment. *Scandinavian Journal of Urology and Nephrology* **15** 331–332

Keuppens F, Denis L, Smith PH *et al* (1990) Zoladex R and flutamide versus bilateral orchiectomy a randomized phase III EORTC 30853 study. *Cancer* **66** 39–51

Knuth UA, Hano R and Nieschlag E (1984) Effect of flutamide or cyproterone acetate on pituitary and testicular hormones in normal men. *Journal of Clinical Endocrinology and Metabolism* **59** 963–969

Kyprianou N and Isaacs JT (1987) Biological significance of measurable androgen levels in the rat ventral prostate following castration. *Prostate* **10** 313–324

Kyprianou N and Isaacs JT (1988) Activation of programmed cell death in the rat ventral prostate after castration. *Endocrinology* **122** 552–562

Kyprianou N and Isaacs JT (1989) Thymine-less death in androgen-independent prostatic cancer cells. *Biochemical and Biophysical Research Communications* **165** 73–81

Kyprianou N, English HF and Isaacs JT (1990) Programmed cell death during regression of PC-82 human prostate cancer following androgen ablation. *Cancer Research* **50** 3748–3753

Labrie F, Dupont A, Belanger A *et al* (1983) New approaches in the treatment of prostate cancer complete instead of partial withdrawal of androgens. *Prostate* **4** 579–594

Labrie F, Belanger A, Veilleux R *et al* (1988) Rationale for maximal androgen withdrawal in the therapy of prostate cancer. *Bailliére's Clinical Oncology* **2** 597–619

Leuprolide Study Group (1984) Leuprolide versus diethylstilbestrol for metastatic prostate cancer. *New England Journal of Medicine* **311** 1281–1286

Lund F and Rasmussen F (1988) Flutamide versus stilbestrol in the management of advanced prostatic cancer. *British Journal of Urology* **61** 140–142

Oesterling JE, Epstein JI and Walsh PC (1986) The viability of adrenal androgens to stimulate the adult human prostate an autopsy, evaluation of men with gonadotropic hypogonadism and panhypopituitarism. *Journal of Urology* **136** 1030–1034

Parmar H, Lightman SL, Allen L, Philips RH, Edwards L and Schally AV (1985) Randomised controlled study of orchidectomy versus long-acting D-TRP-6-LHRH microcapsules in advanced prostatic carcinoma. *Lancet* **ii** 30

Pavone-Macaluso de Voogt HJ, Viggiano G, Barasolo E, Lardennois B, de Pauw M and Sylvester R (1986) Comparison of diethylstilbestrol, cyproterone acetate, medroxyprogesterone acetate in the treatment of advanced prostatic cancer final analysis of a randomized phase II trial of the European Organization for Research on Treatment of Cancer Urological Group. *Journal of Urology* **136** 624–631

Peeling WB (1989) Phase III studies to compare goserelin (zoladex) with orchiectomy and DES in treatment of prostatic carcinoma. *Urology* **33** 45–51

Rittmaster RS, Stoner E, Thompson DL, Nance D and Lasseter KC (1989) Effect of MK-906, a specific 5α-reductase inhibitor, on serum androgens and androgen conjugates in normal men *Journal of Andrology* **10** 259–262

Robinson MRG and Thomas BS (1971) Effect of hormonal therapy on plasma testosterone levels in prostatic carcinoma. *British Medical Journal* **4** 391–394

Robinson MRG and Hetherington J (1986) The EORTC studies Is there an optimal endocrine management for M1 prostatic cancer? *World of Urology* **4** 171–175

Ruizeveld de Winter JA, Trapman J, Brinkmann AO *et al* (1990) Heterogeneity of androgen receptor expression in human prostatic carcinomas visualized by immunohistochemistry. *Journal of Pathololology* **161** 329–332

Schally AV, Arimura A, Baba Y *et al* (1971) Isolation and properties of the FSH and LH-releasing hormone. *Biochemical and Biophysical Research Communications* **43** 393–399

Schröder FH (ed) (1990) *Treatment of Prostatic Cancer, Facts and Controversies: Progress in Clinical and Biological Research* 359 EORTC Genitourinary Group Monograph 8, Wiley-Liss, New York

Schröder FH and Steenbrugge GJ van (1988) Rationale against total androgen withdrawal. *Bailliére's Clinical Oncology* **2** 621–633

Schröder FH and Röhrborn CG Endocrine management of prostate cancer, In: Lytton B, Catalona W (eds). *Advances in Urology* 4 Mosby-Year Book Inc, Chicago (in press)

Schröder FH, Lock MTWT, Chadha DR *et al* (1987) Metastatic cancer of the prostate managed with Buserelin versus Buserelin plus cyproterone acetate. *Journal of Urology* **137** 912–918

Shearer RJ, Hendry WF and Sommerville IF *et al* (1973) Plasma testosterone an accurate monitor of hormone treatment in prostatic cancer. *British Journal of Urology* **45** 668–677

Smith PH, Suciu S, Robinson MRG *et al* (1986) A comparison of the effect of diethylstilbestrol with low dose estramustine phosphate in the treatment of advanced prostatic cancer final analysis of a phase III trial of the European Organization for Research on Treatment of Cancer. *Journal of Urology* **136** 619–623

Sogani PC, Minoo R, Vagaiwala R and Whitmore WS (1984) Experience with flutamide in patients with advanced prostatic cancer without prior endocrine therapy. *Cancer* **54** 744–750

Tannock I, Gospodarowic M, Meakin W, Panzarella T, Stewart L and Rider W (1989) Treatment of metastatic prostatic cancer with low-dose Prednisone evaluation of pain and quality of life as pragmatic indices of response. *Journal of Clinical Oncology* **7** 590–597

van Aubel OGJM, Hoekstra WJ and Schröder FH (1985) Early orchiectomy for patients with stage D1 prostatic carcinoma. *Journal of Urology* **134** 292–294

van Weerden W, van Kreuningen A, Moerings EPCM, de Jong FH, van Steenbrugge GJ and Schröder FH (1991a) The biological significance of low testosterone levels and of adrenal androgens in transplantable prostate cancer lines. *Urological Research* **19** 1–5

van Weerden W, van Steenbrugge GJ, van Kreuningen A, Moerings EPCM, de Jong FH and Schröder FH (1991b) Assessment of the critical level of androgen for growth response of transplantable human prostatic carcinoma (PC-82) in nude mice. *Journal of Urology* **145** 631–634

Veterans Administration Cooperative Urological Research Group (VACURG)(1976) Treatment and survival of patients with cancer of the prostate. *Surgery, Gynecology and Obstetrics* **124** 10–11

Voogt HJ de, Smith PH, Pavone-Macaluso M, Pauw M de, Suciu S and members of the EORTC GU Group (1986) Cardiovascular side effects of diethylstilbestrol, cyproterone acetate, medroxyprogesterone acetate and Estramustine phosphate used for the treatment of advanced prostatic cancer results from European organization for Research on Treatment of Cancer trials 30761 and 30762. *Journal of Urology* **135** 303–307

Voogt HJ de, Klijn JGM, Studer U, Schröder FH, Sylvester R, Pauw M de and members of the EORTC GU Group (1990) Orchidectomy versus buserelin in combination with cyproterone acetate, for 2 weeks or continuously, in the treatment of metastatic prostatic cancer: preliminary results of EORTC trial 30843. *Journal of Steroid Biochemistry and Molecular Biology* **37** 965–971

The author is responsible for the accuracy of the references.

Androgen Receptors and Growth Fraction in Metastatic Prostate Cancer as Predictors of Time to Tumour Progression after Hormonal Therapy

MARCUS V SADI • EVELYN R BARRACK

Department of Urology, The Johns Hopkins University School of Medicine, Baltimore, Maryland 21205

RATIONALE FOR ANDROGEN RECEPTOR STUDIES

Prostate cancer is the most frequently diagnosed cancer and the second leading cause of cancer deaths in men in the USA (100 000 new cases and 28 000 deaths per year) (Carter and Coffey, 1990). About 60% of newly diagnosed prostate cancer patients already have metastatic disease, for which standard treatment is suppression of androgenic stimuli, such as by castration (Scott *et al*, 1980). About 80% of these patients initially show a beneficial response to hormone therapy, but the extent and duration of response are variable and unpredictable, and their prostate cancer eventually relapses to an androgen independent state (Scott *et al*, 1980). This variability among tumours might be due to different proportions of androgen dependent cells, different growth rates, different tumour loads or the acquisition of factors that could override a requirement for androgen.

Cancer Surveys Volume 11: *Prostate Cancer*
© 1991 Imperial Cancer Research Fund. 0-87969-368-1/91. $3.00 + .00

One of our goals has been to define indices that will predict the androgen responsiveness and time to progression of prostate cancer (Diamond and Barrack, 1984; Barrack and Tindall, 1987; Barrack *et al*, 1987; Sadi and Barrack, 1991; Sadi *et al*, 1991a,b). Response probably results from the loss of androgen dependent prostate cancer cells after androgen withdrawal, and relapse probably results from the continued proliferation of androgen independent cells.

If prostate cancer were heterogeneous, containing both androgen dependent and androgen independent cells, then one would predict that the larger the percentage of androgen dependent cells in the tumour the greater the extent of involution after androgen withdrawal, and the longer it would take for the remaining androgen independent cells to repopulate the tumour to a size equal to or greater than that which existed before therapy. The theoretical basis for this concept has been elegantly described and illustrated by Coffey and Isaacs (1981). Because androgens act via androgen receptors, it was proposed that androgen receptors might be a marker of androgen dependent cells and that the androgen receptor (AR) content in prostate cancer might predict its responsiveness to androgen withdrawal (Trachtenberg and Walsh, 1982). The hypothesis evolved that the higher the AR level, the more androgen dependent and the more responsive the tumour to androgen withdrawal, and the longer the time to progression.

The ability of AR assays, based exclusively on radioligand binding, to predict the androgen responsiveness of advanced prostate cancer has been controversial (reviewed in Barrack and Tindall, 1987). Some studies have shown lower levels of nuclear AR associated with a shorter duration of response and vice versa (Trachtenberg and Walsh, 1982; Brendler *et al*, 1984; Fentie *et al*, 1986; Barrack *et al*, 1987; Benson *et al*, 1987), but others have found no correlation (van Aubel *et al*, 1988). In no study has the relation or methodology been accurate enough to predict the response of individual tumours. A major limitation of these previous studies was the use of homogenized tissue, which yields the average AR content of all cells in the homogenized specimen. Contamination of a biopsy specimen by non-malignant cells that are AR positive or AR negative would yield a misleadingly high or low level of "tumour" AR content, respectively. Therefore, differences in AR content between patients due to admixture with different proportions of non-malignant prostate tissue cannot be distinguished from differences in AR content that are due to different percentages of AR positive tumour cells and AR negative tumour cells. Perhaps this accounts for the imperfect relation between AR content and response to androgen ablation.

We therefore devised methods to localize AR at the light microscope level. Autoradiography and immunohistochemistry circumvent the difficulty of admixture of malignant and non-malignant cells by allowing selective evaluation of malignant cell AR status. By quantitative AR autoradiography and AR immunohistochemistry, we were able for the first time to test directly the hypothesis that AR content in the malignant cells themselves correlates with the time to progression after hormonal therapy.

QUANTITATIVE ANDROGEN RECEPTOR AUTORADIOGRAPHY

We developed a new method of ^{3}H-labelled steroid autoradiography that offers several advantages over other such methods and that is applicable to human tissues stored in liquid nitrogen (Peters and Barrack, 1987a,b,c; Barrack
et al, 1988). To localize AR, slide-mounted frozen tissue sections are incubated
with ^{3}H-labelled R1881 (to measure total androgen binding; excess unlabelled
triamcinolone acetonide is also present to block binding of ^{3}H-labelled R1881
to progesterone receptors) or with ^{3}H-labelled R1881 plus excess unlabelled
R1881 (to measure non-specific binding). After incubation, washing and
drying, the labelled slides are apposed to emulsion-coated coverslips (glued at
one end of the slide to ensure registry) and exposed in the dark at 4°C for
about 6 weeks; autoradiograms are then developed and sections are stained
with toluidine blue. Unfortunately, because ^{3}H-labelled steroid binds to non-
specific sites in addition to specific high affinity AR, visualization of an
autoradiogram of bound ^{3}H-labelled steroid does not directly reveal the location of receptors. Rather, analysis of specific nuclear AR location in these
autoradiograms depends on counting the number of grains over nuclei in sections that represent total binding versus in sections that represent non-specific
binding, and subtracting non-specific from total binding.

Because radioactive decay is random, grain densities have a Poisson distribution (Arnold, 1981). Therefore, even if all cells contain the same amount of
AR/nucleus, different nuclei have different numbers of grains; the frequency
distribution of the number of grains/nucleus has the properties of a Poisson
distribution. Therefore, a small number of grains over a specific nucleus is not
necessarily due to the presence of a small number of receptors in that nucleus.
It also follows that it is not possible to discern whether individual nuclei in a
specific population contain different numbers of AR. By contrast, quantitative
AR immunohistochemistry is amenable to this type of analysis (Sadi *et al*,
1991b). Nevertheless, we found that grain count distributions can be analysed
to calculate the following important indices: (a) mean AR content (expressed
as mean number of grains/nucleus) of all nuclei, (b) percentage of nuclei that
are AR positive and (c) mean AR content (number of grains/nucleus) of AR
positive nuclei.

Mean AR Content

Specific AR labelling is the difference between total androgen binding and
non-specific androgen binding, and grain counts representing total binding
and non-specific binding both exhibit Poisson distributions. Statistical analysis
of this difference is therefore done with a one-tailed 1% confidence limit of
the Poisson distribution (Arnold, 1981). The difference (ie specific binding) is
regarded as statistically significant (p <0.01) if the mean of total binding is
greater than the upper 1% tail value of the non-specific binding (grain count)
distribution. Because the upper 1% tail value of the non-specific binding distribution is the number of grains above which 1% of the grain count observa-

tions could occur by chance, grain counts higher than this are regarded as (99% probability of being correct) different from (greater than) non-specific labelling.

When we applied this 1% Poisson criterion to ^{3}H-labelled androgen auto-radiograms of stage D2 human prostate cancers, we found specific AR labelling only in epithelial nuclei; there was no specific AR labelling (ie no statistically significant difference between total and non-specific binding of ^{3}H-labelled R1881) in epithelial cell cytoplasm, stromal cell cytoplasm or stromal nuclei (Chuknyiska RS and Barrack ER, unpublished data). We reached the same conclusions about AR location in human glandular BPH (Peters and Barrack, 1987b) and normal rat prostate (Peters and Barrack, 1987a). Only in fibromuscular BPH did we find statistically significant labelling of both stromal nuclei and epithelial nuclei (Peters and Barrack, 1987c).

Percentage of AR Positive Nuclei

Our conclusion that stromal nuclei in prostate cancer biopsy specimens were AR negative was based on the absence of a difference between the mean grain count of total binding and the upper 1% tail value of the non-specific grain count distribution. However, we realized that although the mean of total binding was not higher, some individual nuclei might have a total binding grain count higher than the 1% criterion for non-specific binding; these nuclei would be regarded as receptor positive (Arnold, 1981). By this type of analysis, we indeed found that some stromal nuclei (18–25%) in stage D2 prostate cancer biopsy specimens were AR positive. This suggests that the non-malignant stroma may have an unexpected supportive role in cancer; for example, it is possible that androgen dependent stromal factors could affect malignant epithelial cells (even those that are AR negative).

We also estimated the percentage of AR positive cancer epithelial nuclei; it varied among several specimens, illustrating the presence of both AR positive and AR negative nuclei in a certain specimen before androgen ablation. At the time we did the grain counting, we were not aware of this heterogeneity; we deliberately chose areas at random, and if they contained malignant epithelium, the number of grains/nucleus was counted. This method of choosing areas at random did not allow us to establish, retrospectively, how these AR positive nuclei were distributed. A limited re-analysis of a small number of samples indicated that the percentage of AR positive nuclei/acinus varied from 0% to 94%, and there were many acini with intermediate levels (Chuknyiska RS and Barrack ER, unpublished data).

Mean AR Content of AR Positive Nuclei

Having identified a way to distinguish between AR positive nuclei versus AR negative nuclei (based on the 1% criterion as described above), we then measured the average number of grains/AR positive nucleus. Interestingly, the average amount of AR per AR positive epithelial nucleus was similar to the average amount of AR per AR positive stromal nucleus. In addition, this value was surprisingly similar among several specimens (Chuknyiska RS and Barrack ER, unpublished data). This type of observation has not been made before and illustrates the power of quantitative autoradiography.

QUANTITATIVE ANDROGEN RECEPTOR IMMUNOHISTOCHEMISTRY

While our studies on AR autoradiography were in progress, polyclonal AR antibodies, prepared in the laboratory of Wilson and French (Lubahn *et al*, 1988; Tan *et al*, 1988; Quarmby *et al*, 1990), became available. One antibody, designated AR-52, was prepared against a synthetic 15 aminoacid peptide sequence located just 5′ of the DNA binding domain of the AR (Tan *et al*, 1988). A second antibody, designated AR-32, recognizes the aminoterminal 21 aminoacid fragment of the AR (Quarmby *et al*, 1990), a different portion of the molecule than that recognized by AR-52. Both antibodies react specifically with AR since both peptide antigen sequences are found only in AR, and both antibodies were shown to be applicable for immunohistochemical studies on frozen sections (Lubahn *et al*, 1988; Tan *et al*, 1988; Quarmby *et al*, 1990).

AR immunohistochemistry offers the advantage over autoradiography that AR positive cells can be visualized directly. In addition, immunohistochemistry is much less time consuming because specimens can be processed in 1 day for immunohistochemistry, compared with about 6 weeks for autoradiography; the time required for data analysis is also substantially less with immunohistochemistry. We therefore used AR immunohistochemistry to measure the percentage of AR positive malignant epithelial cells in stage D2 prostate cancer biopsy specimens, obtained just before castration and correlated this with the time to progression after therapy (Sadi *et al*, 1991a).

Immunohistochemical Staining of AR in Biopsy Specimens

AR positive and AR negative malignant epithelial nuclei are both found in the same field, and occasionally adjacent to each other, demonstrating that ARs are distributed heterogeneously among the epithelial cells in metastatic prostate cancer before androgen ablation. Some stromal nuclei also are AR positive. Specific AR immunostaining is apparent only in nuclei (Sadi *et al*, 1991a). Interestingly, autoradiography yields the same conclusions (see Mean AR Content above; also Peters and Barrack, 1987a,b,c).

Biopsy specimens contained variable proportions of adenocarcinoma and non-malignant (normal or benign hyperplastic [BPH]) prostate tissue. Several specimens contained only cancerous tissue, but even these contained non-malignant stroma in various proportions. Some specimens consisted predominantly of stroma. On the basis of our experience, the presence of non-malignant epithelial and stromal cells could greatly complicate the interpretation of AR assays on homogenized biopsy specimens.

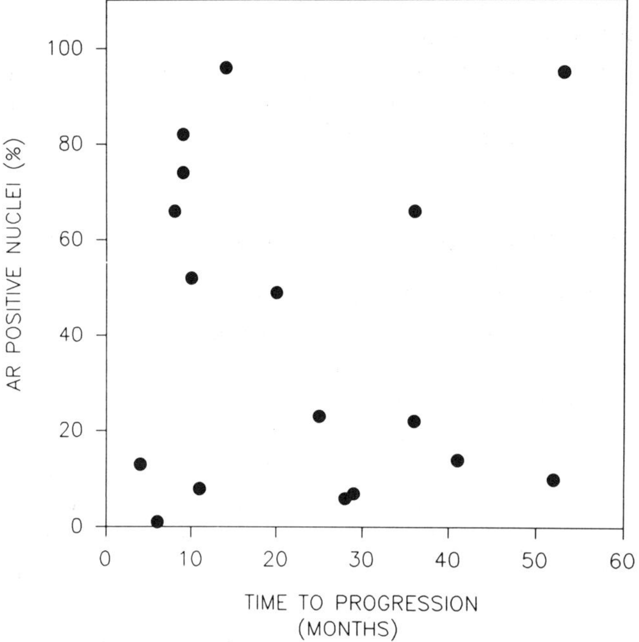

Fig. 1. Relation between the percentage of malignant epithelial nuclei that are AR positive in stage D2 prostate cancer biopsy specimens taken before androgen ablation therapy and the time to tumour progression after therapy. Time to progression is defined as the time between therapy and relapse (deterioration of symptoms)

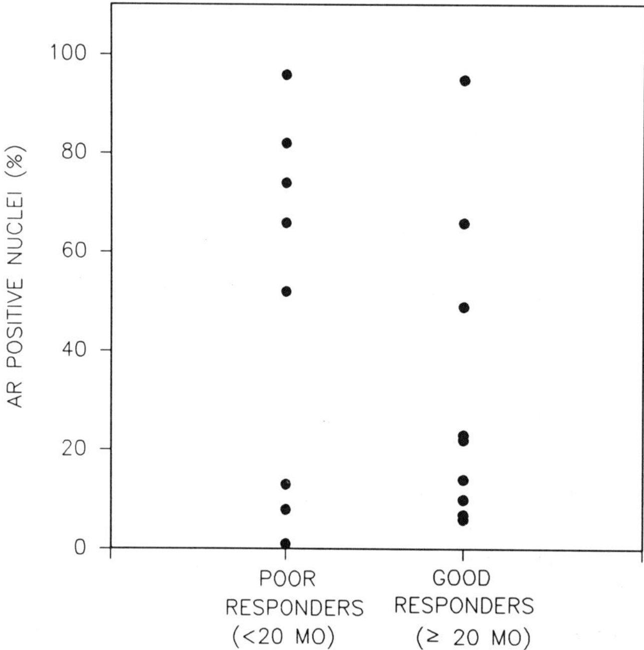

Fig. 2. AR positive malignant epithelial nuclei in poor responders (time to progression <20 months) and good responders (time to progression ≥20 months). The mean percentage of AR positive nuclei is 49 (13)% in the poor responders and 30 (10)% in the good responders

Some specimens contained substantial amounts of BPH (or normal) acinar components; in these, the non-malignant secretory epithelial nuclei were strongly and uniformly AR positive. In contrast, AR staining of prostate cancer epithelial nuclei was generally less intense, and AR staining intensity was variable both within individual specimens and among different patients. Weak or negative AR staining was not likely to be due to experimental artifact because (a) intense staining was seen in non-malignant epithelial nuclei present in the same specimen or (b) intense staining was observed in other specimens subjected concurrently to the immunohistochemical procedure.

There was no apparent relation between the amount of AR staining and the degree of tumour differentiation. Well differentiated tumours were not always AR rich, and poorly differentiated tumours were not always AR negative.

Percentage of AR Positive Nuclei Does Not Predict Time to Progression

Our objective was to evaluate the prognostic value of AR in prostate cancer nuclei in biopsy specimens taken immediately before androgen withdrawal therapy. We quantified the percentage of AR positive malignant prostate epithelial nuclei and compared this to the time to progression after therapy (time between treatment and relapse) (Fig. 1). There is no apparent relation between these indices, even at the extremes. Among patients with the longest time to progression, some are very rich in AR and others are very poor in AR. Four of nine good responders had only 6–14% AR positive nuclei. Similarly, among the worst responders, there were AR poor tumours and AR rich tumours. Five of eight poor responders had more than 50% AR positive nuclei. Recognizing the possibility that poorly stained tumours might contain AR in which the epitope for antibody AR-52 was masked, we reevaluated two AR poor tumours with an AR antibody (AR-32) made against a different portion of the AR molecule. Both tumours (one from a good responder and one from a poor responder) yielded similarly poor staining with either AR antibody. Seeing no apparent correlation, nor any apparent cutoff values that might distinguish two groups of patients, we analysed the data in Fig. 1 in two ways. We divided the patients into two groups on the basis of (a) the median time to progression (Fig. 2) and (b) the median percentage of AR positive nuclei (Fig. 3).

The median time to progression for our 17 patients was 20 months, which is comparable to previous estimates for larger populations of patients and suggests that our sample is representative. The median time to progression divides the patients into two statistically different groups—poor responders with a time to progression of less than 20 months (mean 9 [SEM 1] months, n = eight patients) and good responders with a time to progression 20 months or more (36 [4] months, n = 9). However, the percentage of AR positive malignant epithelial nuclei in these two groups did not differ significantly, as shown by the complete overlap of values (Fig. 2). The mean (SEM) percentage of AR positive nuclei is 49 (13)% in the poor responder group and 30 (10)% in the good responder group (p = 0.37).

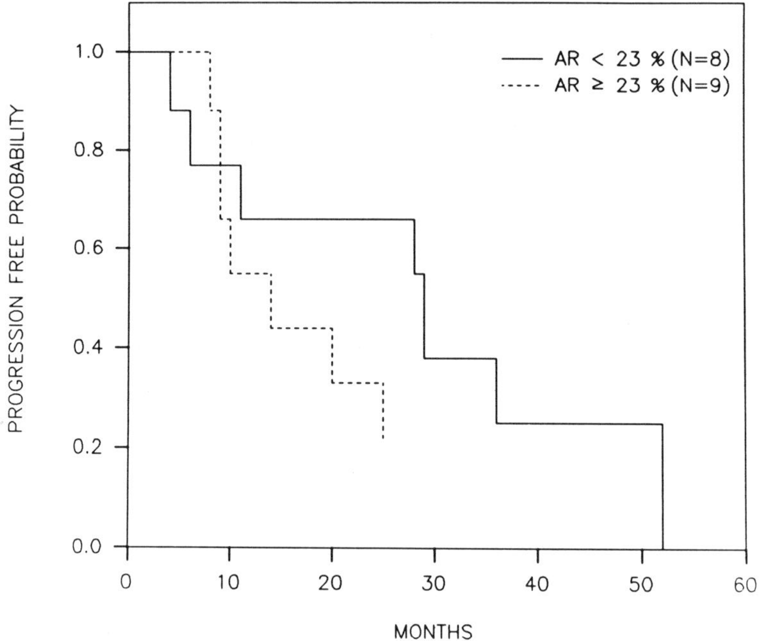

Fig. 3. Kaplan-Meier plots of progression free probability for prostate cancer patients with AR poor tumours (<23% AR positive nuclei) or AR rich tumours (≥23% AR positive nuclei). There is no statistically significant difference between the two curves (p = 0.9)

The median percentage of AR positive nuclei was used to classify tumours as either AR poor (<23% AR positive nuclei) or AR rich (23% or more AR positive nuclei). However, the mean time to progression for these groups did not differ significantly (25 [6] months versus 20 [5] months, respectively). In addition, Kaplan-Meier estimates of the progression free interval are not significantly different for AR poor tumours versus AR rich tumours (Fig. 3).

We also considered other endpoints of response that might better reflect the degree of androgen dependence of a specific tumour. Because secretion of prostatic acid phosphatase (PAP) increases during puberty and adulthood (Mann, 1964), and serum concentrations of PAP decrease after castration of patients with metastatic prostate cancer (Huggins and Hodges, 1941), PAP is frequently referred to as an androgen dependent secretory protein marker of prostate function.

We reasoned that if PAP is androgen dependent, then changes in PAP values might be expected to correlate with the level of AR. Consistent with this, it seems that there is less of a decrease in serum PAP concentrations in patients with AR poor tumours than in patients with AR rich tumours (54 [13]% versus 76 [8]%, respectively); this difference is not statistically significant (p = 0.17) but is suggestive of a trend. When patients are divided into two groups on the basis of the median percentage decrease in serum PAP for all 17 patients (72%), patients with a less than 72% decrease in PAP have 29

(10)% AR positive nuclei, and patients with a decrease in PAP greater than 72% have 55 (13)% AR positive nuclei (p = 0.23). Thus, although changes in serum PAP do not predict clinical outcome (serum PAP decreased 70 [9]% in poor responders versus 63 [12]% in good responders, p = 0.83), there seems to be a trend in the data, suggesting that changes in PAP may reflect the AR positivity of the primary tumour.

Perspectives on AR as a Predictor of Androgen Responsiveness

We were surprised to find no relation between the percentage of AR positive malignant epithelial cells and the time to progression of metastatic prostate cancer after hormone therapy. The hypothesis that the percentage of AR positive cells in prostate cancer might predict the clinical response to androgen ablation is based on the assumption that androgen dependent malignant epithelial cells are AR positive and, conversely, that the presence of AR is a sensitive and specific marker of dependence on androgen for cell survival. Evidence in other systems indicates that this assumption may be invalid because some AR negative cells are androgen dependent and some AR positive cells are androgen independent. For example, AR negative epithelial cells in the fetal mouse prostate undergo androgen dependent proliferation, perhaps caused by an androgen regulated growth factor produced by AR positive stroma (Shannon and Cunha, 1983, 1984). Proteins secreted by rat prostate stromal cells can affect epithelial cell function (Djakiew *et al*, 1990; Swinnen *et al*, 1990), and production of some of these stroma derived proteins is regulated by androgen (Swinnen *et al*, 1990). Thus, it is tempting to speculate that AR positive stromal cells might regulate AR negative prostate cancer epithelial cells explaining why some AR poor tumours respond to androgen withdrawal.

There is also evidence that AR positive cancer cells do not necessarily die after castration. Some normal and malignant rat prostate cells remain AR positive after castration (Lippert and Keefer, 1987; Prins, 1989). Also, progression of an androgen dependent mouse mammary tumour (Shionogi S115) to an androgen independent state takes place despite the continued presence of AR (Darbre and King, 1987). Some specimens of human prostate cancer also seem to be AR positive after castration (Walsh *et al*, 1978; Benson *et al*, 1985); however, those assays were done on homogenized tissue and so do not rule out the possibility that the AR was stroma derived. If some AR positive malignant prostate epithelial cells were not dependent on androgen for their survival, then the AR content of a tumour would not be a reliable predictor of response to androgen withdrawal.

Because immunohistochemical detection of AR requires only the presence of the immunoreactive epitope, AR positive staining does not distinguish between functional versus non-functional AR. Mutations in the hormone binding domain could produce AR molecules that are unable to bind androgen and therefore are inactive in the presence of androgen. Such mutations have been detected in the AR gene of some patients with complete androgen insensitivity syndrome (Brown *et al*, 1988, 1990; Lubahn *et al*, 1989; Marcelli *et al*, 1990). Alternatively, mutations in other parts of the AR molecule, such as in the DNA binding domain, could disrupt androgen dependent transcriptional activity of the AR (Quigley *et al*, 1990). If any of the above types of mutations occurred in prostate cancer, the tumour cells might be immunohistochemically AR positive but already androgen independent before androgen withdrawal. A single example of an AR mutation in a human prostate cancer cell line (LNCaP) has been reported (Harris *et al*, 1990). The mutation is in the hormone binding domain, and it produces AR that can bind and be transcriptionally activated not just by androgen but also by anti-androgen, oestrogen or progesterone (Harris *et al*, 1990). Prostate cancers with such mutant AR would be immunohistochemically AR positive but might continue to proliferate in patients treated with oestrogen or anti-androgen. Other types of mutations in the AR, such that the epitope for the AR antibody was missing or masked, could yield a tumour that is immunohistochemically AR negative but that contains transcriptionally active AR.

There are thus many possible explanations to account for our finding that immunohistochemical measurement of the percentage of AR positive nuclei in a biopsy specimen of metastatic prostate cancer taken just before hormone therapy does not predict the time to progression after therapy. Although we cannot discriminate among these possibilities, we can conclude that knowledge of the percentage of AR positive nuclei is not a sufficient criterion to predict time to progression. In addition, the presence (or absence) of AR should not be assumed to be sufficient and specific as a marker of androgen dependent (or independent) cells. We need ways to detect in a tumour evidence of androgen dependent biological activity of AR and of androgen dependent cell survival.

Image Analysis of AR Immunostaining

In visual evaluation of the AR status of malignant epithelial nuclei as AR positive or AR negative, we could not take into account variations in staining intensity within a specimen or between specimens. Therefore, tumours with the same percentage of AR positive nuclei might have different amounts of AR per cell and possibly different degrees of androgen responsiveness. To investigate this possibility, we quantified the intensity of nuclear AR immunostaining (optical density/unit area) by computer assisted image analysis (Sadi *et al*, 1991b).

Staining intensity proved to vary among nuclei in a certain section, probably at least partly because the proportion of each nucleus that is represented in a tissue section of 8 µm thickness varies. However, this cannot account for all variation in staining intensity because the shape of the frequency distribution of optical density/unit area is frequently different for AR antibody stained sections versus their normal IgG control stained counterpart. In many good responders, the frequency distribution of nuclear AR content was quite uniform, presenting as a single peak. In striking contrast, many poor responders had flattened, highly variable, multimodal distributions, indicating a wide range of nuclear AR content within each tumour. The mean AR concentration was not different in good versus poor responders (p = 0.28), but the variance was significantly greater (p = 0.01) in poor responders than in good responders. The kurtosis was also significantly different (p = 0.03), reflecting the more flattened frequency distribution curves in poor responders. Although the variance and kurtosis of AR content frequency distributions differ, on average, in poor versus good responders, there is some overlap between the groups; therefore, frequency distribution analysis of AR immunostaining intensity cannot by itself predict the clinical outcome of individual patients. Nevertheless, these data indicate that the AR concentration per cell is more heterogeneous in poor responders; this may reflect a greater genetic instability in these patients that is independent of AR content.

RATIONALE FOR KI-67 GROWTH FRACTION STUDIES

Since we found no relation between the percentage of AR positive prostate cancer cells and time to tumour progression after hormone therapy, we considered the possibility that the time to progression might be more dependent on the growth rate of the androgen independent malignant cells than on the percentage of these cells in the tumour. Thus, a tumour with a long doubling time would be expected to have a more favourable clinical course than a tumour with a shorter doubling time (Coffey and Isaacs, 1981).

Little is known about the growth rate of human prostate cancer. Methods that have been used to analyze prostate tumour cell kinetics include crude tumour volume measurement (Haddad *et al*, 1987), mitotic index (Alison and Wright, 1981), [^{3}H]thymidine or 5-bromo-2′-deoxyuridine labelling index (Meyer *et al*, 1982; Nemoto *et al*, 1989), flow cytometry (Lundberg *et al*, 1987; Stephenson *et al*, 1987; Lee *et al*, 1988; Winkler *et al*, 1988; Nativ *et al*, 1989; Haugen and Mjolnerod, 1990) or Ki-67 immunohistochemistry (Gallee *et al*, 1987, 1989; Raymond *et al*, 1988). The use of [^{3}H]thymidine or bromodeoxyuridine requires that these DNA precursors be incubated with fresh tissue in vitro (Meyer *et al*, 1982) or administered in vivo (Nemoto *et al*, 1989). Flow cytometric analysis disrupts the tissue and underestimates the S phase fraction of the tumour cells if the specimen also contains non-malignant cells (Garcia *et al*, 1989; Merkel and McGuire, 1990). Immunohistochemistry with antibodies against proliferating cell nuclear antigens such as PCNA/cyclin (Garcia *et al*, 1989), DNA polymerase α (Yamaguchi *et al*, 1990), topoisomerase II (Nelson *et al*, 1987) and Ki-67 (Gerdes *et al*, 1983, 1984, 1986; Gallee *et al*, 1987, 1989; Raymond *et al*, 1988; Sasaki *et al*, 1988; Kamel *et al*, 1989; Isola *et al*, 1990; Yonemura *et al*, 1990) represents a recent alternative approach to study tumour cell kinetics.

A mouse monoclonal antibody Ki-67 appears to provide an immunohisto-chemical estimate of the growth fraction (Gerdes *et al*, 1983, 1984, 1986;

Sasaki *et al*, 1988; Kamel *et al*, 1989; Isola *et al*, 1990; Yonemura *et al*, 1990). Ki-67 identifies cells that are cycling since it reacts with a nuclear antigen that is present in the G_1, S, G_2 and M phases of the cell cycle, but not in G_0 (Gerdes *et al*, 1983, 1984; Sasaki *et al*, 1987). In studies where an independent estimate of the S phase fraction was compared with the Ki-67 positive growth fraction, the Ki-67 fraction was greater than the S phase fraction, but there was a strong positive correlation between the two variables (Sasaki *et al*, 1988; Silvestrini *et al*, 1988; Kamel *et al*, 1989; Isola *et al*, 1990; Yonemura *et al*, 1990). Thus, it has been suggested that Ki-67 provides an estimate of the growth fraction. Immunohistochemical assay of Ki-67 circumvents many of the disadvantages of other methods described above; it is simple and fast, can be done with frozen tissues stored in liquid nitrogen and allows direct evaluation of cancer cells since tissue morphology is maintained. Although the identity and function of the antigen recognized by Ki-67 are not known (Verheijen *et al*, 1989), several reports suggest that patients with a high percentage of Ki-67 positive nuclei have a worse clinical course than those with a lower growth fraction (Hall *et al*, 1988; Bouzubar *et al*, 1989; Ueda *et al*, 1989).

Only a few workers have used Ki-67 immunohistochemistry in prostate cancer (Gallee *et al*, 1987, 1989; Raymond *et al*, 1988). However, there were no attempts to correlate the Ki-67 growth fraction with clinical response. We therefore set out to investigate whether the tumour growth fraction might predict tumour behaviour in prostate cancer patients (Sadi and Barrack, 1991). Because of availability of tissue and clinical follow-up data, we studied stage D2 prostate cancer patients.

RELATION BETWEEN KI-67 GROWTH FRACTION AND TIME TO TUMOUR PROGRESSION

The Ki-67 growth fraction (measured as the percentage of immunohistochemically Ki-67 positive malignant epithelial nuclei) was quantified in 17 patients with metastatic stage D2 prostate cancer. The mean Ki-67 growth fraction of these stage D2 cancers was 3.3% (range 1.7–7.5%). Raymond et al. (1988) reported a mean Ki-67 growth fraction of 16.3% (range 6–53%) for prostate cancer of different clinical stages, whereas Gallee et al. (1989) reported a mean of 2.9% (range, 0.4–9.1%) for localized prostate cancer. The explanation for the much higher growth fractions reported by Raymond et al. (1988) is not clear; however, their methodology was somewhat different and they evaluated only 200–300 nuclei per patient. We established in our study that it was necessary to evaluate 1000 nuclei to obtain reproducible estimates of the percentage of Ki-67 positive nuclei (Sadi and Barrack, 1991). Investigators using [^{3}H]thymidine or bromodeoxyuridine labelling index (Meyer *et al*, 1982; Nemoto *et al*, 1989) find a low percentage of proliferating cells in prostate cancer (ranges 0.14–3.9% and 1.0–6.3%, respectively), and these data are consistent with the low Ki-67 growth fraction for metastatic prostate cancer found

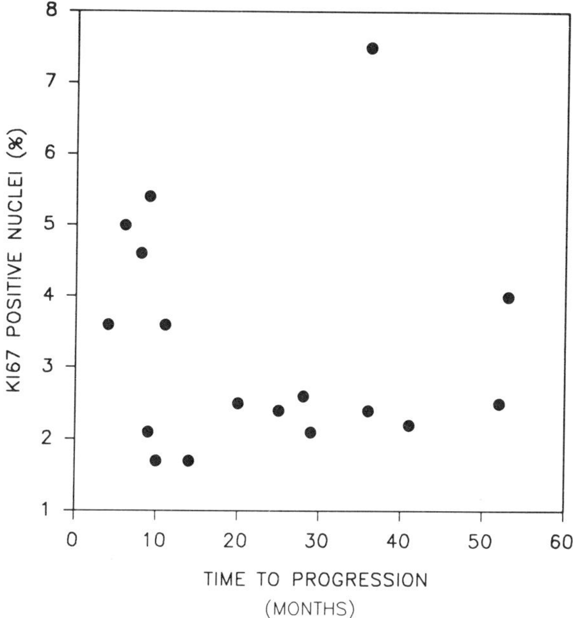

Fig. 4. Relation between the Ki-67 growth fraction of stage D2 prostate cancer before hormone therapy and time to tumour progression after therapy

in our study. This low growth fraction indicates that prostate cancer has a low rate of cell turnover relative to that of other cancers and is consistent with the slow natural history of the disease. The low Ki-67 growth fraction of prostate cancer contrasts with much higher growth fractions in many other tumours, averaging 15–25% for cancers of the breast, uterus, ovary, lung, stomach and colon (Sasaki *et al*, 1988; Kamel *et al*, 1989; Matsumura *et al*, 1989; Isola *et al*, 1990; Yonemura *et al*, 1990).

We had anticipated that tumours with a short time to progression would have a short doubling time, reflected by a high Ki-67 growth fraction, and, conversely, that a long time to progression would be associated with a long doubling time and low growth fraction. There is a trend, such that eight of ten (80%) patients with a good response (ie time to progression of over 12 months) had a Ki-67 growth fraction of less than 3% (see Fig. 4). In addition, five of seven (71%) patients with a high growth fraction (more than 3% Ki-67 positive) had a short time to progression (less than 12 months). Notable exceptions were the patient with the highest growth fraction (7.5%) who nevertheless had an excellent response to therapy, and the three patients with the lowest growth fraction who nevertheless progressed in a short time. With these somewhat arbitrary or visual cut-off values (12 months to progression, 3% Ki-67 positive nuclei), statistical analysis by Fisher's exact test yielded a p value of less than 0.05.

A more rigorous statistical analysis of the data in Fig. 4 was done by dividing the patients into two groups based on the median time to progression (Fig.

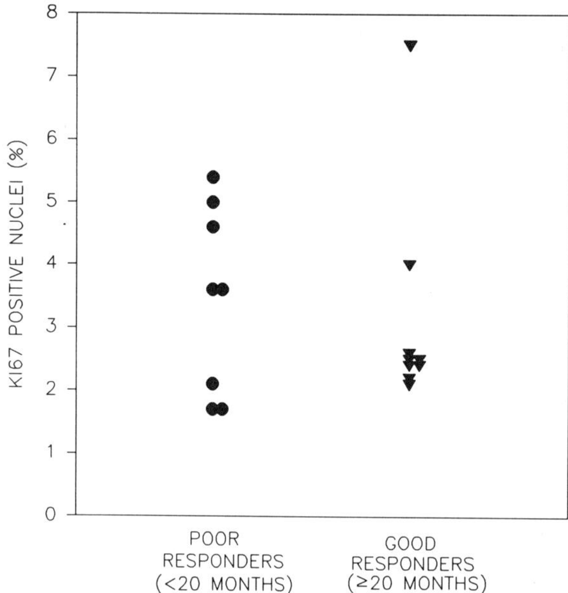

Fig. 5. Ki-67 growth fractions in poor responders (time to progression <20 months) and good responders (time to progression ≥20 months). The mean growth fraction is 3.5 (0.5)% in the poor responders and 3.1 (0.6)% in the good responders

5) or based on the median Ki-67 growth fraction (Fig. 6). The growth fraction did not differ significantly between good responders (3.1 [0.6]%, median 2.5%) and poor responders (3.5 [0.5]%, median 3.6%) (Fig. 5). On the basis of

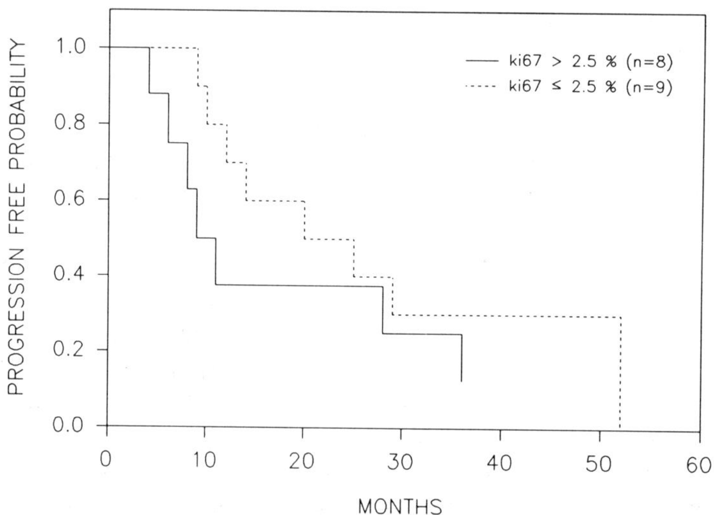

Fig. 6. Kaplan-Meier plots of progression free probability for patients with high growth fraction tumours (>2.5% Ki-67 positive nuclei) or low growth fraction tumours (≤2.5% Ki-67 positive). Patients with a high growth fraction tumour tended to progress sooner than patients with a low growth fraction

median Ki-67 growth fraction (2.5%), patients with a low growth fraction (Ki-67 2.5% or less) had a mean of 2.2 (0.1)% Ki-67 positive nuclei (median, 2.2%), and patients with a high growth fraction (Ki-67 more than 2.5%) had a mean of 4.5 (0.5)% (median, 4.3%). The median time to progression was longer for tumours with a low growth fraction than for tumours with a high growth fraction (25 months versus 10 months, respectively). Statistical comparison of the mean time to progression in these two groups yielded a p value of 0.18 for low growth fraction tumours (mean time to progression 26 [5] months) versus high growth fraction tumours (19 [6] months). Kaplan-Meier estimates of the progression free interval probability for low growth fraction tumours versus high growth fraction tumours are shown in Fig. 6. There is a trend towards a shorter time to progression in tumours with a high growth fraction, but it is not significant for this small sample of patients (p = 0.4).

PERSPECTIVES ON KI-67 GROWTH FRACTION AS A PREDICTOR

There is a trend towards a shorter time to tumour progression in patients with a higher Ki-67 growth fraction, but the Ki-67 growth fraction cannot be used to predict time to progression for individual patients. Although several other studies show a statistically significant correlation between the Ki-67 growth fraction and clinical outcome (Hall *et al*, 1988; Bouzubar *et al*, 1989; Ueda *et al*, 1989), in none is the Ki-67 index accurate enough to predict outcome for individual patients.

Because it is the proliferation of androgen independent cancer cells that accounts for tumour progression, it would be interesting to determine whether there is a closer relation between time to progression and growth fraction of androgen independent cells specifically. To address this question, it would be necessary to obtain prostate cancer biopsy specimens after androgen ablation. In our study, tissue was available only before hormone therapy, and the growth fractions we measured therefore probably represent the sum of both androgen dependent and androgen independent cells.

Although we suspect that the presence of AR is not sufficient evidence of androgen dependence, it would also be interesting to measure the Ki-67 growth fraction separately for AR positive cells and AR negative cells. This would require double antibody immunohistochemistry. So far, we have evaluated Ki-67 positivity without regard to AR status; there is no relation between the percentage of Ki-67 positive malignant epithelial nuclei and that of AR positive nuclei (Fig. 7). Tumours classified as AR poor (<23% AR positive) or AR rich (>23% AR positive) have similar growth fractions (3.5 [0.6]% and 3.1 [0.5]%, respectively). It is notable that in the oestrogen stimulated neonatal mouse uterus, oestrogen receptor negative cells have the same S phase fraction as oestrogen receptor positive cells (Yamashita *et al*, 1990).

Metastatic prostate cancer may be so complex that no single index can give enough information about tumour behaviour to predict individual clinical re-

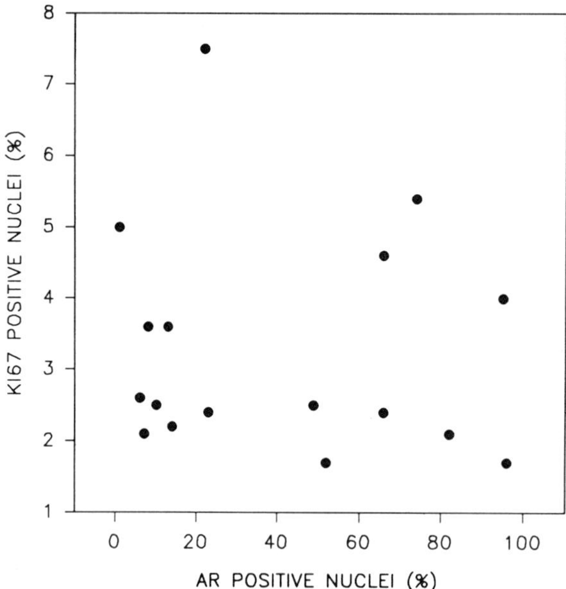

Fig. 7. Relation between the percentages of Ki-67 positive and AR positive nuclei. Ki-67 and AR immunohistochemistry were done on the same biopsy specimens. The mean Ki-67 growth fraction of AR poor tumours (<23% AR positive nuclei) is 3.5 (0.6)% and that of AR rich tumours (>23% AR positive nuclei) is 3.1 (0.5)%

sponse to therapy. For example, total tumour load in the patient may be an important factor that affects time to progression (Coffey and Isaacs, 1981), but these data are not easily obtained. Secondly, if the cell proliferation rate of the primary tumour differed from that of distant metastases, then biopsy of the primary tumour might not predict the overall clinical behaviour of the patient.

Although Ki-67 estimates the growth fraction, actual tumour doubling time depends on the rate of cell proliferation and rate of cell death. If a high proliferation rate were balanced by a high cell death rate, then Ki-67 data alone would overestimate the net growth rate (doubling time) of the tumour. For instance, one of our patients had a tumour growth fraction of 7.5%, three times higher than the median for the whole group of patients, yet he had a very good response to castration; perhaps the apparently high rate of cell proliferation in his tumour was balanced by a high rate of cell death. A study on the growth kinetics of the Dunning R-3327-G rat prostate adenocarcinoma shows the importance of determining the rate of cell death. Tumors in intact and castrated rats have the same rate of proliferation (based on [^{3}H]thymidine incorporation) but different doubling times; this apparent paradox is accounted for by a difference in the rate of cell death (Humphries and Isaacs, 1982). Thus, reliable prediction of prostate cancer growth rates may only be possible when methods are available to measure both cell proliferation and cell death rates.

Rapidly growing tumours generally respond well to chemotherapy, in contrast to slow growing tumours such as prostate cancer, which are known for their lack of response to chemotherapy. It is tempting to speculate that measurement of a high Ki-67 growth fraction could identify a subpopulation of prostate cancer patients who might benefit from chemotherapy.

SUMMARY

Reliable predictors of response for prostate cancer patients undergoing hormone therapy are lacking. Since 80–90% of such patients do respond but the time between therapy and relapse (progression) is variable, our goal has been to predict the time to tumour progression after therapy rather than merely to predict whether a patient would respond. We investigated AR positivity and Ki-67 growth fraction of malignant epithelial cells as potential predictors of the time to progression; these studies are summarized in this chapter.

The percentage of AR positive nuclei has no predictive value; however, the variance of AR immunostaining intensity within a certain specimen is an important discriminator between good responders (patients with a prolonged interval between initiation of therapy and relapse) and poor responders (short time to relapse). There is a trend towards a higher growth fraction in poor responders, but statistical significance is borderline at best. Growth fraction measurement might be more useful as a predictor if the rate of cell death could also be evaluated or if analysis could be limited to the androgen independent cells that continue to proliferate after hormone therapy and that ultimately are responsible for the clinical manifestation of tumour progression and relapse.

Acknowledgements

The work described in this review has been supported by the National Cancer Institute grant CA-16924. We thank our colleague Dr Patrick C Walsh for providing patient specimens and clinical follow-up data, Piroska Bujnovszky and Dalal Tonb for technical assistance, Ruth Middleton for preparing the manuscript, and Dr Elizabeth M Wilson and Dr Frank S French for generously providing us with their AR antibodies.

References

Alison MR and Wright NA (1981) Growth kinetics. *Recent Results in Cancer Research* **78** 29–43
Arnold AP (1981) Quantitative analysis of steroid autoradiograms. *Journal of Histochemistry and Cytochemistry* **29** 207–211
Barrack ER and Tindall DJ (1987) A critical evaluation of the use of androgen receptor assays to predict the androgen responsiveness of prostatic cancer. *Progress in Clinical and Biological Research* **239** 155–187
Barrack ER, Brendler CB and Walsh PC (1987) Steroid receptor and biochemical profiles in

prostatic cancer: correlation with response to hormonal treatment. *Progress in Clinical and Biological Research* **243A** 79–97

Barrack ER, Peters CA and Schulze H (1988) Localization of androgen receptors and estrogen receptors in the prostate, In: Sheridan PJ, Blum K and Trachtenberg MC (eds). *Steroid Receptors and Disease: Cancer, Autoimmune, Bone, and Circulatory Disorders*, pp 329–368, Marcel Dekker Inc, New York

Benson Jr RC, Utz DC, Holicky E and Veneziale CM (1985) Androgen receptor binding activity in human prostate cancer. *Cancer* **55** 382–388

Benson Jr RC, Gorman PA, O'Brien PC, Holicky EL and Veneziale CM (1987) Relationship between androgen receptor binding activity in human prostate cancer and clinical response to endocrine therapy. *Cancer* **59** 1599–1606

Bouzubar N, Walker KJ, Griffiths K *et al* (1989) Ki-67 immunostaining in primary breast cancer: pathological and clinical associations. *British Journal of Cancer* **59** 943–947

Brendler CB, Isaacs JT, Follansbee AL and Walsh PC (1984) The use of multiple variables to predict response to endocrine therapy in carcinoma of the prostate: a preliminary report. *Journal of Urology* **131** 694–700

Brown TR, Lubahn DB, Wilson EM, Joseph DR, French FS and Migeon CJ (1988) Deletion of the steroid-binding domain of the human androgen receptor gene in one family with complete androgen insensitivity syndrome: evidence for further genetic heterogeneity in this syndrome. *Proceedings of the National Academy of Sciences of the USA* **85** 8151–8155

Brown TR, Lubahn DB, Wilson EM, French FS, Migeon CJ and Corden JL (1990) Functional characterization of naturally occurring mutant androgen receptors from subjects with complete androgen insensitivity. *Molecular Endocrinology* **4** 1759–1772

Carter HB and Coffey DS (1990) The prostate: an increasing medical problem. *Prostate* **16** 39–48

Coffey DS and Isaacs JT (1981) Prostate tumor biology and cell kinetics-theory. *Urology* **17** **(Supplement)** 40–53

Darbre PD and King RJB (1987) Progression to steroid insensitivity can occur irrespective of the presence of functional steroid receptors. *Cell* **51** 521–528

Diamond DA and Barrack ER (1984) The relationship of androgen receptor levels to androgen responsiveness in the Dunning R3327 rat prostate tumor sublines. *Journal of Urology* **132** 821–827

Djakiew D, Tarkington MA and Lynch JH (1990) Paracrine stimulation of polarized secretion from monolayers of a neoplastic prostatic epithelial cell line by prostatic stromal cell proteins. *Cancer Research* **50** 1966–1974

Fentie DD, Lakey WH and McBlain WA (1986) Applicability of nuclear androgen receptor quantification to human prostatic adenocarcinoma. *Journal of Urology* **135** 167–173

Gallee MPW, van Steenbrugge G-A, ten Kate FJW, Schroeder FH and van der Kwast TH (1987) Determination of the proliferative fraction of a transplantable, hormone-dependent, human prostatic carcinoma (PC-82) by monoclonal antibody Ki-67: potential application for hormone therapy monitoring. *Journal of the National Cancer Institute* **79** 1333–1340

Gallee MPW, Visser-De Jong E, ten Kate FJW, Schroeder FH and van der Kwast TH (1989) Monoclonal antibody Ki-67 defined growth fraction in benign prostatic hyperplasia and prostatic cancer. *Journal of Urology* **142** 1342–1346

Garcia RL, Coltrera MD and Gown AM (1989) Analysis of proliferative grade using anti-PCNA/cyclin monoclonal antibodies in fixed, embedded tissues: comparison with flow cytometric analysis. *American Journal of Pathology* **134** 733–739

Gerdes J, Schwab U, Lemke H and Stein H (1983) Production of a mouse monoclonal antibody reactive with a human nuclear antigen associated with cell proliferation. *International Journal of Cancer* **31** 13–20

Gerdes J, Lemke H, Baisch H, Wacker H-H, Schwab U and Stein H (1984) Cell cycle analysis of a cell proliferation-associated human nuclear antigen defined by the monoclonal antibody Ki-67. *Journal of Immunology* **133** 1710–1715

Gerdes J, Lelle RJ, Pickartz H *et al* (1986) Growth fractions in breast cancers determined in situ with monoclonal antibody Ki-67. *Journal of Clinical Pathology* **39** 977–980

Haddad FS, Haddad L, Griffin II EE, Haddad R and Haddad Z (1987) Doubling time and annual doubling rate of human prostatic cancer. *Urology* **29** 35–39

Hall PA, Richards MA, Gregory WM, d'Ardenne AJ, Lister TA and Stansfeld AG (1988) The prognostic value of Ki-67 immunostaining in non-Hodgkin's lymphoma. *Journal of Pathology* **154** 223–235

Harris SE, Rong Z, Harris MA and Lubahn DB (1990) Androgen receptor in human prostate carcinoma LNCAP/ADEP cells contains a mutation which alters the specificity of the steroid-dependent transcriptional activation region. *The Endocrine Society 72nd Annual Meeting Program and Abstracts,* **275** 93 [Abstract]

Haugen OA and Mjolnerod O (1990) DNA-ploidy as prognostic factor in prostatic carcinoma. *International Journal of Cancer* **45** 224–228

Huggins C and Hodges CV (1941) The effect of castration, of estrogens and of androgen injection on serum phosphatase in metastatic carcinoma of the prostate. *Cancer Research* **1** 293–297

Humphries JE and Isaacs JT (1982) Unusual androgen sensitivity of the androgen-independent Dunning R-3327-G rat prostatic adenocarcinoma: androgen effect on tumor cell loss. *Cancer Research* **42** 3148–3156

Isola JJ, Helin HJ, Helle MJ and Kallioniemi O-P (1990) Evaluation of cell proliferation in breast carcinoma: comparison of Ki-67 immunohistochemical study, DNA flow cytometric analysis, and mitotic count. *Cancer* **65** 1180–1184

Kamel OW, Franklin WA, Ringus JC and Meyer JS (1989) Thymidine labeling index and Ki-67 growth fraction in lesions of the breast. *American Journal of Pathology* **134** 107–113

Lee SE, Currin SM, Paulson DF and Walther PJ (1988) Flow cytometric determination of ploidy in prostatic adenocarcinoma: a comparison with seminal vesicle involvement and histopathological grading as a predictor of clinical recurrence. *Journal of Urology* **140** 769–774

Lippert MC and Keefer DA (1987) Prostate adenocarcinoma: effects of castration on in situ androgen uptake by individual cell types. *Journal of Urology* **137** 140–145

Lubahn DB, Joseph DR, Sar M *et al* (1988) The human androgen receptor: complementary deoxyribonucleic acid cloning, sequence analysis and gene expression in prostate. *Molecular Endocrinology* **2** 265–1275

Lubahn DB, Brown TR, Simental JA *et al* (1989) Sequence of the intron/exon junctions of the coding region of the human androgen receptor gene and identification of a point mutation in a family with complete androgen insensitivity. *Proceedings of the National Academy of Sciences of the USA* **86** 9534–9538

Lundberg S, Carstensen J and Rundquist I (1987) DNA flow cytometry and histopathological grading of paraffin-embedded prostate biopsy specimens in a survival study. *Cancer Research* **47** 1973–1977

Mann T (1964). *The Biochemistry of Semen and of the Male Reproductive Tract,* pp 183–185, John Wiley, New York

Marcelli M, Tilley WD, Wilson CM, Wilson JD, Griffin JE and McPhaul MJ (1990) A single nucleotide substitution introduces a premature termination codon into the androgen receptor gene of a patient with receptor-negative androgen resistance. *Journal of Clinical Investigation* **85** 1522–1528

Matsumura K, Tsuji T, Shinozaki F, Sasaki K and Takahashi M (1989) Immunohistochemical determination of growth fraction in human tumors. *Pathology Research and Practice* **184** 609–613

Merkel DE and McGuire WL (1990) Ploidy, proliferative activity and prognosis: DNA flow cytometry of solid tumors. *Cancer* **65** 1194–1205

Meyer JS, Sufrin G and Martin SA (1982) Proliferative activity of benign human prostate, prostatic adenocarcinoma and seminal vesicle evaluated by thymidine labeling. *Journal of*

Urology **128** 1353–1356

Nativ O, Winkler HZ, Raz Y *et al* (1989) Stage C prostatic adenocarcinoma: flow cytometric nuclear DNA ploidy analysis. *Mayo Clinic Proceedings* **64** 911–919

Nelson WG, Cho KR, Hsiang Y-H, Liu LF and Coffey DS (1987) Growth-related elevations of DNA topoisomerase II levels found in Dunning R3327 rat prostatic adenocarcinomas. *Cancer Research* **47** 3246–3250

Nemoto R, Uchida K, Shimazui T, Hattori K, Koiso K and Harada M (1989) Immunocytochemical demonstration of S phase cells by anti-bromodeoxyuridine monoclonal antibody in human prostate adenocarcinoma. *Journal of Urology* **141** 337–340

Peters CA and Barrack ER (1987a) A new method for labeling and autoradiographic localization of androgen receptors. *Journal of Histochemistry and Cytochemistry* **35** 755–762

Peters CA and Barrack ER (1987b) Androgen receptor localization in the human prostate: demonstration of heterogeneity using a new method of steroid receptor autoradiography. *Journal of Steroid Biochemistry* **27** 533–541

Peters CA and Barrack ER (1987c) Androgen receptor localization in the prostate using a new method of steroid receptor autoradiography. In: Rodgers CH, Coffey DS, Cunha G, Grayhack JT, Hinman F Jr and Horton R (eds). *Benign Prostatic Hyperplasia*, Volume II, pp 175–187, United States Department of Health and Human Services, NIH Publication No. 87–2881

Prins GS (1989) Differential regulation of androgen receptors in the separate rat prostate lobes: androgen independent expression in the lateral lobe. *Journal of Steroid Biochemistry* **33** 319–326

Quarmby VE, Kemppainen JA, Sar M, Lubahn DB, French FS and Wilson EM (1990) Expression of recombinant androgen receptor in cultured mammalian cells. *Molecular Endocrinology* **4** 1399–1407

Quigley CA, Simental JA, Evans BA, Lubahn DB, Hughes IA and French FS (1990) Androgen insensitivity due to deletion of the second zinc finger of the androgen receptor. *The Endocrine Society 72nd Annual Meeting Program and Abstracts*, **793** 223 [Abstract]

Raymond WA, Leong AS-Y, Bolt JW, Milios J and Jose JS (1988) Growth fractions in human prostatic carcinoma determined by Ki-67 immunostaining. *Journal of Pathology* **156** 161–167

Sadi MV and Barrack ER (1991) Determination of growth fraction in advanced prostate cancer by Ki-67 immunostaining and its relationship to the time to tumor progression after hormonal therapy. *Cancer* **67** 3065–3071

Sadi MV, Walsh PC and Barrack ER (1991a) Immunohistochemical study of androgen receptors in metastatic prostate cancer: comparison of receptor content and response to hormonal therapy. *Cancer* **67** 3057–3064

Sadi MV, Walsh PC and Barrack ER (1991b) Image analysis of androgen receptor (AR) immunostaining in metastatic prostate cancer: greater heterogeneity of AR content predicts short response to hormonal therapy. *Journal of Urology* **145** 295A [Abstract]

Sasaki K, Murakami T, Kawasaki M and Takahashi M (1987) The cell cycle associated change of the Ki-67 reactive nuclear antigen expression. *Journal of Cellular Physiology* **133** 579–584

Sasaki K, Matsumura K, Tsuji T, Shinozaki F and Takahashi M (1988) Relationship between labeling indices of Ki-67 and BrdUrd in human malignant tumors. *Cancer* **62** 989–993

Scott WW, Menon M and Walsh PC (1980) Hormonal therapy of prostatic cancer. *Cancer* **45** 1929–1936

Shannon JM and Cunha GR (1983) Autoradiographic localization of androgen binding in the developing mouse prostate. *Prostate* **4** 367–373

Shannon JM and Cunha GR (1984) Characterization of androgen binding and deoxyribonucleic acid synthesis in prostate-like structures induced in the urothelium of testicular feminized (Tfm/Y) mice. *Biology of Reproduction* **31** 175–183

Silvestrini R, Costa A, Veneroni S, Del Bino G and Persici P (1988) Comparative analysis of different approaches to investigate cell kinetics. *Cell and Tissue Kinetics* **21** 123–131

Stephenson RA, James BC, Gay H, Fair WR, Whitmore Jr WF and Melamed MR (1987) Flow cytometry of prostate cancer: relationship of DNA content to survival. *Cancer Research* **47** 2504–2509

Swinnen K, Cailleau J, Heyns W and Verhoeven G (1990) Prostatic stromal cells and testicular peritubular cells produce similar paracrine mediators of androgen action. *Endocrinology* **126** 142–150

Tan J-a, Joseph DR, Quarmby VE *et al* (1988) The rat androgen receptor: primary structure, autoregulation of its messenger ribonucleic acid, and immunocytochemical localization of the receptor protein. *Molecular Endocrinology* **2** 1276–1285

Trachtenberg J and Walsh PC (1982) Correlation of prostatic nuclear androgen receptor content with duration of response and survival following hormonal therapy in advanced prostatic cancer. *Journal of Urology* **127** 466–471

Ueda T, Aozasa K, Tsujimoto M *et al* (1989) Prognostic significance of Ki-67 reactivity in soft tissue sarcomas. *Cancer* **63** 1607–1611

van Aubel O, Bolt-deVries J, Blankenstein MA and Schroder FH (1988) Prediction of time to progression after orchiectomy by the nuclear androgen receptor content from multiple biopsy specimens in patients with advanced prostate cancer. *Prostate* **12** 191–198

Verheijen R, Kuijpers HJH, Schlingemann RO *et al* (1989) Ki-67 detects a nuclear matrix-associated proliferation-related antigen I Intracellular localization during interphase. *Journal of Cell Science* **92** 123–130

Walsh PC, Greco JM, Tananis CE, Hicks LL, McLoughlin MG and Menon M (1978) The binding of a potent synthetic androgen-methyltrienolone (R1881) - to cytosol preparations of human prostatic cancer. *Transactions of the American Association of Genito-Urinary Surgeons* **69** 78–80

Winkler HZ, Rainwater LM, Myers RP *et al* (1988) Stage D1 prostatic adenocarcinoma: significance of nuclear DNA ploidy patterns studied by flow cytometry. *Mayo Clinic Proceedings* **63** 103–112

Yamaguchi A, Takegawa S, Ishida T *et al* (1990) Detection of the growth fraction in colorectal tumours by a monoclonal antibody against DNA polymerase α. *British Journal of Cancer* **61** 390–393

Yamashita S, Newbold RR, McLachlan JA and Korach KS (1990) The role of the estrogen receptor in uterine epithelial proliferation and cytodifferentiation in neonatal mice. *Endocrinology* **127** 2456–2463

Yonemura Y, Ooyama S, Sugiyama K *et al* (1990) Growth fractions in gastric carcinomas determined with monoclonal antibody Ki-67. *Cancer* **65** 1130–1134

The authors are responsible for the accuracy of the references.

Prostatic Polyamines and Polyamine Targeting as a New Approach to Therapy of Prostatic Cancer

W D W HESTON

Urologic Oncology Research Laboratory, Memorial Sloan-Kettering Cancer Center, New York, New York 10021

INTRODUCTION

Polyamines are polycationic molecules found in all living systems. The human prostate and its secretions are rich in several cations, including zinc, calcium and polyamines. Whereas zinc and calcium are derived from nutritional sources, polyamines are synthesized primarily by the prostatic epithelium. Although structurally simple compared with many organic molecules, their synthesis and function have been the subject of intensive investigation for several decades. Their pathways of formation, degradation and interconversion have been established. As cations, polyamines form ionic bonds with cellular anions, such as the nucleic acid phosphates of DNA and RNA, as well as with cellular phosphoproteins and membrane phospholipids. It is clear that polyamines profoundly affect cell proliferation, yet their precise role remains to be determined. Polyamines also affect embryonic development, cell differentiation and the functioning of several proteins. The involvement of polyamines in cell growth has made them a focus for the development of inhibitors for use as chemotherapeutic agents against parasitic diseases and cancer. The structures of the usual intracellular polyamines are shown in Fig. 1.

Cancer Surveys Volume 11: *Prostate Cancer*
© 1991 Imperial Cancer Research Fund. 0-87969-368-1/91. $3.00 + .00

Putrescine

$$H_3\overset{+}{N}(CH_2)_4\overset{+}{N}H_3$$

Spermidine

$$H_3\overset{+}{N}(CH_2)_3\text{-}\overset{+}{P}utres\overset{+}{c}ine$$

Spermine

$$H_3\overset{+}{N}(CH_2)_3\text{-}\overset{+}{P}utres\overset{+}{c}ine\text{-}(CH_2)_3\overset{+}{N}H_3$$

N^1acetylspermidine

$$H_3C\text{-}\overset{O}{\overset{\|}{C}}\text{-}N\text{-}(CH_2)_3\text{-}\overset{+}{P}utres\overset{+}{c}ine$$

Fig. 1. Structures of the normal intracellular polyamines

HISTORICAL PERSPECTIVE

The prostate and its secretions have played an important part in our understanding of polyamines. The initial identification of a polyamine was made from crystals of spermine phosphate, which became known as Boettcher's crystals. Rosenheim's review (1924) of the discovery and subsequent multiple rediscovery of this substance credits the original discovery to van Leeuwenhoek in 1678. Schreiner in 1878 first identified spermine as a nitrogenous base, but his structural formula proved to be incorrect. Rosenheim (1924) perfected a technique for isolating spermine from the semen and testes. His research group then deduced the correct formula (Dudley *et al*, 1926). Although polyamines are found in all cells, the names given to the most common polyamines (spermidine, spermine) reflect this early history. The other common polyamine, putrescine, got its name from an inaccurate association with decaying tissue. Actually, putrescine has no odour in the salt form that is found at physiological pH. Even as the free base with a pH of 13, its odour, although not pleasant, is distinctly different from that of putrefying decaying dead animals (Russell and Durio, 1978).

A second reason for the importance of the prostate in polyamine biochemistry is that it has one of the highest polyamine concentrations of any tissue (Mann, 1964). Harrison was one of the first to survey human organs for polyamine levels. He found the spermine concentration in immediate postmortem prostate to be 130 mg/100 g, whereas it was 90 mg/100 g in semen, 16 mg/100 g in the pancreas, 5 mg/100 g in the kidney, 1–9 mg/100 g in the testis and 2–11 mg/100 g in the liver. Smaller amounts were identified in the brain, spleen, lung, heart and faeces, and none was detected in the muscle by the methods available at that time (Harrison, 1931). Rosenthal and Tabor (1956) identified differences among human and animal species, with the rat prostate considerably more enriched in polyamine content than that of the dog, and human semen containing substantially more than that of the bull. Indeed, with respect to polyamine content, the rat and human prostates are very similar (Janne *et al*, 1964). Janne and coworkers found polyamine concentrations to be age dependent (Janne *et al*, 1964; Piik *et al*, 1977). Current analytical techniques are able to detect picomolar concentrations of the polyamines (Wagner *et al*, 1982, 1984). However, the original figures generally reflect true organ and species differences. The polyamines can be rapidly formed, interconverted and degraded as required by the needs of the cell. Thus, rather than the static levels of measured polyamines, it is probably the "free" pool of polyamines that is functionally important. High ratios of spermidine to spermine are characteristic of rapidly growing tissues (Janne *et al*, 1964).

POLYAMINE BIOCHEMISTRY AND FUNCTION

Metabolic Pathways

The biosynthetic pathways for the polyamines have been well characterized and the subject of many recent reviews (Pegg, 1988; Heby and Persson, 1990). The biosynthetic and intraconversion pathways of the polyamines are depicted in Fig. 2. The precursor for polyamines in eukaryotic cells is ornithine. Ornithine is generated from arginine by the activity of the enzyme arginase. Although arginase can be considered part of the polyamine biosynthetic pathway, the serum levels of ornithine in most mammals are such that the level of ornithine is not rate limiting for polyamine synthesis. The metabolic pathway for polyamine formation and interconversion is depicted in Fig. 2. The first enzyme in the polyamine biosynthetic pathway is ornithine decarboxylase (ODC; EC 4.1.1.17); ODC acts on ornithine to generate putrescine, N1,N4-diaminobutane, the simplest natural polyamine. This simple aliphatic diamine is fully protonated at physiological pH and therefore has two positive charges. The formation of putrescine is irreversible, and once formed, the activity of the other polyamine synthetic enzymes provides for the sequential formation of spermidine and spermine. Putrescine is converted to spermidine by the action of the aminopropyltransferase spermidine synthase (SPDS; EC 2.5.1.16). Spermidine is converted to spermine by the action of spermine synthase (SPMS; EC 2.5.1.22). Both of these distinct aminopropyltransferases use decarboxylated S-adenosyl-l-methionine as the aminopropyl donor, and each is specific for putrescine (SPDS) and spermidine (SPMS) with respect to their acceptors. The aminopropyl groups are ultimately derived from methionine. The decarboxylated S-adenosylmethionine (dcAdoMet) is produced from S-adenosyl-l-methionine (AdoMet) by the action of the enzyme S-adenosylmethionine decarboxylase (S-AMDC; EC4.1.1.50). The content of dcAdoMet is normally very low and limited by the activity of S-AMDC. The activities of the aminopropyltransferases are thus regulated by the levels of dcAdoMet and the respective acceptor amines. S-AMDC, which produces dcAdoMet, is activated by putrescine (Pegg, 1988).

Polyamines were once thought to be produced and then degraded by

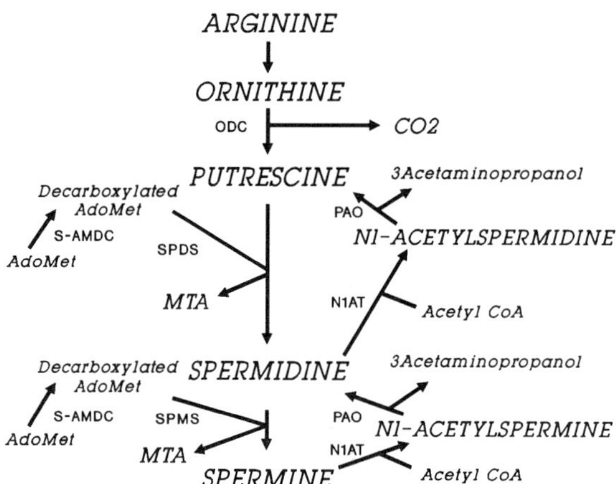

Fig. 2. Flow chart for the metabolic formation and interconversion of polyamines and their respective enzymes (adapted from Pegg, 1988)

amine oxidases, but it was discovered that they are intraconvertible from spermine back to putrescine. This is accomplished by the action of two enzymes. Firstly, spermine or spermidine is acetylated by an acetylase that is specific for the n-propylamine groups of spermidine and spermine, spermidine/spermine N1 acetyltransferase (N1AT). The acetylated spermidine or spermine is then acted upon by a flavin dinucleotide dependent polyamine oxidase (PAO) (see Fig. 2). The product of the N1AT/PAO interaction is the polyamine minus one n-propylamine group, ie spermine becomes spermidine and spermidine becomes putrescine, with the n-propylamine group function appearing as a 3-acetamidopropanal moiety (Fig. 2). Thus, a cycle can occur in which active intracellular cycling of the polyamines can occur without a net change in the concentration of polyamine but with the generation of methylthioadenosine from dcAdoMet and generation of potentially reactive aldehyde groups associated with the 3-acetamidopropanal and hydrogen peroxide (Pegg, 1988).

These pathways (Fig. 3) are controlled mainly by the availability of the three key enzymes ODC, S-AMDC and N1AT. Each of these enzymes is usually present in vanishingly small concentrations in adult tissues, an exception being the prostate, where in the normal adult man or male rat, high polyamine biosynthetic activity of ODC and S-AMDC is associated with high secretory activity and polyamine content is associated with the glandular secretions.

The three important regulatory enzymes in the polyamine synthetic pathway, ODC, S-AMDC and N1AT, have short half lives, being 1 hour or less in most cells (Pegg, 1988; Heby and Persson, 1990). Their synthesis is readily induced by a number of stimuli to the cell and can be the result of an increase in transcription or translation or both. The activity of ODC is increased by decreased intracellular spermidine and spermine content and decreased by increased intracellular spermidine and spermine content. Putrescine seems not

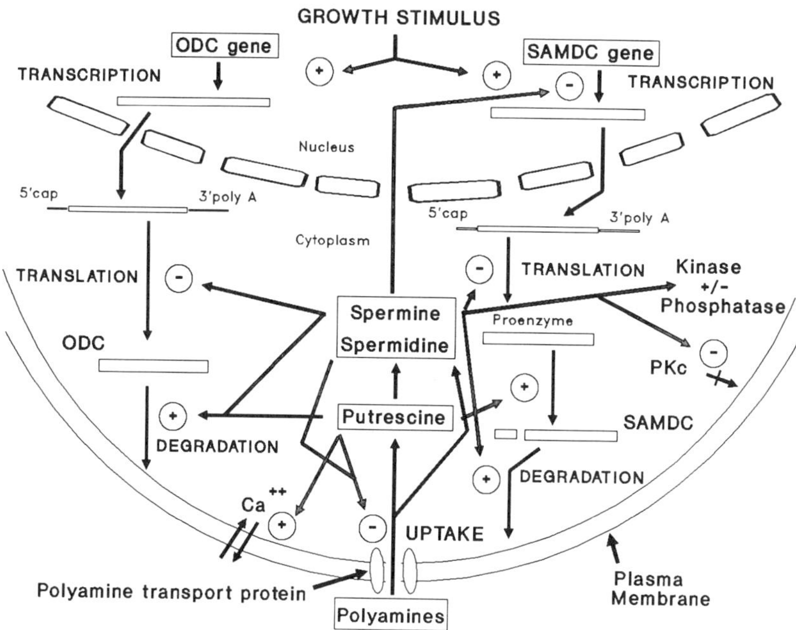

Fig. 3. Intracellular pathways for polyamine regulation (modified from Heby and Persson, 1990)

to play a part in the intracellular regulation of ODC activity at the level of transcription or translation. Putrescine and other diamines do have a role in stimulating the increased production of an intracellular protein termed "antizyme", which binds to and inactivates the enzymatic activity of ODC (Heller and Canellakis, 1981). Although ODC can be posttranslationally modified by phosphorylation, it remains unclear how phosphorylation affects its activity (Pegg, 1988). Still, posttranslational actions appear to play a part in ODC expression. Spermidine and spermine decrease translation of S-AMDC. Putrescine converts precursor S-AMDC to S-AMDC. Putrescine also acts on S-AMDC directly to increase its enzymatic activity (Pegg, 1988). N1AT is induced manyfold by the administration of spermidine or spermine. Putrescine is ineffective, as the induction requires an n-propylamine group and putrescine is a butyldiamine. With N1AT, the increased rate of protein production results from both an increased rate of synthesis and a decreased rate of degradation. In terms of protein degradation, both ODC and S-AMDC have sequences corresponding to "PEST regions" associated with rapid protein turnover (Pegg, 1988; Heby and Persson, 1990).

In humans, ODC genes reside on chromosomes 2 and 7. The ODC message on chromosome 2 resides near the message for the N-*myc* gene. The M2 subunit of ribonucleotide reductase is also localized on the short arm of chromosome 2 and has been found to be co-amplified in cells selected for resistance to hydroxyurea (Heby and Persson, 1990). The leader sequences of ODC mRNA are unusual in that they are very long (300 nucleotides in length) and extremely rich in GC content. In mitogenic induction of ODC, nuclear runoff transcriptional analysis can account for the increase in mRNA, whereas the androgen induction of ODC activity in mouse kidney results in a combination of increased transcription and mRNA processing and/or turnover (Heby and Persson, 1990). S-AMDC sequences have been found on human chromosomes 6 and X (Heby and Persson, 1990). Whether both are active or one is a pseudogene is not known. Like ODC, the mRNA leader sequence is GC rich and forms stable secondary structures. ODC is a typical pyridoxal phosphate requiring decarboxylase. S-AMDC, on the other hand, is unique in that its active moiety is a pyruvate group.

Inhibitors of Polyamine Metabolism

The characterization of the various enzyme activities involved in the synthesis of the polyamines and the apparent importance of polyamines in cell growth have enabled inhibitors selective for the various enzymes to be synthesized (Porter and Sufrin, 1986; Pegg, 1988). The problem with trying to inhibit the key regulatory polyamine biosynthetic enzymes is their rapid inducibility and high turnover rate. They also tend to become stabilized and protected from degradation in the presence of inhibitors, so that competitive inhibitors of their activity become readily circumvented by the increased level of enzyme activity. The development of mechanism based inhibitors or "suicide substrates" allowed the development of polyamine synthesis inhibitors with the potential to be therapeutically active. These inhibitors are inactive until the enzyme transforms them as it acts on them as potential substrates and generates a reactive species that irreversibly inactivates the enzyme. A number of compounds that are suicide substrates of ODC have been synthesized, and these include α-difluoromethylornithine (DFMO, eflornithine), (E)-α-fluoro-methyl-dehydro-ornithine methyl ester and (R)-α-ethynyl-(R)-γ-methyl-putrescine. The most studied of these inhibitors of ODC is DFMO (Pegg, 1988). Treatment with DFMO eliminates the cell's ability to make polyamines from ornithine. As cells divide in the presence of DFMO, their content of polyamines drops. The first polyamines to be depleted are putrescine and spermidine. The last polyamine to be depleted is spermine (Pegg, 1988). As expected, without putrescine to serve as a polyamine substrate for the n-propylamine groups provided by S-AMDC for spermidine synthase, there is a build up of dcAdoMet. Depletion of a cell's spermidine pool leads to its loss of ability to progress through the cell cycle.

Inhibitors of S-AMDC have also been synthesized. Methylglyoxal bis(guanylhydrazone) (MGBG) is the classic inhibitor, which served as the basis for development of a number of structural analogues. None of these proved specific, and most inhibited a number of other enzyme systems as well. S-(5′-Deoxy-5′-adenosyl) methylthioethyl hydroxylamine is an irreversible inhibitor (Pegg, 1988). Treatment with this inhibitor and structurally similar inhibitors synthesized by Secrist leads to a reduction of spermidine and spermine and dcAdoMet, with a tremendous accumulation of putrescine. Cell growth is inhibited as spermidine becomes depleted and is restored with addition of exogenous spermidine. This is consistent with the hypothesis that spermidine, but not putrescine, is the polyamine required for cell growth. Specificity of inhibition of spermidine synthase and spermine synthase has been achieved with the multisubstrate adduct inhibitors ADODATO and ADODATAD, respectively, synthesized by Coward (Coward and Pegg, 1987). Specific inhibitors of N1AT are being developed; however, the polyamine oxidase that utilizes the acetylated polyamine as substrate to generate the smaller polyamine is inhibited potently and selectively by agents such as N1,N4-bis-(2,3-butanedienyl)-1,4-butandiamine (MDL72527) (Claverie *et al*, 1987). This agent prevents the interconversion of polyamines without interfering with their acetylation. MDL72527 also allows the importance of polyamine interconversion in the growth and maintenance of cell function to be determined.

Polyamine Function

Intense interest has been focused on the activity of these enzymes, because polyamine synthesis is tightly regulated in concert with cell growth. Also, anything that causes a cell to increase its metabolic activity, such as mitogens and carcinogens, will often yield an increase in ODC, S-AMDC and N1AT activity. Because of the close association between cell proliferation and polyamine synthesis, it was expected that ODC would turn out to be an oncogene. Such has not proven to be the case, and the overexpression of ODC has not produced cellular transformation. What did become apparent, however, was that overexpression of ODC in transformed cells can confer a growth advantage. With mouse myeloma and leukaemia cell lines that were selected for ODC overproduction, the cloning efficiency in soft agar of the ODC overproducers was dramatically increased (Polvinen *et al*, 1988). Parental L1210 cells yielded 13 colonies per 700 cells plated, and the ODC overproducers L1210/10DC produced 439 colonies per 700 plated cells. Parental X63 myeloma cells produced 0 colonies per 1000 cells plated, whereas the X63/20D ODC overproducer yielded 17 colonies per 1000 cells (Polvinen *et al*, 1988). These investigators have observed that, in vivo, ODC overproducer carcinoma cells are also more aggressive (Alhonen-Hongisto, 1985). Polyamine production may produce a growth advantage in increases of the clonogenic potential of the cell even in highly malignant cells.

In carcinogen transformed cells, it appears that a common property of tumour promoters is induction of ODC and that the resulting increase in putrescine is critical for the induction of tumours (Nakadate *et al*, 1985; Verma and Boutwell, 1987). Inhibition of tumour formation can be brought about by inhibition of ODC, often by lower concentrations of inhibitor than are required to inhibit the growth of established tumours (Malt *et al*, 1985; Manni and Wright, 1986; Thompson *et al*, 1986).

Although polyamines appear necessary for cell growth and tumour promotion, the exact mechanism of action is unknown. As they are positively charged cations at physiological pH, they bond ionically with a large number of cellular anions, such as DNA and RNA, membrane phospholipids and phosphoproteins. In each instance, this interaction can result in an alteration of the functional activity of the anion. The template activity of DNA can be reduced, RNA translation rates increased or decreased depending on the mRNA, membrane fluidity altered and the activity of phosphoproteins, phosphokinases and phosphatases increased or decreased (Tung *et al*, 1985; Ahmed *et al*, 1986; Pegg and McCann, 1988; Celano *et al*, 1989; Schuber, 1989). For example, Celano *et al* (1989) have demonstrated that polyamines differentially modulate the transcription of growth associated genes such as *myc* and *fos* relative to other genes, supporting the hypothesis that this may be one mechanism by which polyamines modulate growth. Still, because of the ionic nature of these interactions, it is difficult to ascertain the extent to which these operate intracellularly. The parameter most sensitive to polyamine depletion appears to be protein synthesis (Pegg and McCann, 1988). Protein synthesis is often depressed with polyamine depletion. Further polyamines become incorporated in the protein initiation complex eIF-4D and become part of the modified unique aminoacid hypusine of eIF-4D (Cooper *et al*, 1983).

Because of the amine functional groups on the polyamines, they are involved in cross linking reactions through the activity of transglutaminases. In psoriasis, an abnormal growth condition associated with increased polyamine synthesis, N1,N8-bis(γ-glutamyl) spermidine cross linking in epidermal cell envelopes has been shown to be increased relative to that of the normal γ-glutamyl-lysine cross links (Martinet *et al*, 1990). Often, the activity of the polyamines in these interactions is proportional to their charges. Spermine is often more effective than spermidine, which is more active than putrescine. Spermine strongly inhibits the activity of protein kinase C by blocking its translocation to the cell membrane. Spermidine is much less active, and putrescine is almost without effect (Moruzzi *et al*, 1987, 1990). Similarly, spermine has activity as a calcium independent antagonist of calmodulin. Spermine is nearly 100 times more active as an antagonist than spermidine, and putrescine has negligible activity (Walters and Johnson, 1988). Spermine, but not spermidine nor putrescine, has also been found to bind to the neuronal glycine site associated with the N-methyl-D-aspartate receptor complex (Sacaan and Johnson, 1989). Polyamines also affect the activity of other cations. An early effect of testosterone stimulation of kidney cells is the formation of polyamines and a subsequent alteration of calcium fluxes at the cell membrane (Koenig *et al*, 1983). These investigators found dramatic ODC increases within seconds in the kidney cortex in response to exogenous testosterone both in vivo and in vitro. This resulted in increases in putrescine and the other polyamines and was followed by changes in calcium fluxes and subsequent membrane transport processes such as hexose and aminoacid transport. The calcium fluxes and transport changes could be inhibited by ODC inhibition with DFMO and restored by putrescine. This activity of polyamines at the cell membrane is further accentuated by the ability of exogenously added putrescine to reverse the growth inhibition of interleukin-1 (IL-1) of A375 human melanoma cells, to enhance IL-1 stimulated growth of the D10.G4.1 helper T cell line and to reverse the growth inhibitory activity of tamoxifen on carcinogen induced mammary tumours (Manni and Wright, 1984; Endo *et al*, 1988).

Because high ODC activity is associated with growth, it is often observed that the tissues of the fetus and newborn are higher in ODC activity than are those of the adult. ODC activity has also been observed to be higher in tumours than in adjacent normal tissue. Heston *et al* (1982) observed a positive correlation between the activity of ODC and the growth rate of the Dunning prostatic tumour variants, as seen in Table 1.

Table 1 shows that ODC activity in the slow growing well differentiated, androgen sensitive tumour is higher than that of the normal dorsal prostate, which is the prostatic lobe of origin of the Dunning tumour. This is in keeping with the observation that activity in tumour tissue is often greater than that of normal tissue. In the rat, the dorsal lobe of the prostate is one of intermediate ODC activity and is thought to represent an activity more closely related to DNA synthetic activity. This contrasts with the lobe of the highest ODC activity, the ventral prostate, in which activity may be more associated with secretory activity (Fuller *et al*, 1975). The ODC activity of the normal ventral prostate is nearly ten times greater than that of the dorsal lobe. The activity in the dorsal lobe is in turn greater than that found in most other adult tissues. As the tumour progresses from slow hormone sensitive growth to anaplastic rapid growth, the ODC levels change and correlate with the increased growth rate. The R-3327-AT and MAT-LU tumours have very short doubling times and have nearly 20 times the ODC activity of the R-3327-H tumour. The R-3327-AT and R-3327-MAT-LU tumours are anaplastic hormone insensitive tumours.

Another characteristic of the prostate is the sensitivity of its ODC activity to inhibition by DFMO in vivo relative to other tissues (Danzin *et al*, 1979a,b). At every dose, DFMO inhibited the activity of prostatic ODC to a greater extent than the ODC activity found in other tissues. The amount of DFMO in the prostate did not differ from that in other tissues. In the intact male rat, DFMO administration also resulted in a more rapid polyamine depletion in the prostate relative to other tissues. In the castrated rat, androgen induced restoration of the gland was inhibited by DFMO, but the inhibition was characterized by reduced RNA content and protein secretions but not reduced DNA content (Danzin *et al*, 1979a,b). Without putrescine and spermidine to serve as substrates for spermidine and spermine synthase, there is a dramatic increase in intracellular dcAdoMet, rising from 1 to 888 nmol/g wet weight in 3 days in the ventral prostate (Wagner *et al*, 1982). (E)-α-(fluoromethyl) dehydro-ornithine methyl ester is a more potent enzyme activated irreversible inhibitor of ODC than DFMO, and it appears to be more able to enter cells than DFMO. Its effect is also more pronounced and its inhibition of ODC

TABLE 1. Association between tumour doubling time and ODC activity in Dunning R-3327 prostate derived tumors

Tissue	Doubling time (days)	ODC activity[a] (mean ± SEM)
R-3227-AT	2	4920 ± 510
R-3327-MAT-Lu	2	4610 ± 470
R-3327-HIF	5	480 ± 60
R-3327-H	23	240 ± 20
Dorsal prostate	–	110 ± 15

[a]ODC activity values represent mean picomoles of $^{14}CO_2$ released from ^{14}C-carboxyl-L-ornithine per hr/mg protein at room temperature. There were ten controls and ten tumours per group

more prolonged in the prostate than in most other tissues (Mamont *et al,* 1986). Prostatic ODC activity seems to be more sensitive to inhibition. In the Dunning series of prostate derived tumours, when DFMO is administered intraperitoneally at a dose of 100 mg/kg and various tissues assayed for remaining ODC activity 3 hours later, this activity was decreased by 90% in the prostate, whereas in most other tissues, it has fallen by only 10%. The ODC activity of prostate derived tumours was also reduced by 90%. However, if high doses of DFMO are administered to a rat bearing a prostate tumour and the growth of the tumour is measured over time, one observes a slowing of growth, but not as dramatic as one would expect, given the degree of inhibition of ODC (Heston *et al,* 1982). In vivo, this is probably the result of the very active transport by the prostate of polyamines from the serum. In vitro, the prostatic cell lines are very sensitive to growth inhibition by DFMO; yet, if polyamines are added to the medium, the inhibition is overcome. In vivo, the serum contains polyamines from nutritional and non-suppressed metabolic sources. Therefore, it will be more difficult to inhibit growth in vivo because the cells can use these serum polyamines to bypass the blockade of ODC. This can be used to advantage, since polyamine depleted cells will take up an increased amount of polyamines from external sources.

POLYAMINE TRANSPORT AND THERAPY

Transport Characteristics

It is well known that all cells will take up polyamines from the extracellular fluid. Because of the highly charged nature of the polyamines, their translocation across the cell membrane into the cell requires a transport protein. This is reported to be an energy requiring active transport process. A problem in distinguishing active transport from a facilitated diffusion mechanism resides in the aspect that the polyamines are probably not free in solution inside the cell, but bound. This would effectively serve to drive the uptake and give the appearance of active transport (Kashiwagi *et al,* 1986). Still, it has been reported

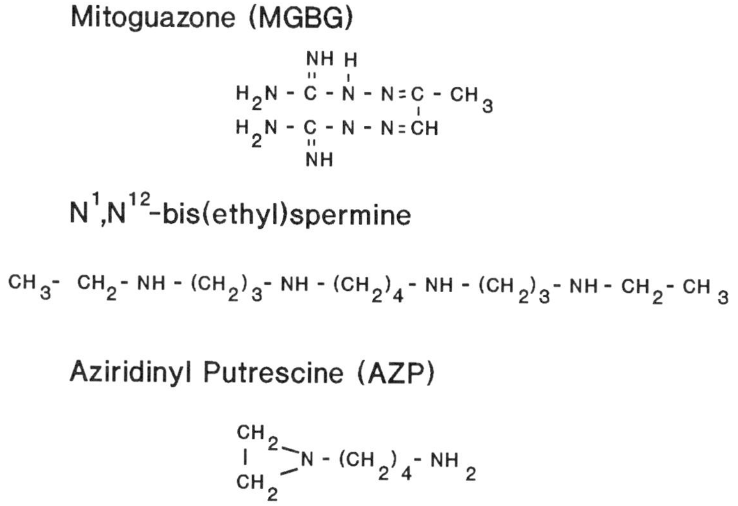

Mitoguazone (MGBG)

$$H_2N-\overset{\overset{\displaystyle NH}{\|}}{C}-\overset{\overset{\displaystyle H}{|}}{N}-N=\overset{\overset{\displaystyle }{|}}{C}-CH_3$$
$$H_2N-\underset{\underset{\displaystyle NH}{\|}}{C}-N-N=CH$$

N^1,N^{12}-bis(ethyl)spermine

$$CH_3-CH_2-NH-(CH_2)_3-NH-(CH_2)_4-NH-(CH_2)_3-NH-CH_2-CH_3$$

Aziridinyl Putrescine (AZP)

$$\begin{array}{c} CH_2 \\ | \diagdown \\ N-(CH_2)_4-NH_2 \\ | \diagup \\ CH_2 \end{array}$$

Fig. 4. Structures of cytostatic (bis-ethylspermine) or cytotoxic agents (MGBG, AZP) that utilize the polyamine transporter

that depletion of cellular energy sources or disruption of membrane potential will reduce transport, consistent with an active transport process.

The early papers characterizing the polyamine transporter focused not on polyamines but on the cytotoxic chemotherapeutic agent methylglyoxal-bis-guanylhydrazone (MGBG) (Fig. 4). Block and colleagues (Block *et al*, 1964; Field *et al*, 1964) observed what has since been identified in all eukaryotic cells, a temperature dependent, energy requiring saturable transport system with, at high concentrations, a non-saturable diffusion component that was dependent on a potential gradient. All cells appeared to have this transport system except for cells that were metabolically quiescent. Because of the charged character of MGBG, these authors examined a number of structurally related charged compounds and found that the polyamines were competitive inhibitors and surmised that they shared the same transporter (Field *et al*, 1964). MGBG has been found to affect many polyamine related systems, being a potent inhibitor of S-AMDC. Structurally, MGBG has been considered similar to spermidine. Clinically, MGBG was an effective agent against acute myelogenous leukaemia but was substantially toxic and has been replaced by other agents. It did serve to demonstrate that the polyamine transporter could be used as a vector for delivering toxic compounds to the cell.

Recently, papers have begun to define further and characterize this transporter. Many of the parameters of polyamine transport were described by Rinehart and Chen (1984). Utilizing the NB-15 mouse neuroblastoma cell line, these investigators observed that putrescine uptake was sodium dependent and that iso-osmotic replacement of sodium with either choline or lithium resulted in a linear decrease in uptake. The channel former gramicidin abolished uptake. Parachloromercuribenzene sulphonate and n-ethylmaleimide abolished uptake, and glutathione and 5,5′-dithiobis-(2-nitrobenzoic acid) stimulated uptake. This established a sulphydryl sensitivity of the transporter. Cells grown in the absence of aminoacids and then fed various aminoacids demonstrated that aminoacids which utilized the sodium dependent transport system A stimulated putrescine uptake nearly tenfold. This was not by a cotransport or countertransport mechanism but appeared to be the result of activating the sodium requiring mechanism. Although this study emphasized the Na^+ requiring aspect of putrescine, other studies have purported to show sodium requirement differences in the the polyamine transport process for the various polyamines. Some studies suggest that spermidine and spermine may be transported in a sodium independent process (Feige and Chambaz, 1985; Nicolet *et al*, 1990; Parys *et al*, 1990). Explanations for the differential sodium transport can be raised. It may be that there are different transporters or it may be the same receptor but coupled differently, as noted previously for sodium dependent and sodium independent polyamine transport processes. We observed that the transport of putrescine in PC-3 prostatic cancer cells in vitro was inhibited by calmodulin antagonists (Heston and Charles, 1988). Thus, calmodulin may have a role in the sodium dependent or apparent differential aspects of the observed uptake. The ability of the transporter to undergo phosphorylation and dephosphorylation may also be involved, for we have found that the phosphatase inhibitor okadaic acid inhibits polyamine transport (Heston WDW, unpublished observations).

Aminoacids, sugars, nucleic acids and other agents that utilize transport systems to enter the cell do not compete for or affect polyamine transport. Nearly identical observations have been observed in other cell systems (Gawel-Thompson and Greene, 1988). When the NB-25 neuroblastoma cells were induced to differentiate, it was observed that polyamine transport was dramatically decreased, whereas transport of the aminoacid aminoisobutyric acid was not affected (Chen and Rinehart, 1981).

The structural requirements for polyamine uptake have been examined. The basic structure consists of at least a diamine separated by four carbon atom lengths (Heston *et al*, 1984). Interest in the structural requirements for polyamine transport has been spurred by the finding that the quaternary bipyridyl herbicides of the paraquat (methyl viologen) family are toxic to the lung, and accidental poisonings have been reported. Paraquat has been reported to utilize the polyamine transporter for its uptake into lung cells (Ross and Krieger, 1981; Gordonsmith *et al*, 1983; Saunders *et al*, 1987; Wyatt, 1988). In the lung, the alveolar type one and two epithelial cells and Clara cells were found to accumulate paraquat and oligoamines (Wyatt *et al*, 1988). It was hoped that a polyamine like compound would be able to block the uptake of paraquat and prevent its toxicity. This hope has yet to be realized (Dunbar *et al*, 1988). These studies helped to identify characteristics of the polyamine for the polyamine transporter in terms of competition for uptake. Maximum uptake or inhibition of polyamine uptake required at least two positively charged groups spaced a minimum of four carbons apart as diaminopropane was substantially less effective than putrescine. Anything that would reduce the positive charge of the amine reduced the ability of the compound to interact with the transporter. In these studies, the ability of the compound to inhibit polyamine transport was studied rather than the utilization of the transporter for entry into the cell.

Following the earlier approach of Israel and to approach more exactly the structure associated with the normal polyamines, Bergeron and colleagues have synthesized an exceedingly large number of oliogoamine derivatives of the normal polyamines spermidine and spermine and tested them for their ability to use the polyamine transporter and to alter intracellular polyamine pools and substitute for polyamine functions (Israel *et al*, 1964; Porter and Bergeron, 1983; Porter and Sufrin, 1986; Bergeron *et al*, 1988, 1989). If the terminal amines were modified by acylation, which eliminated their charge function, their affinity and utilization of the transporter were dramatically reduced. However, the central nitrogens of spermidine and spermine could be modified to carry fairly bulky groups and still utilize the transporter. Bis ethyl derivatives of the end terminal nitrogens used the transporter for cellular uptake. These compounds, like polyamines, decreased the activity of ODC and S-AMDC. As with spermidine and spermine, uptake of these compounds by the cell also further reduces polyamine transport. Unlike the normal polyamines, they did not subserve the mitogenic function, and cell growth was decreased in their presence. Growth inhibition appeared to be reversible, and these compounds are considered to be cytostatic.

Agents that stimulate cellular activity, especially mitogens, will usually increase polyamine uptake. These include epidermal growth factor stimulation of fibroblasts and embryonic palate mesenchymal cells (Dipasquale *et al*, 1978; Gawel-Thompson and Greene, 1989), corticotrophin stimulation of adrenocortical cells. (Feige and Chambaz, 1985), concanavalin A stimulation of lymphocytes (Kakinuma *et al*, 1988), serum stimulation of the basolateral surface of colon carcinoma cells or fibroblasts (Pohjanpelto, 1976; McCormack and Johnson, 1989), insulin and prolactin stimulation of mammary tissue (Kano and Oka, 1976) and testosterone stimulation of the prostate (Kadmon *et al*, 1982; Kapyaho *et al*, 1984). Abnormal growth control and abnormal growth factor production are often associated with transformation of cells. This is also the case with putrescine uptake following transformation. Putrescine uptake no longer responded to cell confluence with a decrease in polyamine transport, and it became less responsive to serum stimulation (Bethell and Pegg, 1981). Transfection of cells with different oncogenes also differentially altered polyamine transport (Chang *et al*, 1988).

The ability of cells to take up toxic MGBG with a transporter was used to generate polyamine transporter deficient cells (Heaton and Flintoff, 1988). These cells have been used for transfection with human DNA from colon carcinoma cells (Byers *et al*, 1989). Selection for cells expressing human polyamine transporter was accomplished in the presence of DFMO and polyamines because mutants lacking polyamine transport, being unable to use exogenous putrescine, cannot grow in the presence of DFMO. A number of clones were identified that differed in their transport characteristics, suggesting that multiple transporters may be involved (Byers *et al*, 1987, 1989). DFMO increased the level of transport activity, which decreases with the uptake of exogenous polyamines but does not decline in activity with MGBG uptake (Byers and Pegg, 1990). In addition, novel polyamine like derivatives have been identified, such as bis(benzyl)polyamine analogues, which appear to use a mechanism different from the polyamine transporter for cellular uptake (Byers, 1990). The identification of these clones by their *Alu* containing human sequences is proceeding and is expected to reveal the nature and genetic identification of the proteins involved in polyamine transport.

Transport Targeted Therapy

MGBG has been tested as a single agent in the treatment of prostatic cancer, and it appears to have minimal activity (Scher *et al*, 1985). Interest in this agent continued because of the observation by Herr *et al* (1984) that animals bearing the Dunning R-3327G tumour that received a combination of DFMO and MGBG exhibited a synergistic response, complete tumour regression being frequently observed. This was accomplished at a very toxic dose level of MGBG, with the lethal toxicity reduced in the group receiving both DFMO and MGBG; DFMO and MGBG also slowed the growth of human prostatic xenografts PC-93 and PC-82 (Romijn *et al*, 1984). However, a recent trial of MGBG and DFMO in human androgen refractory prostatic cancer has been disappointing (Scher HI, unpublished observations). The concentration of MGBG was less in the combination trial than in its trial as a single agent. Also, measurements of tissue parameter of polyamines suggested that at the tissue level, polyamine parameters had not been altered by the therapy (Scher HI, unpublished observations).

There are many possibilities as to why DFMO and MGBG were not effective. One possible explanation is that the prostate has a very active polyamine transporter and DFMO was not effective in suppressing intracellular polyamine levels because of increased uptake of serum polyamines. This has been encountered in model systems. Persson *et al* (1988) have demonstrated that suppression of ODC by DFMO will not cure an animal of L1210 leukaemia in vivo even though it can totally suppress tumour growth in vitro. A mutant of L1210 that lacks the polyamine transporter is cured by DFMO in vivo, suggesting the critical aspect of exogenous source of polyamines in rescuing the tumour (Persson *et al*, 1988). This possibility is further supported by the observation by Seiler *et al* (1990) that a diet deficient in polyamines, but containing antibiotics to rid the colon of polyamine producing bacteria and a polyamine oxidase inhibitor to block the ability of intracellular polyamines to be recycled, increased the activity of polyamine depletion therapy by DFMO.

Our group was not convinced that MGBG like (spermidine like) compounds were the best agents to use in prostatic cancer. This was based on the initial observation of the findings of Clark and Fair (1975). They observed that putrescine injected intravenously tended to localize to the prostate to a greater degree (Clark and Fair, 1975). This was a modest difference in uptake but different enough for visualization using the radiolocalization detection methodologies of positron emission transaxial tomography (PET) (Welch *et al*, 1977; Fair *et al*, 1978). We and others had observed in vitro that depletion of intracellular polyamines with DFMO resulted in increased uptake of polyamines from the extracellular space (Alhonen-Hongisto *et al*, 1980; Heston *et al*, 1984; Porter and Sufrin, 1986; Pegg and McCann, 1988b). Because it appeared that the prostate was especially sensitive to the action of DFMO, we treated castrate and non-castrate males with the androgen dihydrotestosterone propionate (DHTP) with and without pretreatment with DFMO. The combination of DHTP and DFMO dramatically increased the amount of putrescine taken up by the prostate relative to other tissues following an intravenous injection (Kadmon *et al*, 1982). This was also true of the Dunning R-3327-H tumour, whether non-castrate or castrate animals were used and whether exposed to oestrogen treatment or not (Kadmon *et al*, 1985b; Heston and Kadmon, 1986). In this instance, the tumour without any pretreatment tended to have a higher uptake in the castrate animals than the normal prostate.

We examined the nature of the ability of DFMO to increase the uptake of the various polyamines, such as ethylenediamine; 1,4 diaminobutane (putrescine); 1,5-diaminopentane (cadaverine); spermidine; spermine and MGBG. We observed differential tissue uptake of the different polyamines, suggestive of different transporters (Heston *et al*, 1984). Kidney and intestine had high uptake activity of all the polyamines, and the uptake activity during this brief exposure to DFMO was not stimulated. Liver had low uptake activity of all the polyamines except MGBG, and DFMO treatment did not increase uptake into the liver. DFMO stimulated uptake of MGBG into the kidney and minimally into the androgen stimulated ventral prostate but not into the dorsal prostate. The most dramatic stimulation of polyamine uptake by DFMO occurred with the diamine putrescine in the prostate and in the R-3327-MAT-LU androgen independent prostate derived tumour. This suggested that, in vivo, the prostate may be susceptible to manipulation in terms of putrescine, or diamine, targeting or imaging. This uptake was saturable in vivo, which is consistent with a membrane transport system (Kadmon D, unpublished observations). The diamine cadaverine was also shown to be retained in the prostate. It had been observed in other systems that putrescine could be metabolized to γ-aminobutyric acid, which is also concentrated by a transport system. To determine whether this was operating in the prostate, we administered aminoguanidine (AMG) to the animals before giving the radioactively labelled putrescine. Aminoguanidine thoroughly eliminates the metabolism of putrescine to γ-aminobutyric acid. The results on the effect of AMG on putrescine uptake are shown in Table 2 (Kadmon *et al*, 1985a). Similar findings were observed with the Dunning R-3327-H tumour.

TABLE 2. Effect of polyamine depletion and androgen stimulation of the castrated rat on the retention of putrescine by the prostate

Treatment[a]	Putrescine uptake ratio[b] (mean ± SEM)
Castrated control	3.3+/−0.4
+DHTP	3.5+/−0.6
+DFMO	4.0+/−0.5
+AMG	4.2+/−0.5
+DHTP and DFMO	18.5+/−3.2
+DHTP and DFMO and AMG	83.6+/−12.6

[a]Animals were castrated, and after 7 days, they received the androgen DHTP 2 mg per rat subcutaneously per day for 3 days, or DFMO 2% (an irreversible inhibitor of ODC) in the drinking water for 3 days or both, or AMG (an inhibitor of diamine oxidase) 1 hr before the injection of ^{14}C-labelled putrescine or all three and assayed for putrescine uptake, 3 hr after putrescine injection
[b]Uptake relative to skeletal muscle

Previous work examining the potential toxicity of Nylon-66 demonstrated that the diamine 1,6 hexane-diamine also accumulated in the prostate. If it is eventually established that there are different polyamine transport proteins, then it may be that the prostate has a diamine preferring form. Kadmon and colleagues have continued the development of a positron emitting putrescine and have observed that 18F-propylputrescine behaves like putrescine (Kadmon D, personal communication). 19F-Fluorinated polyamines may prove useful for studying intracellular polyamine function and metabolism by conventional means and by magnetic resonance imaging, but the fluorine atom if in close proximity to the end amines tends to reduce the positively charged character of the polyamine, which reduces its utilization of the transporter for uptake into the cell (Danzin *et al*, 1982; Baillon *et al*, 1988; Seiler *et al*, 1988).

Because of the apparent ability of the prostate to accumulate putrescine to a greater extent than other tissues, and this accumulation could be increased dramatically by DFMO pretreatment, we were encouraged to develop putrescine based toxins.

In the literature, we found that monoaziridinylputrescine (AZP) (Fig. 4) had been synthesized as a precursor used for the synthesis of anti-irradiation compounds (Piper *et al*, 1969). It had not yet been tested for toxicity. It represented a minimal change in the molecule, which could possess both transport utilizing capability and alkylating (toxin) capability. We tested it in vitro against the PC-3 prostatic cancer cell line. This cell line is androgen independent and was derived from a bony metastatic deposit. We found that it was a competitve inhibitor of polyamine uptake with a K_I less than that of the K_m of putrescine and that DFMO pretreatment increased the accumulation of AZP by the cell (Heston *et al*, 1987b). It was cytotoxic towards the cell and the cytotoxicity was dose and time dependent. Its cytotoxicity was synergistically increased with DFMO pretreatment as can be seen in Table 3 (Heston *et al*, 1987b).

TABLE 3. Effect of AZP on the growth of PC-3 cells with or without DFMO pretreatment

Treatment[a]	Cell number (mean x 10^4 ± SEM)
Control	414+/−17
DFMO	360+/−10
AZP	123+/−10
DFMO+AZP	7+/−0.2

[a]Thirty-thousand PC-3 cells were plated and allowed to attach to the petri dish overnight. The following day, the medium was aspirated and replaced with RPMI 1640, 10% FCS, 100 μM aminoguanidine with or without 1 mM DFMO. Forty eight hours later, the medium was aspirated, and the cells were rinsed with Hanks' balanced salt solution (HBSS) and exposed to aziridinylputrescine (AZP) or solvent (H_2O) for 1 hr at 37°C, in the above mentioned RPMI medium. After 1 hr, the medium was aspirated, the cells were rinsed with HBSS, and fresh RPMI that did not contain the AMG was added. Six days following exposure to AZP, the cells were lifted from the plate by gentle trypsinization and enumerated by counting of Trypan blue excluding cells with the aid of a haemocytometer

As cytotoxicity of alkylating agents increases dramatically when increased from a monofunctional to a difunctional alkylating moiety, we synthesized N1,N4-diaziridinyl putrescine. It was a very weak inhibitor of polyamine transport and did not have its cytotoxic activity increased by DFMO pretreatment(Heston *et al*, 1987a). Similarly, when we investigated the ability of N1,N4-diethylputrescine to compete for the transporter, it was greatly reduced relative to putrescine or even N1,N1-diethylputrescine. This suggests that with the small putrescine molecule, modification of both aminofunctional groups will reduce its ability to utilize the polyamine transporter. Keeping this in mind, we are currently attempting to synthesize N1,N1-dichloro-ethylputrescine to serve as the bifunctional alkylating agent.

SUMMARY

The prostate is a rich factory of polyamine production. In spite of this, the prostate is also able to accumulate polyamines from the circulation. Intracellular polyamine depletion has been observed to enhance the accumulation of diamines such as putrescine. This needs to be taken advantage of either as a means for imaging prostatic tumour spread to the lymph nodes or as a means of targeting toxins to the prostatic tumour. Putrescine is a small molecule that may prove difficult for use for synthesizing stable toxin derivatives that can take advantage of the targeting potential of the polyamine transporter. The cloning and sequencing characterization of the transporter is under way. When the prostatic transporter is identified, it will be possible to understand the role of the transporter in normal and cancerous prostatic cell growth and functioning and should serve to aid our understanding of how we can better optimize agents to use the transporter for delivery of antitumour agents.

Acknowledgements

This work was supported in part by a grant CA-39203 from the National Cancer Institute of the National Institutes of Health.

References

Ahmed K, Goueli SA and Williams-Ashman HG (1986) Mechanisms and significance of polyamine stimulaton of various protein kinase reactions. *Advances in Enzyme Regulation* **25** 401–421

Alhonen-Hongisto L, Seppanan P and Janne J (1980) Intracellular putrescine and spermidine derivation induces increased uptake of the natural polyamines and methylglyoxal bis (guanyl hydrazone). *Biochemical Journal* **192** 941–945

Alhonen-Hongisto L, Kallio A, Sinervita R, Janne OA, Gahmberg CG and Janne J (1985) Tumorigenicity, cell-surface glycoprotein changes and ornithine decarboxylase gene pattern in Ehrlich ascites-carcinoma cells. *Biochemical Journal* **299** 711–715

Baillon JG, Mamont PS, Wagner J, Gerhart F and Lux P (1988) Fluorinated analogues of spermidine as substrates of spermine synthase. *European Journal of Biochemistry* **710** 237–242

Bethell DR and Pegg AE (1981) Uptake of putrescine by 3T3 and SV3T3 cells and its effect on ornithine decarboxylase activity. *Journal of Cellular Physiology* **109** 461–468

Bergeron RJ, Neims AH, McManis JS *et al* (1988) Synthetic polyamines as antineoplastics. *Journal of Medicinal Chemistry* **31** 1183–1190

Bergeron RJ, Hawthorne TR, Vinson RT, Beck DE and Ingeno MJ (1989) Role of methylene backbone in the antiproliferative activity of polyamine analogues on L1210 cells. *Cancer Research* **49** 2959–2964

Block JB, Field M and Oliverio VT (1964) Cellular accumulation of methyl-bis-guanylhydrazone *in vitro*. II. Studies on the mechanism of accumulation in leukemic leukocytes. *Cancer Research* **24** 1947–1951

Byers TL and Pegg AE (1990) Regulation of polyamine transport in Chinese hamster ovary cells. *Journal of Cellular Physiology* **143** 460–467

Byers TL, Kameji R, Rannels DE and Pegg AE (1987) Multiple pathways for uptake of paraquat, methylglyoxal bis- (guanylhydrazone) and polyamines. *American Journal of Physiology* **252** *(Cell Physiology)* C663–C669

Byers TL, Wechter R, Nuttall ME and Pegg AE (1989) Expression of a human gene for polyamine transport in Chinese-hamster ovary cells. *Biochemical Journal* **263** 745–752

Byers TL, Bitonti AJ and McCann PP (1990) Bis(benzyl)polyamine analogues are substrates for a mammalian cell-transport system which is distinct from the polyamine-transport system. *Biochemical Journal* **269** 35–40

Celano P, Baylin SB and Casero RA (1989) Polyamines differentially modulate the transcription of growth associated genes in human colon carcinoma cells. *Journal of Biological Chemistry* **264** 8922–8927

Chang BK, Libby PR, Bergeron RJ and Porter CW (1988) Modulation of polyamine biosynthesis and transport by oncogene transfection. *Biochemical and Biophysical Research Communications* **157** 264–270

Chen KY and Rinehart CA (1981) Difference in putrescine transport in undifferentiated versus differentiated mouse NB-15 neuroblastoma cells. *Biochemical and Biophysical Research Communications* **101** 243–249

Clark RB and Fair WR (1975) The selective *in vivo* incorporation and metabolism of radioactive putrescine in the adult male rat. *Journal of Nuclear Medicine* **16** 337–342

Claverie N, Wagner J, Knodgen B and Seiler N (1987) Inhibition of polyamine oxidase improves the antitumoral effect of ornithine decarboxylase inhibitors. *Anticancer Research* **7** 765–772

Cooper HL, Park MH, Folk JE, Safer B and Braverman R (1983) Identification of the hypusine-containing protein Hy+ as translation initiation factor eIF-4D. *Proceedings of the National Academy of Sciences of the USA* **80** 1854–1857

Coward JK and Pegg AE (1987) Specific multisubstrate adduct inhibitors of aminopropyltransferases and their effect on polyamine synthesis in cultured cells. *Advances in Enzyme Regulation* **26** 107–113

Danzin C, Jung MJ, Claverie N, Grove J, Sjoerdsma A and Koch-Weser J (1979a) Effects of α-difluoromethylornithine, an enzyme-activated irreversible inhibitor of ornithine decarboxylase, on testosterone-induced regeneration of prostate and seminal vesicle in castrated rats. *Biochemical Journal* **180** 507–513

Danzin C, Jung MJ, Grove J, Bey P (1979b) Effect of α-difluoromethylornithine, an enzyme-activated inhibitor of ornithine decarboxylase, on polyamine levels in rat tissues. *Life Sciences* **24** 519–524

Danzin C, Bey P, Schirlin D and Claverie N (1982) α-Monofluoromethyl and α-difluoromethyl putrescine as ornithine decarboxylase inhibitors: *in vitro* and *in vivo* biochemical properties. *Biochemical Pharmacology* **31** 3871–3878

DiPasquale A, White D and McGuire J (1978) Epidermal growth factor stimulates putrescine transport and ornithine decarboxylase activity in cultivated human fibroblasts. *Experimental Cell Research* **116** 317–323

Dudley HW, Rosenheim O and Starling WW (1926) The chemical constitution of spermine. *Biochemical Journal* **20** 1092–1094

Dunbar JR, DeLucia AJ, Acuff RV and Ferslew KE (1988) Prolonged, intravenous paraquat infusion in the rat. *Toxicology and Applied Pharmacology* **94** 221–226

Endo Y, Matsushima K, Onozaki K and Oppenheim JJ (1988) Role of ornithine decarboxylase in the regulation of cell growth by IL-1 and tumor necrosis factor. *Journal of Immunology* **141** 2342–2348

Fair WR, Miller TR, Siegel BA and Welch MJ (1978) Radionuclide imaging of dog prostate. *Urology* **12** 575–578

Feige JJ and Chambaz EM (1985) Polyamine uptake by bovine adrenocortical cells. *Biochimica et Biophysica Acta* **846** 93–100

Field M, Block JB, Oliverio VT and Rall DP (1964) Cellular accumulation of methylglyoxal-bis-guanylhydrazone *in vitro*. *Cancer Research* **24** 1939–1946

Fuller DJM, Donaldson LH and Thomas GH (1975) Ornithine decarboxylase activity and 125^{I}-iododeoxuridine incorporation in rat prostate. *Biochemical Journal* **150** 5570–5572

Gawel-Thompson K and Greene RM (1988) Characterization of a polyamine transport system in murine embryonic palate mesenchymal cells. *Journal of Cellular Physiology* **136** 237–246

Gawel-Thompson K and Greene RM (1989) Epidermal growth factor modulator of murine embryonic palate mesenchymal cell proliferation, polyamine biosynthesis and polyamine transport. *Journal of Cellular Physiology* **140** 359–370

Gordonsmith RH, Brooke-Taylor S, Smith LL and Cohen GM (1983) Structural requirements of compounds to inhibit pulmonary diamine accumulation. *Biochemical Pharmacology* **32** 3701–3709

Harrison GA (1931) Spermine in human testis. *Biochemical Journal* **25** 1885–1892

Heaton MA and Flintoff WF (1988) Methylglyoxal- bis(guanylhydrazone) resistant Chinese hamster ovary cells: genetic evidence that more than a single locus controls uptake. *Journal of Cellular Physiology* **136** 133–139

Heby O and Persson L (1990) Molecular genetics of polyamine synthesis in eukaryotic cells. *Trends in Biochemical Sciences* **15** 153–158

Heller JS and Canellakis ES (1981) Cellular control of ornithine decarboxylase activity by its antizyme. *Journal of Cellular Physiology* **107** 209–217

Herr HW, Kleinert EL, Relyea NM and Whitmore WF (1984) Potentiation of methylglyoxal-bis-guanylhydrazone by alpha-difluoromethylornithine in rat prostate cancer. *Cancer* **53** 1294–1298

Heston WDW and Charles M (1988) Calmodulin antagonist inhibition of polyamine transport in prostatic cancer cells *in vitro*. *Biochemical Pharmacology* **37** 2511–2514

Heston WDW and Kadmon D (1986) Alpha-difluoromethylornithine enhancement of ^{14}C-putrescine uptake by an androgen-dependent prostatic tumor. *Journal of Urology* **136** 944–948

Heston WDW, Kadmon D, Lazan DW and Fair WR (1982) Copenhagen rat prostatic tumor ornithine decarboxylase activity (ODC) and the effect of the ODC inhibitor alpha-difluoromethylornithine. *Prostate* **3** 383–389

Heston WDW, Kadmon D, Covey DF and Fair WR (1984) Differential effect of α-difluoromethylornithine on the *in vivo* uptake of ^{14}C-labelled polyamines and methyl-glyoxal bis(guanylhydrazone) by a rat prostate-derived tumor. *Cancer Research* **44** 1034–1040

Heston WDW, Watanabe KA, Pankiewicz KW and Covey DF (1987a) Cytotoxic and non-cytotoxic N-alkyl derivatives of putrescine effect on polyamine uptake and growth of prostatic cancer cells *in vitro*. *Biochemical Pharmacology* **36** 1849–1852

Heston WDW, Yang C-R, Pliner L, Russo P and Covey DF (1987b) Cytotoxic activity of a polyamine analogue, monoaziridinyl-putrescine, against the PC-3 human prostatic carcinoma cell line. *Cancer Research* **47** 3627–3631

Israel M, Rosenfeld JS and Modest EJ (1964) Analogues of spermidine and spermine. I. Synthesis of polymethylene polyamines by reduction of cyanomethylated α,o-alkene-diamines. *Journal of Medicinal Chemistry* **7** 710–716

Janne J, Raina A and Siimes M (1964) Spermidine and spermine in rat tissues at different ages. *Acta Physiologica Scandinavica* **62** 352–358

Kadmon D, Heston WDW, Lazan DW and Fair WR (1982) Difluoro-methylornithine enhancement of putrescine uptake into the prostate: concise communication. *Journal of Nuclear Medicine* **23** 998–1002

Kadmon D, Heston WDW, Mahle C and Hahn DA (1985a) Prostatic cancer: imaging feasibility with radiolabelled polyamines. *Journal of Urology* **133** 121A

Kadmon D, Mahle C, Heston WDW and Hahn DA (1985b) Effect of estrogen and androgen administration on α-difluoromethylornithine enhanced putrescine uptake by the rat prostate. *Prostate* **6** 343–349

Kakinuma Y, Hoshino K and Igarashi K (1988) Characterization of the inducible polyamine transporter in bovine lymphocytes. *European Journal of Biochemistry* **176** 409–414

Kano K and Oka T (1976) Polyamine transport and metabolism in mouse mammary gland. *Journal of Biological Chemistry* **251** 2795–2800

Kapyaho K, Kallio A and Janne J (1984) Differential effects of 2-difluoromethylornithine and methylglyoxal bis-(guanyl-hydrazone) on the testosterone-induced growth of ventral prostate and seminal vesicles of castrated rats. *Biochemical Journal* **219** 811–817

Kashiwagi K, Kobayashi H and Igarashi K (1986) Apparently unidirectional polyamine transport by proton motive force in polyamine-deficient *Escherichia coli*. *Journal of Bacteriology* **165** 972–977

Koenig H, Goldstone A and Lu CY (1983) Polyamines regulate calcium fluxes in a rapid plasma membrane response. *Nature* **305** 530–534

Malt RA, Kingsworth AN, Lamuraglia GM, Lacaine F and Ross JS (1985) Chemopreventive and chemotherapy by inhibition of ornithine decarboxylase activity and polyamine synthesis colonic, pancreatic, mammary and renal carcinomas. *Advances in Enzyme Regulation* **24** 93–102

Mamont PS, Danzin C, Kolb M, Gerhart F, Bey P and Sjoerdsma A (1986) Marked and prolonged inhibition of mammalian ornithine decarboxylase *in vivo* by esters of (E)-2-(fluoromethyl)dehydro-ornithine. *Biochemical Pharmacology* **35** 159–165

Mann T (1964) *Biochemistry of Semen and of the Male Reproductive Tract*, pp 193–200, John Wiley, New York

Manni A and Wright C (1984) Reversal of the antiproliferative effect of the antiestrogen tamoxifen by polyamines in breast cancer cells. *Endocrinology* **114** 836–839

Martinet N, Beninati S, Nigra TP and Folk JE (1990) N^1N^8-bis(gamma-glutamyl)spermidine cross-linking in epidermal- cell envelopes. *Biochemical Journal* **271** 305–308

McCormack SA and Johnson LR (1989) Putrescine uptake and release by colon cancer cells. *American Journal of Physiology* **256** G868-G878

Moruzzi M, Barbiroli B, Monti MG, Tadolini B, Hakim G and Mezzetti G (1987) Inhibitory action of polyamines on protein kinase C association to membranes. *Biochemical Journal* **247** 175–180

Moruzzi M, Monti MG, Piccinini G, Marverti G and Tadolini B (1990) Effect of spermine on association of protein kinase C with phospholipid vesicles. *Life Sciences* **47** 1475–1482

Nakadate T, Aizu E, Yamaamoto S, Fujiki H, Sugimura T, and Kato R (1985) Inhibition of teleocidin-caused epidermal ornithine decarboxylase induction by phospholipase A, cycloxygenase- and lipoxygenase inhibitors. *Japanese Journal of Pharmacology* **37** 253–258

Nicolet TG, Scemama J-L, Pradayrol L, Seva C and Vaysse N (1990) Characterization of putrescine and spermidine transport systems of a rat pancreatic acinar tumoral cell line (AR4-2J). *Biochemical Journal* **269** 629–632

Parys JB, DeSmedt H, van den Bosch L, Geuns J and Borghgraef R (1990) Regulation of the Na^+-dependent and the Na^+-independent polyamine transporters in renal epithelial cells (LLC-PK_1). *Journal of Cellular Physiology* **144** 365–375

Pegg A (1988) Polyamine metabolism and its importance in neoplastic growth and as a target for chemotherapy. *Cancer Research* **48** 759–774

Pegg A and McCann PP (1988) Polyamine metabolism and function in mammalian cells and protozoans. *ISI Atlas of Science Biochemistry*, pp 11–18, Institute Scientific Information, Philadelphia

Persson L, Holm I, Ask A and Heby O (1988) Curative effect of dl-2-difluoromethylornithine on mice bearing mutant L1210 leukemia cells deficient in polyamine uptake. *Cancer Research* **48** 4807–4811

Piik K, Rajamaki P, Guha SK and Janne J (1977) Regulation of L-ornithine decarboxylase and S-adenosyl-L-methionine decarboxylase in rat ventral prostate and seminal vesicle. *Biochemical Journal* **168** 379–385

Piper JR, Stringfellow CR, Elliot RD and Johnston TP (1969) S-2-(o-aminoalkylamino)ethyldihydrogen phosphorthioates and related compounds as potential antiradiation agents. *Journal of Medicinal Chemistry* **12** 236

Pohjanpelto P (1976) Putrescine transport is greatly increased in human fibroblasts initiated to proliferate. *Journal of Cell Biology* **68** 512–520

Polvinen K, Sinervirta R, Alhonen L and Janne J (1988) Overproduction of ornithine decarboxylase confers an apparent growth advantage to mouse tumor cells. *Biochemical and Biophysical Research Communications* **155** 373–378

Porter CW and Bergeron RJ (1983) Spermidine requirement for cell proliferation in eukaryotic cells: structural specificity and quantitation. *Science* **219** 1083–1085

Porter CW and Sufrin JR (1986) Interference with polyamine biosynthesis and/or function by analogs of polyamines or methionine as a potential anticancer chemotherapeutic strategy. *Anticancer Research* **6** 525–542

Rinehart CA and Chen KY (1984) Characterization of the polyamine transport system in mouse neuroblastoma cells. *Journal of Biological Chemistry* **259** 4750–4756

Romijn JC, van Steenbrugge G-J and Schroder FH (1984) Effects of polyamine antimetabolites on the growth rate of human prostatic tumors transplantable into nude mice. *Immune Deficient Animals. 4th International Workshop on Immune-Deficient Animals in Experimental Research*, pp 370–373, Karger, Basel

Rosenheim O (1924) The isolation of spermine phosphate in semen and testis. *Biochemical Journal* **18** 1253–1262

Rosenthal SM and Tabor CW (1956) The pharmacology of spermine and spermidine. Distribution and excretion. *Journal of Pharmacology and Experimental Therapeutics* **116** 131–138

Ross JH and Krieger RI (1981) Structure-activity correlations of amines inhibiting active uptake of paraquat (methyl viologen) into rat lung slices. *Toxicology and Applied Pharmacology* **59** 238–249

Russell DH and Durie GM (1978) Polyamines as biochemical markers of normal and malignant growth. *Progress in Cancer Research and Therapy* **8** 3

Sacaan A and Johnson KM (1989) Spermine enhances binding to the glycine site associated with the N-methyl-D-aspartate receptor complex. *Molecular Pharmacology* **36** 836–839

Saunders NA, Ilett KF and Minchin RF (1987) Uptake, efflux and metabolism of the polyamine putrescine in rabbit lung slices. *Biochimica et Biophysica Acta* **927** 170–176

Scher H, Yagoda A and Ahmed T (1985) Phase II trial of mitoguazone in patients with hormone resistant adenocarcinoma of the prostate. *Journal of Clinical Oncology* **3** 224

Schuber F (1989) Influence of polyamines on membrane functions. *Biochemical Journal* **260** 1–10

Seiler N, Sarhan S, Knodgen B and Gerhart F (1988) Chain-fluorinated polyamines as tumor markers. *Journal of Cancer Research and Clinical Oncology* **114** 71–80

Seiler N, Sarhan S, Grauffel C, Jones R, Knodgen B and Moulinoux J-P (1990) Endogenous and exogenous polyamines in support of tumor growth. *Cancer Research* **50** 5077–5083

Thompson HJ, Herbst EJ and Meeker LD (1986) Chemoprevention of mammary carcinogenesis a comparative review of the efficacy of a polyamine antimetabolite, retinoids and selenium. *Journal of the National Cancer Institute* **77** 595–598

Tung HYL, Pelech S, Fisher MJ, Pogson CI and Cohen P (1985) The protein phosphates involved in cellular regulation Influence of polyamines on the activities of protein phosphatase-1 and protein phosphatase-2A. *European Journal of Biochemistry* **149** 305–313

Verma A and Boutwell RK (1987) Inhibition of carcinogenesis by inhibitors of putrescine biosynthesis, In: McCann PP, Pegg AE and Sjoerdsma A (eds). *Inhibition of Polyamine Metabolism Biological Significance and Basis for New Therapies*, pp 249–258, Academic Press, Orlando, Florida

Wagner J, Danzin C and Mamont P (1982) Reversed-phase ion-pair liquid chromatographic procedure for the simultaneous analysis of S-adenosylmethionine, its metabolites and the natural polyamines. *Journal of Chromatography* **227** 349–368

Wagner J, Claverie N and Danzin C (1984) A rapid high- performance liquid chromatographic procedure for the simultaneous determination of methionine, ethionine, S-adenosylmethionine, S-adenosylethionine and the natural polyamines in rat tissues. *Analytical Biochemistry* **140** 108–166

Walters JD and Johnson JD (1988) Inhibition of cyclic nucleotide phosphodiesterase and calcineurin by spermine, a calcium-independent calmodulin antagonist. *Biochimica et Biophysica Acta* **957** 138–142

Welch MJ, Coleman RE, Straatmann MG *et al* (1977) Carbon-11-labelled methylated polyamine analogs: uptake in prostate and tumor in animal models. *Journal of Nuclear Medicine* **18** 74–78

Wyatt I, Soames AR, Clay MF and Smith LL (1988) The accumulation and localisation of putrescine, spermidine, spermine and paraquat in the rat lung. *Biochemical Pharmacology* **37** 1909–1918

The author is responsible for the accuracy of the references.

Mechanism Based Chemotherapy for Prostate Cancer

V R SHERIDAN • K D TEW

Department of Pharmacology, Fox Chase Cancer Center, Philadelphia, Pennsylvania 19111

Introduction
    History of estramustine
    Structure and function of microtubules
    Estramustine's effects on microtubules and microtubule associated
    proteins
    Analysis of estramustine's effects on living cells
Future perspectives
Summary

INTRODUCTION

Prostatic cancer is the leading cause of death from cancer in elderly men. In addition to a high mortality rate, prostatic cancer has a high annual incidence in males, accounting for 17% of the total annual incidence of all forms of cancer in males in the USA (Silverberg, 1982). Unfortunately, present therapeutic approaches to prostate cancer treatment are not satisfactory—few patients are cured of the disease. The most common treatment for prostatic carcinoma is orchiectomy followed by oestrogen therapy. This treatment frequently yields a substantial beneficial response (Scott *et al*, 1980). However, nearly all patients eventually relapse to a hormone insensitive state and succumb to progression of the disease (Menon and Walsh, 1979; Scott *et al*, 1980). Thus, the annual death rate from prostatic cancer has remained virtually unchanged in the past 40 years (Devera and Silverman, 1978).

The purpose of this chapter is to review a novel compound, estramustine (also known as Estracyt or Emcyt), currently in clinical use in the treatment of prostatic carcinoma. Although estramustine initially was used because of its presumed steroidal activity, it is now clear that the drug acts by a unique mechanism and offers a promising alternative therapy in the treatment of prostatic cancer.

History of Estramustine

Estramustine was synthesized in the mid 1960s (Fex *et al*, 1967) as a compound that could improve specificity for the treatment of breast cancer. It is1 noteworthy that the rationale for the design of the drug has resulted in a drug with considerable target specificity and biological activity. However, such char-

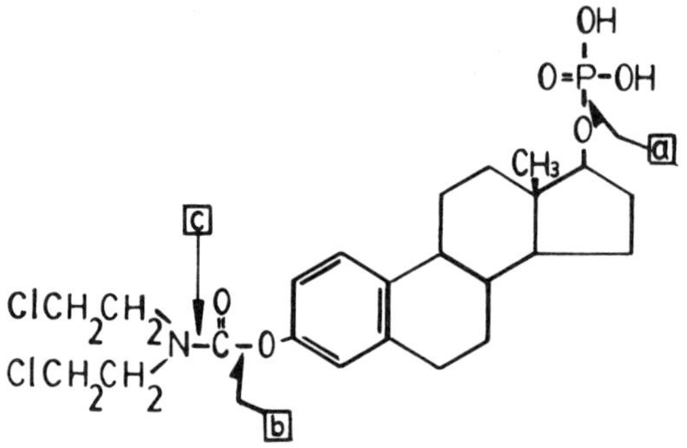

Fig. 1. Structure of estramustine phosphate. Arrows indicate bonds that are available for cleavage by (a) phosphatases, (b) esterases, (c) carbaminidases or proteases

acteristics arise for reasons unrelated to conceptual considerations in the drug's design.

Figure 1 illustrates the structure of estramustine phosphate. The molecule is an oestradiol attached to nor-nitrogen mustard by a carbamate ester linkage. In proprietary form, the drug has a phosphate at the 17β position of the steroid D ring to enhance its solubility in water. Treatment of animals or cells with the compound results in a rapid dephosphorylation and subsequent production of estramustine or its oxidized metabolite, estromustine (Andersson *et al*, 1981; Gunnarsson *et al*, 1981).

The initial rationale dictated that the steroid moiety would facilitate selective uptake of estramustine in oestrogen receptor positive tumours, producing a raised concentration of the drug in malignant tissue. Subsequent to uptake, the drug would undergo intracellular cleavage, by hydrolytic enzymes, to form its constitutive oestradiol and nor-nitrogen moieties. The release of the nor-nitrogen mustard would then presumably result in covalent drug induced damage to cellular nucleophilic sites contained in nucleic acids and proteins.

Although release of oestrogens does occur after estramustine administration (Anderson *et al*, 1977; Gunnarsson *et al*, 1984; Gunnarsson and Forshell, 1984), the drug has been shown to be pharmacologically active in a number of cell lines that lack oestrogen receptors (Tew, 1983). In earlier studies, several observations indicated that an unusual mechanism of action underlaid the drug's pharmacological properties (Tew and Stearns, 1989). In addition to showing activity in receptor negative cell lines, estramustine binding was not inhibited competitively by greater than 1000-fold excess concentrations of oestradiol (Tew, 1983). Furthermore, the drug had no alkylating activity in vitro at concentrations that induced cytotoxicity (Tew, 1983; Tew *et al*, 1983).

Data from a large number of clinical experiences are also consistent with a lack of alkylating activity since toxicity to rapidly dividing tissues such as bone marrow and gastrointestinal epithelia was not apparent (Groupe European du Cancer du Sein, 1969; Benson, 1988). A clue to the possible mechanism of action of estramustine was revealed when the drug was shown to cause the accumulation of cells in metaphase (Hartley-Asp, 1984; Tew and Hartley-Asp,

1984). Since that time, it has become apparent that the pharmacological activity of estramustine results from its effects on the cytoskeleton—specifically microtubules—rather than via covalent interactions with proteins and/or nucleic acids (Tew and Hartley-Asp, 1984; Stearns and Tew, 1985, 1988; Wallin *et al*, 1985; Friden *et al*, 1987; Wang *et al*, 1987).

Structure and Function of Microtubules

Microtubules are long, rigid polymers formed by the energy dependent assembly of heterodimer subunits composed of α and β tubulins (Dustin, 1978; Darnell *et al*, 1986). Microtubules are present in all eucaryotic cells and are implicated in several diverse functions, including cell division, cell motility, secretion and maintenance of cell polarity. Partial or complete loss of microtubule structures after treatment with colchicine or vinca alkaloids has been shown to effect dramatic inhibition of these cellular processes (Hyams and Stebbings, 1979; Inoue, 1981).

A group of diverse proteins, collectively referred to as microtubule associated proteins (MAPs), has been described on the basis of the proteins' ability to associate physically with microtubules, stimulate microtubule assembly and/or stabilize microtubules under conditions that lead to disassembly (Kim *et al*, 1979; Albertini *et al*, 1984; Olmsted, 1986). The most abundant source of and best characterized MAPs are in brain tissue and include a group of high molecular weight proteins, MAP1 and MAP2 (330 and 300 kDa, respectively) and a group of intermediate molecular weight proteins (55–68 kDa), collectively referred to as tau. The MAPs in both non-neuronal tissue and cell lines have been less well characterized but appear to include MAP1 and a group of proteins with molecular weights between 120 kDa and 210 kDa, which vary according to cell and tissue type (Olmsted, 1986; Wiche *et al*, 1986). Both the high molecular weight MAP1 and tau have been shown to be phosphorylated under certain conditions (Lindwal and Cole, 1984; Diaz-Nido *et al*, 1990;). Furthermore, MAP2 and tau are known to exist in various forms because of different processing of their respective mRNAs (Himmler, 1989). In summary, a diverse group of MAPs exist that varies in cell and tissue specificity and presumably is responsible, at least in part, for the regulation of microtubule assembly and functions in various cellular processes. The following section describes how estramustine is thought to interact with MAPs and to affect microtubule regulated processes.

Estramustine's Effects on Microtubules and Microtubule Associated Proteins

Experiments on the human prostatic carcinoma cell lines DU-145 and PC-3 demonstrated that the cytotoxic activity of estramustine did not involve steroidal or alkylating activity. The drug was shown, however, to inhibit cell growth, clonogenic survival and induce mitotic arrest in these cell lines (Tew and Hartley-Asp, 1984). These studies suggested that estramustine was exerting an effect on cell division, a microtubule regulated process. This was confirmed in subsequent experiments with immunofluorescent localization of microtubules in cell lines treated with estramustine. The drug was shown to effect rapid disassembly of microtubules at concentrations between 30 and 120 μmol/l. Both interphase and mitotic microtubules were shown to be disrupted by estramustine. The only subset of microtubules that seemed to be resistant to the drug were those composing the intracellular bridge between daughter cells during telophase and cytokinesis (Stearns and Tew, 1985; Wang *et al*, 1987).

In vitro experiments showed that estramustine inhibits microtubule assembly (Stearns *et al*, 1985; Wallin *et al*, 1985), binds MAP2 and tau (Friden *et al*, 1987; Stearns and Tew, 1988) and causes the dissociation of MAP1 and MAP2 from taxol stabilized microtubules (Stearns and Tew, 1988). Thus, it seems reasonable to interpret the cytotoxic effects of estramustine as being mediated through the dissociation of MAPs from microtubules which results in the subsequent disassembly of microtubules and the resultant disruption of critical microtubule dependent cellular processes.

Although there are now convincing data, both in vivo and in vitro, that estramustine exerts a cytotoxic effect on cells by means of microtubule disruption, the precise mechanism of action of the drug remains to be elucidated. Firstly, it is not yet known whether estramustine has a primary cytotoxic effect on one phase (eg mitosis) of the cell cycle or, instead, exerts a multiplicity of effects on several microtubule regulated processes. In fact, Mareel *et al* (1988) have shown that the drug also inhibits the invasive activity of malignant mouse MO_4 cells and human DU-145 cells, suggesting that estramustine inhibits cell motility and/or secretory processes, presumably by effecting the disassembly of interphase microtubules. Secondly, the concentrations of estramustine used in most studies to date range from 10 to 120 μmol/l, which are relatively high for a compound with a target specificity. Estramustine concentrations approaching millimolar levels could possibly exert pleiotropic effects on metabolic processes, such as creating an imbalance in the thiol-disulphide balance within cells. Indeed, studies by Tew *et al* (1986) indicate that estramustine affects both the level of intracellular glutathione as well as glutathione S-transferase activity. Other antimitotic agents such as the vinca alkaloids have been shown to cause a shift in the thiol-disulphfide balance in cells (Beck, 1980). It therefore seems critical to understanding estramustine's mechanism(s) of action to determine whether the drug acts in a specific way in the cell cycle, and, if so, what concentration is necessary for this activity.

Analysis of Estramustine's Effects on Living Cells

We have used video-enhanced differential-interference contrast (DIC) microscopy of living DU-145 cells to examine the effects of estramustine on cell division. The progression of DU-145 cells from metaphase through cytokinesis

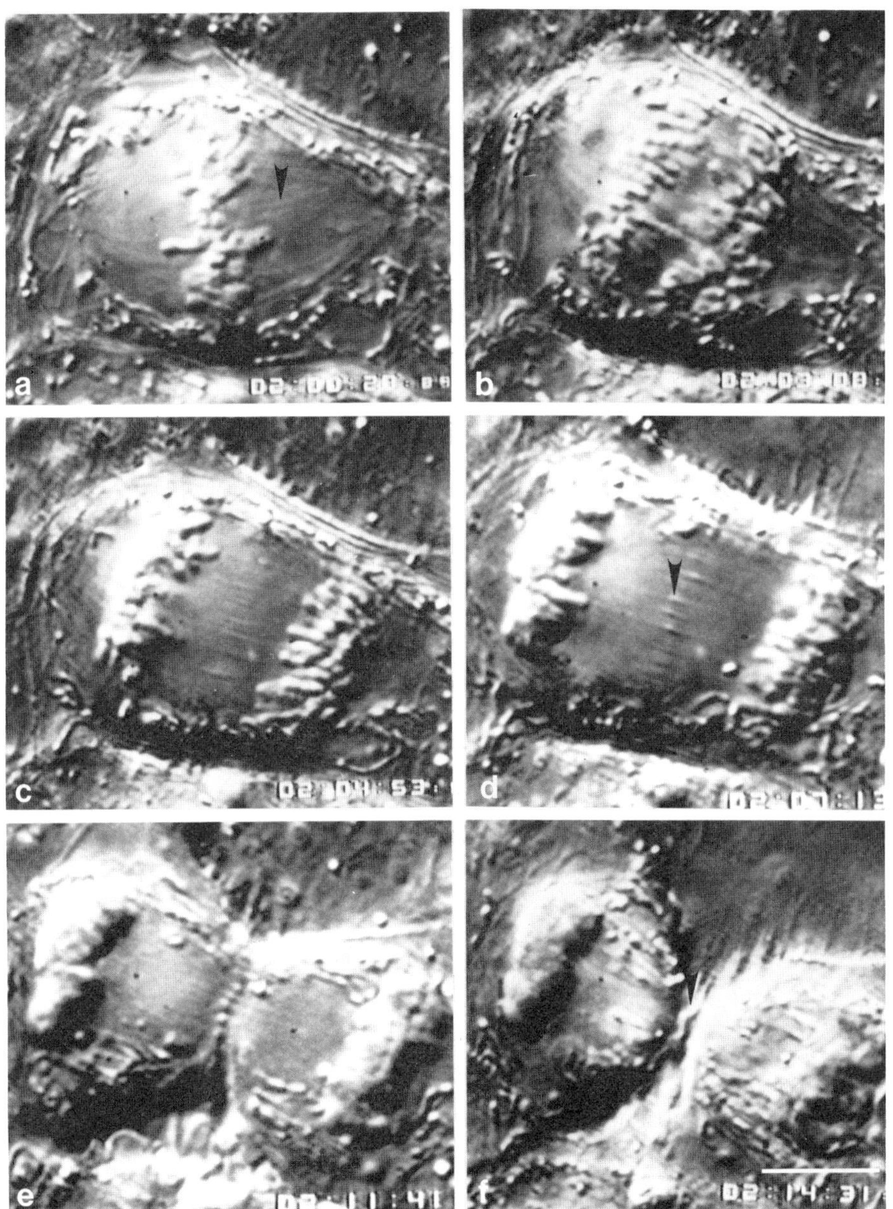

Fig. 2. Living DU-145 cell in the absence of drug, visualized with DIC optics. Time is displayed in lower right (hours, minutes, seconds, hundredths of seconds). (a) Metaphase showing spindle fibers (arrowhead); (b–d) anaphase, interzonal microtubule bundles in d indicated by arrowhead; (d) telophase, stembodies indicated by arrowhead; (e–f) cytokinesis, midbody indicated in f by arrowhead. (bar = 10 μm) (Sheridan *et al*, 1991)

is illustrated in Fig. 2; DIC optics clearly show the metaphase mitotic apparatus surrounded by mitochondria and other organelles, with the chromosomes aligned along the equatorial region of the spindle. Individual microtubule bundles also are visible (Fig. 2a). Following anaphase onset, chromosomes move to each spindle pole (anaphase A), and the distance between spindle poles increases (anaphase B) until telophase (Fig. 2b–d). The duration of anaphase is 6–7 minutes. During telophase, individual bundles of microtubules (stembodies) are visible in the equatorial region of the spindle (Fig. 2d). As cytokinesis progresses, individual stembodies coalesce to form the midbody (Fig. 2e,f), a structure physically delineating the daughter cells. Cytokinesis also is 6–7 minutes in duration.

Exposure of cells in division to estramustine has two major results depending on the phase of mitosis in which the cell is exposed to drug and the concentration of drug used. Figure 3 shows the effects of 10 μmol/l estramustine on metaphase which results in a gradual reduction of spindle size and in chromosome disorganization. After 15 minutes exposure to estramustine, the chromosomes have lost equatorial alignment (Fig. 3d) and anaphase is not initiated. This result is obtained with concentrations of estramustine as low as 2.5 μmol/l (Sheridan *et al*, 1991). Large organelles, however, are excluded from the reduced spindle region, indicating that some structural organization of the mitotic apparatus persists after drug treatment. This is shown conclusively by electron microscopy. Figure 4 illustrates a cell treated for 16 hours with 10 μmol/l estramustine. Bundles of microtubules in association with spindle poles and chromosomes are apparent. Figures 5 and 6 are higher magnification images of microtubules in association with centromeres and the centriole, respectively, demonstrating that numerous microtubules remain in association with these structures in the presence of drug.

The second major effect on cell division is observed when cells were treated with drug after anaphase had begun. Figure 7 demonstrates the effect of 60 μmol/l estramustine on anaphase and cytokinesis. After drug treatment, chromosome-to-pole movement proceeded at rates identical to those of untreated cells (Fig. 7b–d). The extent of spindle pole separation, however, was considerably less than that observed in control cells (Fig. 7d versus Fig. 2d). In contrast to what was seen in untreated cells, mitochondria and other membranous organelles were observed in the spindle interzone, whereas microtubule bundles were absent (Fig. 7d,e). Finally, cleavage furrow formation and progression were strikingly delayed and midbodies did not form (Fig. 7f). Table 1 (Sheridan *et al*, 1991) demonstrates the relation between estramustine concentration and inhibition of anaphase B (the extent of spindle pole elongation). The extent of chromosome separation at the end of anaphase was reduced substantially in each treated population with respect to the control population. In addition, a clear trend was apparent between increased estramustine concentration and decreased chromosome separation.

In summary, DIC studies on living cells suggest that estramustine selectively interferes with specific classes of microtubules and mitotic stages. Metaphase spindles are disorganized but not completely disassembled by micromolar concentrations of estramustine. Onset of anaphase is either inhibited or strikingly delayed. Electron microscopy demonstrates that microtubules in

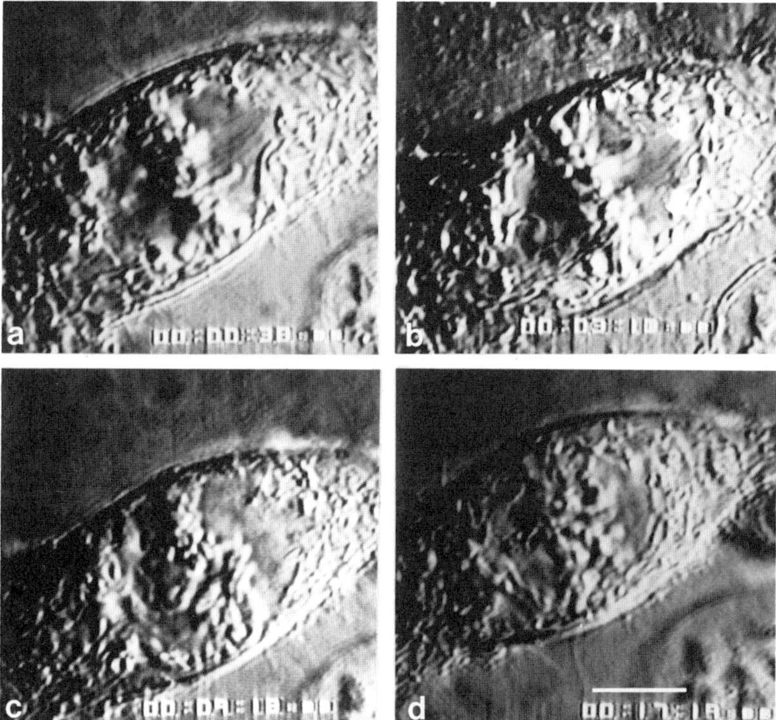

Fig. 3. Metaphase cell treated with 10 µmol/l estramustine at 00:01:45:00 (between panels a and b) showing a gradual reduction in spindle size accompanied by chromosome disorganization. (bar = 10 µm) (Sheridan *et al.*, 1991)

association with spindle poles and chromosomes are not disassembled by estramustine. Treatment of cells with estramustine after anaphase onset indicates that chromosomes are still able to move to the spindle poles, yet pole-to-pole separation is inhibited. Interzonal microtubules present during anaphase B appear to be disassembled by estramustine. Notably, the concentrations of estramustine used in these studies had little effect on organelle motility and microtubule organization in interphase DU-145 cells as judged by DIC studies on living cells and immunofluorescent localization of microtubules in cells fixed after drug treatment (unpublished observations). Estramustine therefore appears to inhibit selectively certain classes of microtubules in cell division, presumably by binding to one or more MAPs that are crucial to the dynamic organization of microtubules during mitosis.

FUTURE PERSPECTIVES

Most clinical studies so far have tested estramustine as a single agent and compared its efficacy with that for hormonal therapy. Although in general terms, estramustine has proved more effective, the drug has not been used as one that has antimitotic activity. It is unlikely that any antimicrotubule agent would

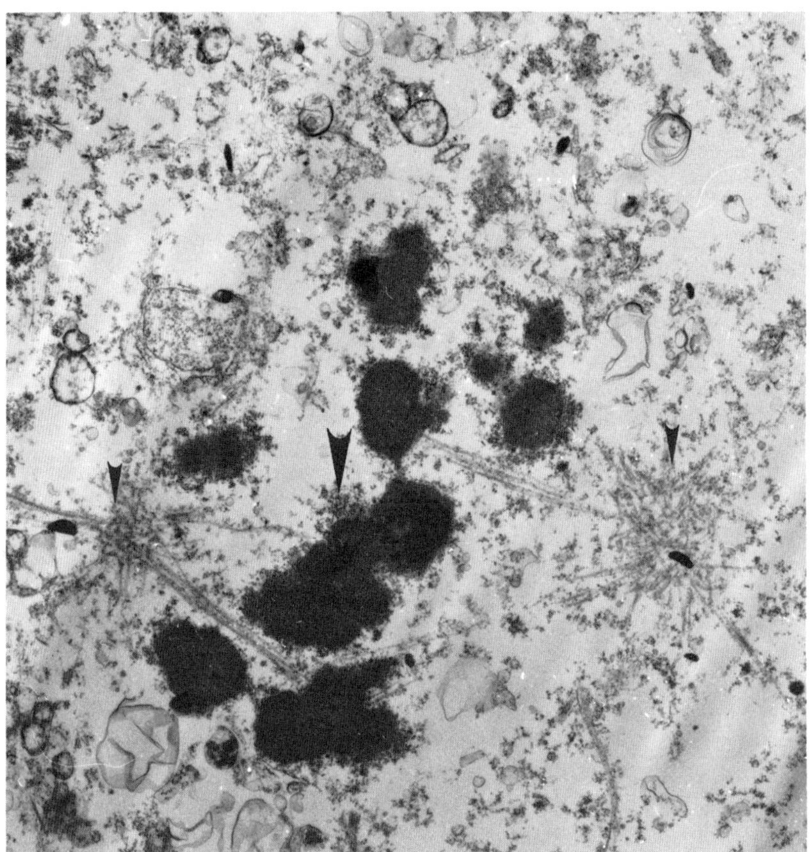

Fig. 4. Electron micrograph of a cell treated with 10 μmol/l estramustine for 16 hr before fixation. Arrowheads indicate spindle poles and microtubule bundles associated with chromosomes (x 4600)

have impressive antitumour potential when used clinically as a single agent.

Conceptually, the principle of combining two antimicrotubule drugs would not appear to be an attractive approach to enhancement of the therapeutic index, especially in a relatively chemoresistant disease such as prostate cancer. However, a number of factors have contributed to the design of clinical trials with estramustine and vinblastine. From a mechanistic standpoint, although both cause antimicrotubule and antimitotic effects, the targets of estramustine and vinblastine are distinct. Since both tubulin and MAPs are critical to interphase microtubules and the mitotic spindle, a "sequential blockade" could logically produce the reported synergistic cell kill observed in vitro (Mareel *et al*, 1988). The different protein targets of the two drugs also contribute to the reduced likelihood of the development of collateral resistance. Indeed, vinblastine resistance can be expressed in a number of ways, either through mutations in tubulin isoforms (Cabral *et al*, 1986) or through enhanced efflux of the drug. The latter predominantly involves the classic multidrug resistant (MDR) phenotype where the overexpression of membrane p-glycoprotein gives resis-

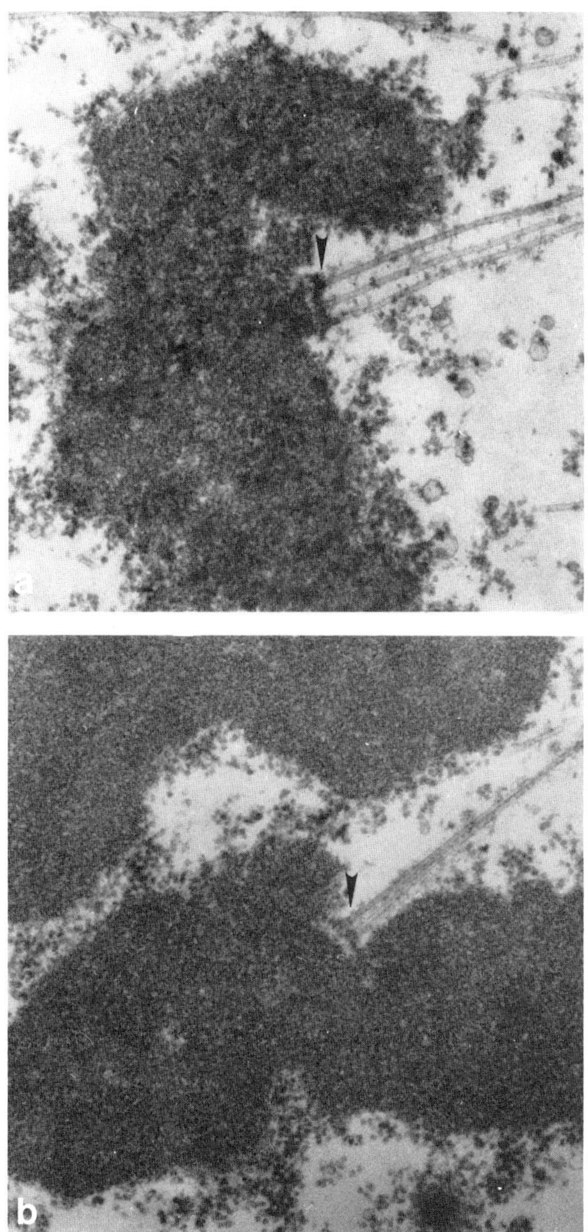

Fig. 5. Electron micrographs of (a) untreated cell and (b) a cell treated with 10 μmol/l estramustine for 16 hr. Arrowheads indicate centromeres with associated microtubules. (a) x 13 600, (b) x 10 400

tance to a broad range of hydrophobic natural products (Bech-Hansen *et al*, 1976). Estramustine is not part of the MDR phenotype. Cell lines made resistant to vinca alkaloids remain sensitive to estramustine. In addition, estramustine resistant cell lines do not show cross resistance to vinca alkaloids. Nor do they overexpress the p-glycoprotein (Speicher *et al*, in press), a factor

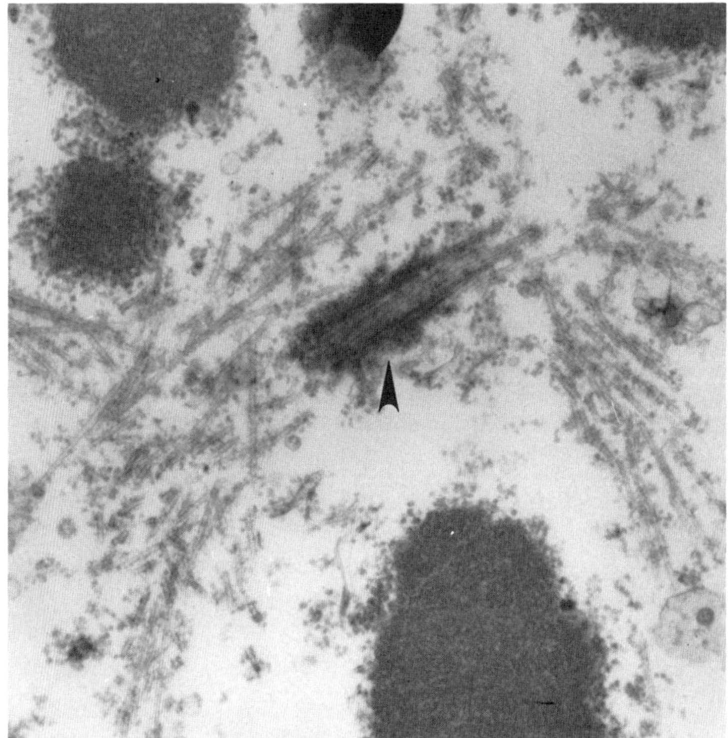

Fig. 6. Electron micrograph of a cell treated with 10 μmol/l estramustine for 16 hr. Arrowhead indicates tangential section through a centriole (x 13 000)

of some consequence in determining the potential usefulness of estramustine as a therapeutic agent.

Selectivity of estramustine for prostate cancer has primarily been based on high prostatic levels of estramustine binding protein (EMBP), a protein with a high affinity for estramustine and the ability to concentrate the drug in the organ; human ventral prostate has substantially less EMBP than rat (Forsgren *et al*, 1979; Bjork *et al*, 1982), but nonetheless, there is still a slight "concentration gradient" effect. It is noteworthy that other organs such as colon and brain have also been shown to express the EMBP at reasonably high levels, suggesting a potentially broader oncological use for estramustine in combination drug therapy. Also of some consequence is the long clinical half life ($t_{1/2}$ = 16 hr) of estramustine, which indicates that serum availability of the drug is not a limiting factor. Either estramustine or its primary oxidized metabolite estromustine has antimitotic activity. Since in vitro studies have demonstrated the reversibility of estramustine's antimicrotubule effects (Sheridan *et al*, 1991), the continued presence of the drug will be critical to the enactment of its pharmacological effects. Figure 8 demonstrates the reversal of mitotic arrest following removal of drug as determined by immunofluorescence microscopy.

Host toxicities for estramustine and vinblastine are also non-overlapping.

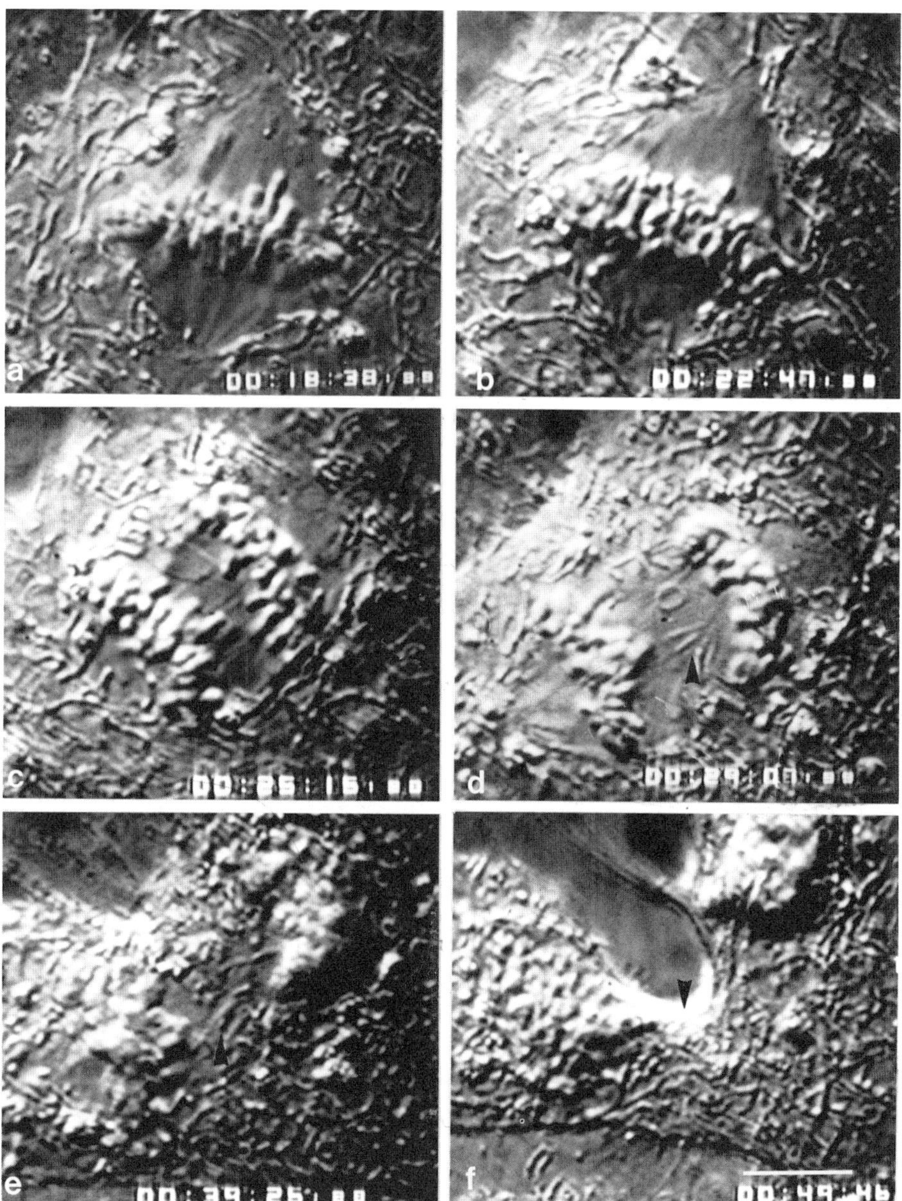

Fig. 7. Cell treated at 00:21:00 (between panels a and b) with 60 µmol/l estramustine after anaphase onset. (a) Metaphase; (b–d) anaphase, mitochondria in spindle interzone indicated by arrowhead in d; (e) telophase, vesicles in spindle interzone indicated by arrowhead; (f) cytokinesis, cleavage furrow indicated by arrowheads (bar = 10 µm)

For example, estramustine causes mainly mild gastrointestinal toxicity, with increased risk of cardiac complications in patients with heart problems. The primary dose limiting tissues for vinblastine include bone marrow and central nervous tissue. Thus, the combination of the two should not produce synergistic host toxicities.

TABLE 1. Relation between estramustine concentration and inhibition of anaphase B

	Mean metaphase pole-to pole distance (μmol/l) before addition of drug[a]	Mean anaphase spindle pole separation (μm)[b,c]	Individual high/low values for anaphase chromosome separation (μm)
Control	19.5 ± 2.19 (n = 7)	28.7 ± 2.39 (n = 8)	32.5/25.3
2.5 μmol/l	19.1 ± 1.97 (n = 5)	25.0 ± 2.20 (n = 8)	27.7/21.7
10 μmol/l	19.1 ± 1.09 (n = 8)	22.0 ± 2.10 (n = 8)	24.1/17/6
30 μmol/l	18.6 ± 0.94 (n = 7)	20.1 ± 2.27 (n = 8)	24.1/17.6
60 μmol/l	18.9 ± 1.43 (n = 8)	18.7 ± 3.08 (n = 8)	22.9/14.5

[a]Means of controls v. each treated population did not differ (>0.05)
[b]Means of controls v. each treated population significantly different (p<0.05)
[c]Anaphase spindle pole separation was measured as distance from centrosomal side of each separated chromosome set before onset of cytokinesis

Through the combined efforts of the Fox Chase and Sloan-Kettering Cancer Centers, a phase I/II clinical trial has been instigated in hormone refractory prostate cancer. So far, 23 patients with hormone refractory prostate cancer were treated with a combination of 4 μg/m^2 intravenous vinblastine (18 patients), 2–3 μg/m^2 (5 patients) via weekly or biweekly bolus injection, and estramustine at 10–15 μg/kg per day orally. All patients had progressive disease, and conventional and adequate hormonal therapy had failed. Patients were 56–80 years old (median 68) with Karnofsky performance status 50–100% (mean 70). Initial serum prostate specific antigen (PSA) concentrations were between 0.6 and 1570 μg (median 40; mean 479). During the course of therapy, where the total number of vinblastine doses received per patient was between 2 and 23 (median 8), 11 of the 23 patients showed a reduction in PSA levels of greater than 50% on the basis of at least two consecutive weekly measurements. The duration of these reductions was 4 to over 32 weeks (mean 17), with a median decrease in PSA of 62% (mean 70). Although there is still some controversy about the accuracy of PSA as a response predictor, it is generally accepted that large reductions in circulating PSA represent good progression criteria. The side-effects of the treatment were limited and generally well tolerated by the patients: leukopenia, 8.6%; gastrointestinal disturbances (predominantly nausea/constipation), 26%; peripheral neuropathy, 3%; and painful gynaecomastia, 8.6%.

These results are encouraging from a number of standpoints. Primarily, this group of patients has no other standard alternative therapy. Because of the disease and average age of the patients, the fact that the drugs were well tolerated is surprising. The PSA responses were frequently accompanied by alleviation of pain, and in some cases, regression of lesions and/or metastatic nodules.

In view of the preliminary indications of activity of such concerted antimicrotubule therapy, it may be of value to screen for other agents that target MAPs, especially since tumour cells can vary in their MAP components from normal tissues. It is also of interest that tumour cells developing resis-

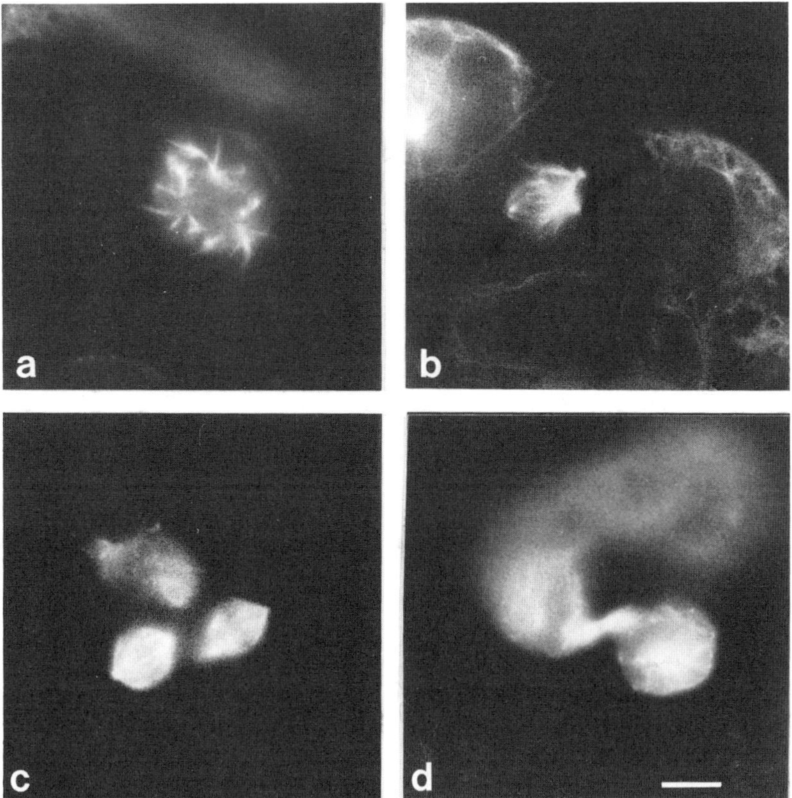

Fig. 8. Immunofluorescent localization of tubulin in mitotic cells in the presence of (a) 10 μmol/l estramustine; (b) 10 μmol/l estramustine treatment, 30 min after removal of drug; (c) 10 μmol/l estramustine treatment, 1 hr after drug removal and (d) 10 μmol/l estramustine treatment, 4 hr after drug removal (bar = 10 μm)

tance to tubulin binding drugs, such as podophyllotoxins, have been shown to overexpress a protein with a molecular weight of 66 kDa that has been suggested to be a MAP (Gupta *et al*, 1986). The somewhat limited information presently available on tumour specific MAPs and the possibility that differential expression exists between tumour and normal tissues suggest that this may be a fruitful arena for research.

Overall, prostate cancer remains a difficult tumour to treat by chemotherapy. Hormonal manipulation will remain a front line therapy in most instances. The encouraging early results of the estramustine/vinblastine combination in hormone refractory disease (Seidman *et al*, 1991) may form a basis for extending such an approach, either in early treatment or as a fulcrum for drug additions to such a protocol. The search for better means of early detection and for markers of response would greatly enhance the chances of successful chemotherapy. Certainly, there are many reasons to reassess the potential extended usefulness of drugs such as estramustine in clinical management. Because of the growth characteristics of prostate cancer and the nature of the patients who are subject to treatment, chemotherapy will not always be the simplest of therapies. However, a further encouraging aspect of microtubule targeted chemotherapy has been the success of taxol in the treatment of refractory ovarian cancer. As a single agent at dose ranges from 110 to 250 mg/m^2, taxol induced patient disease remissions lasting from 3 to 15 months. Dose limiting toxicity was myelosuppression, with leukocytes being more sensitive than thrombocytes or reticulocytes. Conclusions from this non-randomized, prospective phase II trial were that taxol studies should be extended to combination therapies (McGuire *et al*, 1989). Unfortunately, the supply of this natural product is limited by the lack of the yew tree source and its geographical distribution. Consequently, extensive trials or trials in diseases such as prostate cancer must await the elucidation and implementation of large scale chemical synthesis.

The overall approach of targeting cellular structural proteins has provided a reasonably successful mechanism for chemotherapeutic control of cancer cells. As is always the case, selectivity remains a major obstacle in the improvement of therapeutic index. Although tubulin per se has, to this time, been a primary target, some novelty has been invoked by the use of taxol to stabilize microtubules, and this may be the forerunner of other stabilizing agents. In addition, the expanding knowledge of MAPs and those drugs that bind to these proteins may provide a fertile area for drug development.

SUMMARY

Estramustine offers a mechanistically novel therapy for the treatment of prostatic cancer. The drug is composed of oestradiol coupled to nor-nitrogen mustard. The cytotoxic properties of estramustine act independently of its constituent molecules. In vivo and in vitro studies indicate that the drug binds microtubule associated proteins and inhibits microtubule regulated processes. We have lately shown that micromolar levels of estramustine inhibit selected processes in mitosis, suggesting that certain classes of microtubules and/or MAPs are differentially sensitive to the drug. New clinical trials using estramustine and vinblastine on patients with advanced hormone refractory disease suggest that the combination of two antimicrotubule agents acting by means of different target molecules may be important clinically.

References

Albertini DF, Herman B and Sherline P (1984) In vivo and in vitro studies on the role of HWM-MAPs in taxol-induced microtubule bundling. *European Journal of Cell Biology* 33 134–143

Anderson L, Edsmyr F, Jonason G and Konyves I (1977) Estramustine phosphate therapy in carcinoma of the prostate, In: Grundmann E and Vahlensieck W (eds). *Recent Results in Cancer Research*, pp 73–77, Springer Verlag, Berlin

Andersson SB, Gunnarsson PO, Nilsson T and Plym-Forshell G (1981) Metabolism of estramustine phosphate (Estracyt) in patients with prostatic carcinoma. *European Journal of Metabolism and Pharmacokinetics* **6** 149–154

Bech-Hansen NT, Till JE and Ling V (1976) Pleiotropic phenotype of colchicine-resistant CHO cells: cross- resistance and collateral sensitivity. *Journal of Cellular Physiology* **88** 23–39

Beck WT (1980) Increase by vinblastine of oxidized glutathione in cultured mammalian cell. *Biochemical Pharmacology* **29** 2333–2337

Benson RC (1988) Role of estramustine phosphate in the treatment of prostate cancer, In: H Schafers (ed). *Estracyt, Scientific edition 2*, pp 35–64, Eguipage, Utrecht

Bjork P, Forsgren B, Gustafsson J-A, Pausette A and Hogberg B (1982) Partial characterization and "quantitation" of a human prostatic estramustine-binding protein. *Cancer Research* **42** 1935–1942

Cabral FR, Brady RC and Schibler MJ (1986) A mechanism of cellular resistance to drugs that interfere with microtubule assemply, In: D Soifer (ed). *Annals of the NY Academy of Science*, pp 745–756,

Darnell JE, Lodish H and Baltimore D (1986) *Molecular Cell Biology* Part III Scientific American Books, Inc, New York

Devera SS and Silverman DT (1978) Cancer incidence and morbidity trends in the United States: 1935–1974. *Journal of the National Cancer Institute* **60** 545–571

Diaz-Nido J, Serrano L, Hernandez MA and Avila J (1990) Phosphorylation of microtubule proteins in rat brain at different developmental stages: comparison with that found in neuronal cultures. *Journal of Neurochemistry* **54** 211–222

Dustin P (1978) *Microtubules* Springer Verlag, New York

Fex HJ, Hogberg KB, Konyves I and Kneip PHOJ (1967) Certain steroid N-bis-(halo-ethyl)-carbamates. US Patent No 3 299 104, 17.1

Forsgren B, Bjork P, Carlstrom K, Gustafsson J-A, Pausette A and Hogberg B (1979) Purification and distribution of a major protein in the rat prostate that binds estramustine, a nitrogen mustard derivative of estradiol-17b. *Proceedings of the National Academy of Sciences of the USA* **76** 3149–3152

Friden B, Wallin M, Deinum J, Prasade V and Luduena R (1987) Effect of estramustine phosphate on the assembly of trypin-treated microtubules and microtubules reconstituted from purified tubulin with either tau, MAP-2 or the tubulin binding fragment of MAP-2. *Archives of Biochemistry and Biophysics* **257** 123–130

Garner CC and Matus A (1988) Different forms of microtubule-associated protein 2 are encoded by separate mRNA transcripts. *Journal of Cell Biology* **106** 779–783

Groupe Europeen du Cancer du Sein (1969) Essai clinique du phenol bis(2-chloroethyl)carbamate d'estradiol dans le cancer mammale en phase avancee. *European Journal of Cancer* **5** 1–4

Gunnarsson PO and Forshell GP (1984) Clinical pharmacokinetics of estramustine phosphate. *Urology* **23** 22–27

Gunnarsson PO, Forshell GP, Fritjofsson A and Norlen BJ (1981) Plasma concentrations of estramustine phosphate and its major metabolites in patients with prostatic carcinoma treated with different doses of estramustine phosphate (Estracyt). *Scandinavian Journal of Urology and Nephrology* **15** 201–205

Gunnarsson PO, Andersson SB, Johansson SA, Nilsson T and Plym-Forshell G (1984) Pharmacokinetics of estramustine phosphate (Estracyt) in prostatic cancer patients. *European Journal of Clinical Pharmacology* **26** 113–119

Gupta RS (1986) Cross-resistance of nocodazole-resistant mutants of CHO cells toward other microtubule inhibitors: similar mode of action of benzimidazole carbamate derivatives and NSC 181928 and TN- 16. *Molecular Pharmacology* **30** 142–148

Hartley-Asp B (1984) Estramustine-induced mitotic arrest in two human prostatic carcinoma cells lines, DU 145 and PC-3. *Prostate* **5** 93–100

Himmler A (1989) Structure of the bovine tau gene: alternatively spliced transcripts generate a protein family. *Molecular and Cellular Biology* **9** 1389–1396

Hyams JS and Stebbings H (1979) Microtubule associated cytoplasmic transport, In: Roberts K and Hyams JS (eds). *Microtubules*, pp 487–530, Academic Press, New York

Inoue S (1981) Cell division and the mitotic spindle, In: *Discovery in Cell Biology. Journal of Cell Biology* **91** 132s–147s

Kim H, Binder LI and Rosenbaum JL (1979) The periodic association of MAP2 with brain microtubules in vitro. *Journal of Cell Biology* **80** 266–276

Lindwall G and Cole RD (1984) The purification of tau protein and the occurrence of two phosphorylation states of tau in brain. *Journal of Biological Chemistry* **259** 12241–12245

McGuire WP, Rowinsky EK, Rosenshein NR *et al* (1989) Taxol: a unique antineoplastic agent with significant activity in advanced ovarian epithelial neoplasms. *Annals of Internal Medicine* **111** 273–279

Mareel MM, Storme GA, Dragonetti CH *et al* (1988) Antiinvasive activity of estramustine on malignant MO_4 mouse cells and on DU-145 human prostate carcinoma cells in vitro. *Cancer Research* **48** 1842–1849

Menon M and Walsh PC (1979) Hormonal therapy for prostatic cancer, In: Murphy GP (ed). *Prostatic Cancer* pp 175–200, PSG, Littleton, Massachusetts

Olmsted JB (1986) Microtubule-associated proteins. *Annual Reviews in Cell Biology* **2** 421–457

Schulze H and Isaacs JT (1986) Biology and therapy of prostatic cancer. *Cancer Surveys* **5** 487–503

Scott WW, Menon M and Walsh PC (1980) Hormonal therapy of prostatic cancer. *Cancer* **45** 1929–1936

Seidman A, Scher H, Petrylak D *et al* (1991) Estramustine and vinblastine: effects on serum prostate specific antigen in hormone-refractory prostate cancer. *Proceedings of the American Association Cancer Research* **32** 187

Sheridan VR, Speicher LA and Tew KD (1991) The effects of estramustine on mitotic progression in DU 145 prostatic carcinoma cells. *European Journal of Cell Biology* **54** 268–276

Silverberg F (1982) Cancer statistics. *Cancer* **32** 15–35

Speicher LA, Sheridan VR and Tew KD Establishment and characterization of estramustine-resistant human prostatic carcinoma cell lines. *British Journal of Cancer* (in press)

Stearns ME and Tew KD (1985) Antimicrotubule effects of estramustine, an antiprostatic tumor drug. Cancer Research **45** 3891–3897

Stearns ME and Tew KD (1988) Estramustine binds MAP-2 to inhibit microtubule assembly in vitro. *Journal of Cell Science* **89** 331–342

Tew KD (1983) The mechanism of action of estramustine. *Seminars in Oncology* **10** 21–26

Tew KD and Hartley-Asp B (1984) Cytotoxic properties of estramustine unrelated to alkylating and steroid constituents. *Urology* **23** 28–33

Tew KD and Stearns ME (1989) Estramustine—a nitrogen mustard/steroid with antimicrotubule activity. *Pharmacology and Therapeutics* **43** 299–319

Tew KD, Erickson LC, White G, Wang AL, Schein PS and Hartley-Asp B (1983) Cytotoxicity of estramustine, a steroid-nitrogen mustard derivative, through non-DNA targets. *Molecular Pharmacology* **24** 324–328

Tew KD, Woodworth A and Stearns ME (1986) Antimitotic properties of estramustine are accompanied by a depletion in intracellular glutathione and an inhibition in glutathione S-transferase. *Cancer Treatment Reports* **70** 715–720

Wallin M, Deinum J and Friden B (1985) Interaction of estramustine phosphate with microtubule-associated proteins. *Federation of the European Biochemical Society Letters* **179** 289–293

Wang M, Tew KD and Stearns ME (1987) Immunofluorescent studies of the antimicrotubule effects of the anticancer drug estramustine. *Anticancer Research* **7** 1165–1172

Wiche G, Herrman H, Dalton JM *et al* (1986) Molecular aspects of MAP1 and MAP2: microheterogeneity, in vitro localization and distribution in neuronal and nonneuronal cells, In: Soifer D (ed). *Annals of the New York Academy of Sciences*, pp 180–198

The authors are responsible for the accuracy of the references.

Cell Motility as a Chemotherapeutic Target

KENNETH J PIENTA • DONALD S COFFEY

Department of Oncology and Department of Urology, Johns Hopkins University School of Medicine, Baltimore, Maryland 21205

Introduction: The metastatic phenotype and cell motility
Stimulation of cell motility
Structural basis of cell motility
Cell motility as a chemotherapeutic target
Summary

INTRODUCTION: THE METASTATIC PHENOTYPE AND CELL MOTILITY

One of the most life threatening aspects of cancer is the ability of tumour cells to metastasize. The multistep transformation of a normal diploid population of cells to a tumorigenic cell population exhibiting the metastatic phenotype is a complex and poorly understood process. To accomplish the many steps in metastasis successfully, cells must be able to leave the primary tumour by invading the local host tissue and entering the circulation and lymphatics, arrest at the distant vascular bed of another tissue, invade the new tissue and proliferate as a new colony of cells (Liotta *et al*, 1991). An obligatory component at multiple steps of this process is cell motility. Therefore, if we understood how a cell generates locomotion, we might be able to devise treatment strategies to prevent the metastatic process.

Rudolph Virchow in 1863 suggested that cell motility is important in the cancer process, and this was first documented with time lapse cinematography in 1955 by George Gey. In 1968, Sumner Wood used a transparent rabbit ear chamber to study the in vivo motility of V2 carcinoma cells. He demonstrated that the carcinoma cells migrated at velocities comparable to those of leucocytes and 200 times faster than macrophages. In the past decade, time lapse videomicroscopy and in vitro motility assays have revolutionized the study of cell movement and have allowed the relationship between cell motility and metastatic potential to be explored (Hosaka *et al*, 1978; Haemmerli and Strauli, 1981; Mohler *et al*, 1987a). Although tumour cell populations are generally heterogeneous, cells that exhibit increased motility in vitro show an increased propensity to metastasize in vivo (Mohler *et al*, 1987a).

The relationship between tumour cell motility and metastatic potential has been most clearly demonstrated in the prostate. The Dunning R-3327 rat prostatic adenocarcinoma model has provided many histologically indistinguishable sublines of varying metastatic potential that originated from a single tumour (Isaacs *et al*, 1986). No studied biological, biochemical or morphological discriminator had previously been capable of identifying the individual sublines or predicting their metastatic potential. However, Mohler *et al* (1987b) demonstrated that five sublines of varying metastatic potential as well as normal rat prostate cells could be identified by a visual grading system of cell motility. Partin *et al* (1989) then developed a system for quantitating all aspects of cell motility that was able to correlate cell motility changes with an increase in metastatic potential in the Dunning tumours. These studies have established that increased cell motility is an important aspect of metastatic potential. Although these studies demonstrate a correlation between cell motility and metastasis, the mechanisms that lead to increased cellular motility remain unclear. However, clues to what stimulates motility are emerging.

STIMULATION OF CELL MOTILITY

Cell motility appears to be mediated in part through classical signal transduction pathways, which include activation of protein kinase C, tyrosine kinases and guanine triphosphate (GTP) binding proteins. Platelet derived growth factor, transforming growth factors, insulin and epidermal growth factor are thought to act through these pathways, and all have induced motility in normally quiescent cells (Heine *et al*, 1981; Goshima *et al*, 1984; Myrdal and Auersperg, 1986; Myrdal *et al*, 1986). Lassing and Linberg (1988) directly demonstrated the linkage of the phosphatidylinositol, a common second messenger in signal transduction pathways, to cell motility. In addition, Liotta and Schiffman (1988) have identified an autocrine motility factor secreted by tumour cells, which activates the GTP pathway and increases tumour cell motility.

Tumour promoting agents and oncogenes have also been shown to increase cell motility directly. Normal cells demonstrated transient enhanced motility and ruffling after treatment with phorbol ester, a tumour promoter that activates protein kinase C (Feuerstein and Cooper, 1984). Bar-Sagi and Feramisco (1986) induced a transient increase in cell motility when they injected into cells the p21 *ras* protein product, which stimulates the GTP pathway. Partin *et al* (1988) demonstrated that motility and metastatic potential can be induced in the Dunning tumours by transfection and expression of the v-Ha-*ras* oncogene. Furthermore, Taniguchi *et al* (1989) demonstrated that tumour cells transfected with *src* (tyrosine kinase pathway) and *fos* oncogenes exhibited augmented motility. Therefore, the altered regulation of multiple different signal transduction pathways may be involved in the stimulation of cell motility. How these altered signals act within the cell to increase cell locomotion is unclear.

Tissue Matrix System

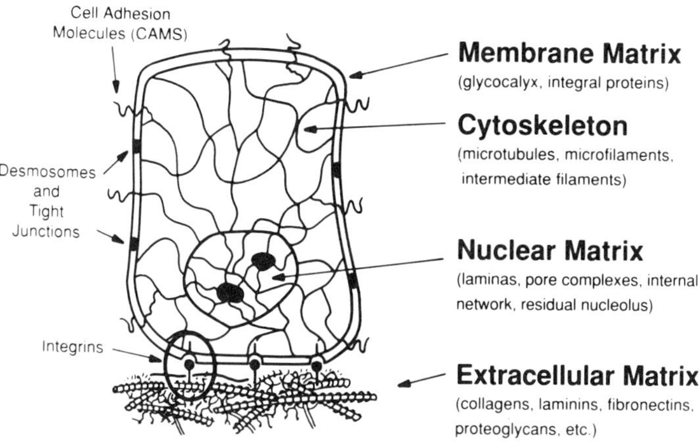

Fig. 1. The tissue matrix system. The cell is composed of a major insoluble framework that remains after extraction of the lipids and soluble proteins. The shape of the cell depends primarily on interactions of these structural components. The nuclear matrix is connected to the cytoskeleton, which in turn is attached to the ECM via the membrane matrix through integrins, cell adhesion molecules and tight junctions

STRUCTURAL BASIS OF CELL MOTILITY

The structures and complex cellular mechanisms involved in integrating cell motility are still poorly understood. It is now clear that cell locomotion is the result of a complex series of interactions between the dynamic skeleton of the cell and the intracellular and extracellular environments. As depicted in Fig. 1, the dynamic skeleton of the cell is made up of a tissue matrix system consisting of linkages and interactions between the nuclear matrix, the cytoskeleton and the extracellular matrix (ECM) (Pienta *et al*, 1989, in press b). The tissue matrix system is capable of undergoing dynamic shifts in structure and conformation through polymerization, cross linking, biochemical modifications and chemomechanical contractile and vibratory movements that result in cell locomotion (Pienta *et al*, in press a).

More specifically, it is thought that the generation of motility involves the generation of vector force by the interaction of intracellular actin microfilaments and microtubules coupled by transmembrane receptors to the external ECM (see Fig. 2) (Getzenberg *et al*, 1990). This interaction is mediated in part by cell adhesion molecules such as the integrin family. Ingber and Jamieson (1985) and Pienta *et al* (in press a) have suggested a tensegrity model as a theoretical system to explain how cells composed of structural elements such as actin and microtubules may be capable of motility. Tensegrity was defined by Buckminster Fuller in 1975 as a structural system composed of discontinuous compression elements, ie microtubules, connected by continuous tension cables (actin microfilaments), which continually interact in a dynamic fashion. Tensegrity structures allow great motility as each part is in coupled equilibri-

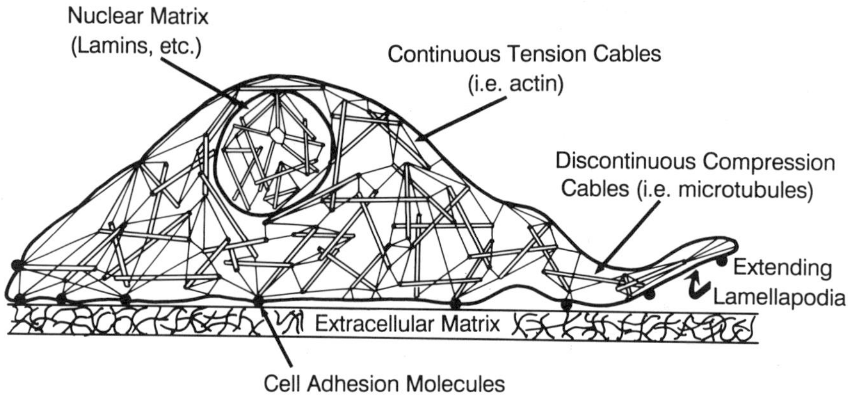

Fig. 2. The structural basis of cell motility. This simplified schematic of the cell skeleton is a first approximation of the tissue matrix system acting as a tensegrity structure (see text). The cytoskeletal elements are under tension and during cell locomotion exhibit complex dynamic changes and interactions. For directional movement to occur, overall vector tension must be generated, and both binding and uncoupling of cell adhesion molecules with the ECM must occur in a synchronized manner to permit traction, release and directional movement

um, so that mechanical forces can be transferred throughout the entire system. There is gathering evidence for this type of dynamic force generating structure within the cell. Both muscle and non-muscle cells are capable of generating tension, and James and Taylor (1969) calculated that a single fibroblast could generate a tensile force of 1.65×10^{-7} newtons. It had previously been hypothesized that within the cell, the actin-myosin-fibrillar network served as a tension producing element and that microtubules formed a scaffold that resisted this stress (reviewed in Getzenberg *et al*, 1990). Dennerll and colleagues (1988, 1989) were the first to measure directly such a tension and compression system in neurites. A tension derived tensegrity structure may be a more appropriate way to view cell structure than a rigid scaffold framework system, but it is unclear how this system is changed in the metastatic cancer cell. However, viewing motility in this framework allows us to devise strategies for inhibition.

CELL MOTILITY AS A CHEMOTHERAPEUTIC TARGET

The structures and mechanisms involved in cell motility can be divided into three broad categories: stimulation of motility, interaction of the cell with the ECM and the cytoskeletal components involved in cellular locomotion (see Fig. 3). The majority of previous work has focused on inhibiting the stimulation of motility, but we and others are currently studying inhibitors in each of these categories to determine their effects on cell motility in vitro and in vivo.

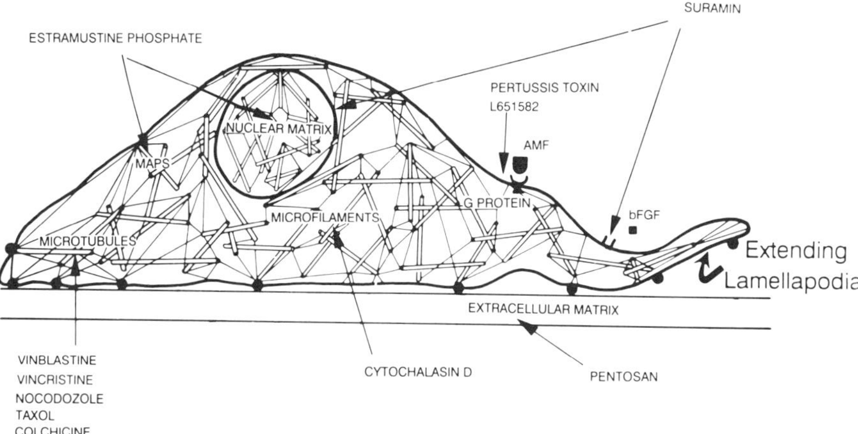

Fig. 3. Inhibition of cell motility may be accomplished at several different levels of cell structure and function (see text). Agents such as suramin and pertussis toxin can interfere with autocrine and paracrine growth factors that stimulate motility. Cell-ECM interactions can be targeted by drugs such as pentosan or by specific antibodies that recognize cell adehesion molecules. Microtubule or microfilament inhibitors can alter the cytoskeleton and inhibit motility as well as other cell processes such as mitosis

Stimulation of cell motility has been studied for at least two different systems. Liotta and colleagues, in a series of elegant experiments, have characterized the autocrine motility factor (Liotta and Schiffman, 1988; Kohn and Liotta, 1990). This factor stimulates cell motility and is coupled to the G protein signal transduction pathway. The effects of autocrine motility factor can be inhibited with pertussis toxin and the coccidiostat L651,582. Kohn and Liotta (1990) demonstrated that L651,582 inhibited melanoma cell motility in vitro and prolonged survival of nude mice injected intraperitoneally with OVCAR-2, a human ovarian carcinoma line.

Pienta *et al* (1991) observed that basic fibroblast growth factor (bFGF) stimulated the motility of Dunning prostate carcinoma cells, MAT-LyLu, in vitro. Basic FGF is a potent mitogen and angiogenic factor, which has been found in both normal and transformed prostate cells. Suramin, a trypan red derivative currently undergoing clinical trials, was found to block this growth factor effect. Suramin inhibited cell motility at a log lower concentration than growth inhibition (see Fig. 4). This suggests that part of the therapeutic action of suramin may be to inhibit cell motility, thereby possibly reducing the establishment of new metastatic lesions. Moreover, Pienta *et al* (1991) found that suramin had an inhibitory effect on cancer cell motility but not on endothelial cell motility. Suramin may represent a new class of chemotherapeutic agents with growth factor antagonist properties.

The interaction of the cell with the ECM is crucial for cell motility. To move, a cell must break the existing connection with the ECM, move forward and then form a new connection with the ECM, ie walk. It is possible that this process could also become a target for chemotherapeutic agents. Pienta *et al*

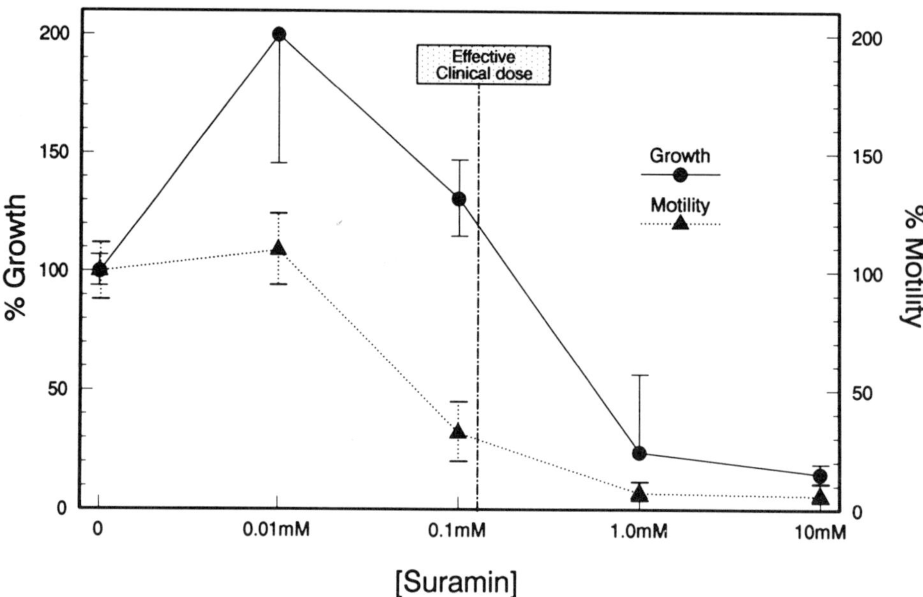

Fig. 4. Comparison of effect of suramin on the Dunning rat prostate adenocarcinoma cell line, the MAT-LyLu, on growth and motility at 48 hr. Cell growth was significantly increased at 0.01 mmol/l suramin without significant effect on cell motility. At 0.1 mmol/l suramin, cell growth was significantly increased, while cell motility was significantly decreased. At 1.0 mmol/l and 10 mmol/l suramin, both cell growth and cell motility were significantly decreased. Error bars represent standard error of the mean for three experiments, ten cells per experiment (from Pienta *et al*, 1991)

(in press c) have demonstrated that pentosan, a highly sulphated polysaccharide also currently in clinical trials, may work through such a mechanism. This drug, which has been shown to cross link vitronectin, a cell adhesion molecule, inhibits cell motility in vitro without inhibiting cell growth. Furthermore, pentosan does not appear to be a growth factor antagonist or to interfere with the integrity of the cytoskeleton. Therefore, pentosan may represent another new class of chemotherapeutic agents—those that interfere with cell-ECM interactions.

Another way to block cell-ECM interactions is with antibodies directed against cellular or ECM components involved in locomotion. The ECM exerts its effect via specific molecular interactions with the cell surface. The two major molecules associated with these interactions appear to be the adhesive glycoproteins laminin and fibronectin. Fibronectin has been shown to promote migration of cells (Norris *et al*, 1982; McCarthy *et al*, 1985), and Situ *et al* (1984) demonstrated that laminin stimulates murine tumour cell motility. Yamada *et al* (1990) have demonstrated that antibodies directed against integrin receptors on the cell surface, which mediate binding to fibronectin and laminin, could inhibit tumour cell migration. Since expression of these receptors changes with the cancer phenotype, this is a promising area for potential therapies.

Several chemotherapeutic agents that interfere with cytoskeletal structure are already in use. The microtubule inhibitors vincristine, vinblastine and taxol are all used as cytotoxic agents. They have multiple effects on cancer cells, and their effects on motility are not well characterized. However, Mareel *et al* (1988) have demonstrated that estramustine phosphate, a microtubule associated protein inhibitor, inhibits the invasion of prostate tumour cells into isolated chick heart cells. These findings suggest that an underappreciated mechanism of microtubule inhibitors is inhibition of motility as well as interference with the mitotic apparatus. The effect on motility of agents such as cytochalasin D, which interfere with actin microfilaments, have also not been well characterized. It is possible that these cytoskeletal structure inhibitors may be potent antimetastasis agents, but this is yet to be explored.

SUMMARY

The major cause of failure in the treatment of patients with solid malignancies is failure to prevent or control the spread of metastases. The metastatic process is a series of interrelated steps that must be accomplished before distant tumour foci can be established. Tumour cell motility is a complex process, which is involved in many of these steps. The mechanisms by which motility is stimulated and physically generated are complex and as yet poorly understood. Viewing the cell as a chemomechanical engine that relies on a tension based system for movement allows us to design chemotherapeutic strategies to inhibit tumour cell motility directly. Chemotherapeutic agents that block stimulation, interfere with cell-ECM interactions and interfere with cytoskeletal mechanics are already being tested. Further studies will be needed to define their efficacy.

Acknowledgements

This work was supported by National Institutes of Health grant CA-15416.

References

Bar-Sagi D and Feramisco JR (1986) Induction of membrane ruffling and fluid-phase pinocytosis in quiescent fibroblasts by *ras* proteins. *Science* **233** 1061–1068

Dennerll TJ, Joshi MC, Steel JL, Buxbaum RE and Heidemann SR (1988) Tension and compression in the cytoskeleton of PC-12 neurites II Quantitative measurements. *Journal of Cell Biology* **107** 665–674

Dennerll TJ, Lamoureaux P, Buxbaum RE and Heidemann SR (1989) The cytomechanics of axonal elongation and retraction. *Journal of Cell Biology* **109** 3073

Feuerstein N and Cooper HL (1984) TI studies of the differentiation of promyelocytic cells by phorbol ester I Induction of discrete membrane proteins characteristic of monocytes and expression of motility functions in HL-60 cells following differentiation by phorbol ester. *Biochima Biophysica Acta* **781** 239–246

Fuller RB (1975) *Synergetics,* p 395, Macmillan Publishing Co, New York

Getzenberg RH, Pienta KJ and Coffey DS (1990) The tissue matrix: cell dynamics and hormone action. *Endocrine Reviews* **11** 399–417

Gey GO (1955) Some aspect of the constitution and behavior of normal and malignant cells maintained in continuous culture, In: *The Harvey Lectures*, Series L, pp 154–229, 1954–1955

Goshima K, Masuda A and Owaribe K (1984) Insulin-induced formation of ruffling membranes of KB cells and its correlation with enhancement of amino acid transport. *Journal of Cell Biology* **88** 82–90

Haemmerli G and Strauli P (1981) In vitro motility of cells from human epidermoid carcinomas: a study by phase-contrast and reflection-contrast cinematography. *International Journal of Cancer* **27** 603–610

Heine UI, Kesi O-A and Wetzel B (1981) Rapid membrane changes in mouse epithelial cells after exposure to epidermal growth factor. *Journal of Ultrastructural Research* **77** 335–343

Hosaka S, Suzuki M, Goto M and Sato H (1978) Motility of rat ascites hepatoma cells with reference to malignant characteristics in cancer metastasis. *Gann* **69** 273–276

Ingber DE and Jamieson J (1985) Cells as tensegrity structures, architectural regulation of histodifferentiation by physical forces transduced over basement membrane, In: Andersson LL, Gahmberg CG and Kblom PE (eds). *Gene Expression during Normal and Malignant Differentiation*, pp 13–32, Academic Press, New York

Isaacs JT, Isaacs WB, Feitz WFJ and Scheres J (1986) Establishment and characterization of seven Dunning rat prostatic cancer cell lines and their use in developing methods for predicting metastatic abilities of prostatic cancer. *Prostate* **9** 261–281

James DW and Taylor JF (1969) The stress developed by sheets of chick fibroblasts *in vitro*. *Experimental Cell Research* **54** 107–112

Kohn EC and Liotta LA (1990) L651S82: A novel antiproliferative and antimetastasis agent. *Journal of the National Cancer Institute* **82** 54–60

Lassing I and Linberg V (1988) Evidence that the phosphatidylinositol cycle is linked to cell motility. *Experimental Cell Research* **174** 1–15

Liotta L and Schiffmann E (1988) Tumor autocrine motility factors. *Important Advances in Oncology* **17** 30–47

Liotta LA, Steeg PS and Stetler-Stevenson WG (1991) Cancer metastasis and angiogenesis: an imbalance of positive and negative regulation. *Cell* **64** 327–336

Mareel MH, Storme GA, Dragonetti CH *et al* (1988) Antiinvasive activity of estramustine on malignant MO_4 mouse cells and DU 145 human prostate carcinoma cells in vitro. *Cancer Research* **48** 1842–1849

McCarthy JB, Basara ML, Palm SL, Sas DF and Furcht LT (1985) The role of cell adhesion proteins—laminin and fibronectin—in the movement of malignant and metastatic cells. *Cancer and Metastasis Reviews* **4** 125–152

Mohler JL, Partin AW and Coffey DS (1987a) Prediction of metastatic potential by a new grading system of cell motility: validation in the Dunning R-3327 prostatic adenocarcinoma model. *Journal of Urology* **138** 168–170

Mohler JL, Partin AW, Isaacs WB and Coffey DS (1987b) Time lapse videomicroscopic identification of Dunning R-3327 adenocarcinoma and normal rat prostate cells. *Journal of Urology* **137** 544–547

Myrdal SE and Auersperg N (1986) An agent or agents produced by virus-transformed cells cause unregulated ruffling in untransformed cells. *Journal of Cell Biology* **102** 1224–1229

Myrdal SE, Twarzdzik DR and Auersperg N (1986) Cell-mediated coaction of transforming growth factors: incubation of type (β) with normal rat kidney cells produces a soluble activity that prolongs the ruffling response to type (α). *Journal of Cell Biology* **102** 1230–1234

Norris DA, Clark RAF, Swigard LM, Huff JC, Weston WL and Howell SE (1982) Fibronectin fragment(s) are chemotactic for human peripheral blood monocytes. *Journal of Immunology* **129** 1612–1618

Partin AW, Isaacs JT, Treiger B and Coffey DS (1988) Early cell motility changes associated with an increase in metastatic ability in rat prostatic cancer cells transfected with the v-

Harvey-*ras* oncogene. *Cancer Research* **48** 6050–6053

Partin AW, Schoeniger JS, Mohler JL and Coffey DS (1989) Fourier analysis of cell motility: correlation of motility with metastatic potential. *Proceedings of the National Acadamy of Sciences of the USA* **86** 1254–1258

Pienta KJ and Coffey DS (1991) Harmonic information transfer through a tissue tensegrity-matrix system. *Medical Hypothesis* **34** 88–95

Pienta KJ, Partin AW and Coffey DS (1989) Cancer as a disease of DNA organization and dynamic cell structure. *Cancer Research* **49** 2525–2532

Pienta KJ, Isaacs WB, Vindivich D and Coffey DS (1991) The effects of basic fibroblast growth factor and suramin on cell motility and growth of rat prostate cancer cells. *Journal of Urology* **145** 199–202

Pienta KJ, Partin AW and Coffey DS Cell motility and structural harmonics in prostate cancer, In: Karr JP, Tindall DJ, Coffey DS, Smith RG (eds). *Molecular and Cellular Biology of Prostate Cancer*, Springer Verlag, New York (in press a)

Pienta KJ, Getzenberg RH, and Coffey DS Cell structure and DNA organization. *CRC Reviews* (in press b)

Pienta KJ, Murphy BC, Isaacs WB, Isaacs JT and Coffey DS Pentosan, a new cancer chemotherapeutic agent, inhibits prostate cancer cell growth and motility. *Proceedings of American Urological Association Annual Meeting* (in press c)

Situ R, Lee EC, McCoy JP Jr and Varani J (1984) Stimulation of murine tumor cell motility by laminin. *Journal of Cell Science* **19** 167–176

Taniguchi S, Tatsuka M, Nakamatsu K *et el* (1989) High invasiveness associated with augmentation of motility in a fos-transferred highly metastatic rat 3Y1 cell line. *Cancer Research* **49** 6738–6744

Virchow R (1863) Ueber bewegliche thierische zellen. *Archives Pathology Anatomy Physiology Kliniche Medicine* **28** 237–240

Wood S Jr, Baker RR and Marzocchi B (1968) *In vivo* studies of tumor behavior: locomotion of and interrelationships between normal cells and cancer cells, In: Frei III E (ed). *The Proliferation and Spread of Neoplastic Cells*, pp 495–510, Williams & Wilkins Co, Baltimore

Yamada KM, Kennedy DW, Yamada SS, Gralnick H, Chen WT and Akiyama SK (1990) Monoclonal antibody and synthetic peptide inhibitors of human tumor cell migration. *Cancer Research* **50** 4485–4496

The authors are responsible for the accuracy of the references.

Programmed Cell Death as a New Target for Prostatic Cancer Therapy

NATASHA KYPRIANOU[1] • PAULA MARTIKAINEN[1]
LAWRENCE DAVIS[2] • HUGH F ENGLISH[3] • JOHN T ISAACS[1,4]

[1]Johns Hopkins Oncology Center, Baltimore Maryland 21205; [2]Johns Hopkins University School of Medicine; [3]Division of Endocrinology and Urology, Pennsylvania State University College of Medicine, Hershey Medical Center, Hershey, Pennsylvania 17033; [4]James Buchanan Brady Urological Institute, Johns Hopkins Medical Institution

INTRODUCTION

The Problem with Prostatic Cancer

Adenocarcinoma of the prostate varies widely in its clinical aggressiveness. In some patients, prostatic cancer metastasizes rapidly, killing the patient within 1 year of initial clinical presentation, whereas other patients may live for many years with localized disease without apparent metastases (Catalona and Scott, 1979). If prostate cancer is truly localized, then radical prostatectomy can be used to cure the patient (Walsh and Jewett, 1980). Unfortunately, about 60% of the 100 000 new cases of prostate cancer detected each year in the USA are non-organ confined at the time of initial diagnosis (Carter and Coffey, 1988). Thus, the majority of prostate cancer patients are not candidates for curative local surgery.

Patients with non-organ confined disease eventually require systemic androgen ablation therapy. The annual death rate from prostatic cancer has not fallen at all over the 50 years since androgen ablation became standard therapy for metastatic disease (Silverberg and Lubera, 1988). The superficially benign nature of androgen ablation has tended to disguise the fact that metastatic prostatic cancer is still a fatal disease for which no therapy that effectively increases survival is available (Lepor *et al*, 1982; Raghaven, 1988). Nearly all men with metastatic prostatic cancer treated by androgen ablation do respond initially, demonstrating that at least a proportion of their cancer cells are androgen responsive (Scott *et al*, 1980). Unfortunately, almost all these patients eventually relapse to a state unresponsive to further anti-androgen therapy, no matter how aggressive their secondary treatment (Schulze *et al*, 1987a). The major reason for the inability of androgen ablation therapy to be curative is that the cancer within an individual patient is composed of clones of androgen dependent and androgen independent prostatic cancer cells even before therapy is initiated (Prout *et al*, 1976; Sinha et al, 1977; Smolev *et al*, 1977; Isaacs and Coffey, 1981).

Therapeutic Implications of the Tumour Cell Heterogeneity of Prostatic Cancer

Development of such tumour cell heterogeneity can occur by a variety of mechanisms, eg multifocal origin of the tumour, adaptation or genetic instability (Isaacs, 1981). Regardless of the mechanism of development, once androgen independent cancer cells are present, the patient is no longer curable by androgen withdrawal therapy alone, no matter how complete, because this therapy kills only the androgen dependent cells without eliminating androgen independent prostatic cancer cells (Schulze *et al*, 1987a). To affect all the heterogeneous prostatic cancer cell populations within an individual patient, effective chemotherapy, specifically targeted against the pre-existing androgen independent cancer cells, must be simultaneously combined with androgen ablation directed against the androgen dependent cells. The validity of each of these points has been demonstrated by a series of studies in animals (Isaacs, 1984a; Ellis and Isaacs, 1985; Redding and Schally, 1985; Kung *et al*, 1988) and humans (Schulze *et al*, 1987b). The animal studies demonstrated that only by giving such a combined chemohormonal treatment is it possible to produce any reproducible level of cures in animals bearing a transplantable prostatic cancer (Isaacs, 1989). To produce cures, however, treatment must be started early in the course of the disease, the chemotherapy must have definitive efficacy against androgen independent cancer cells, it must be given for a crucial period and it must be begun simultaneously with, not subsequently to, androgen ablation (Isaacs, 1989). Although the concept of early combination chemohormonal therapy for prostatic cancer is valid, for such an approach to be therapeutically effective in humans, a chemotherapeutic agent must be available that can effectively control the growth of the androgen independent prostatic cancer cells.

Inability of Present Modalities to Eliminate Androgen Independent Prostatic Cancer Cells

Unfortunately, there are no chemotherapeutic agents that can effectively control the growth of human androgen independent prostatic cancer cells (Raghaven, 1988). This has led to a search for new approaches. The growth of any cancer is determined by the relationship between its rate of cell proliferation and death. Successful treatment for androgen independent cancer cells can be obtained by lowering the rate of cell proliferation and/or by raising the rate of cell death to a point where this exceeds the rate of cell proliferation.

There are a variety of antiproliferative chemotherapeutic agents that are cytostatic and/or cytotoxic to sensitive target cells. Unfortunately, these agents usually lead to death of cancer cells only if they subsequently undergo cell division (Shackney *et al*, 1978). Interphase cancer cells not proliferating at the time of, or soon enough after, exposure are resistant to such cytotoxic agents, since the cell has sufficient time to repair the damage induced (Schackney *et al*, 1978). Unfortunately, more than 90% of prostatic cancer cells within an individual patient are in interphase (Helpap *et al*, 1974; Meyers *et al*, 1982; Nemoto *et al*, 1990) and are thus resistant to standard cytotoxic chemotherapy (Raghaven, 1988).

NEW APPROACH TO THERAPY

What is needed is some type of cytotoxic therapy that induces the death of androgen independent prostatic cancer cells during interphase and thus does not require cell proliferation. Is it possible to induce the death of cells without requiring them to attempt to divide? The answer to this question is yes, as demonstrated by the rapid involution of the normal prostate following androgen ablation. Only about 2% of the cells in the normal adult prostate of intact male rats are undergoing cell proliferation on any day (Isaacs, 1984b). Androgen ablation (ie castration) of the male rat leads to a decrease in cell proliferation and to an increase in the rate of cell death such that 20% of the cells present die each day between 2 and 7 days after castration (Isaacs, 1984). By 7 days, more than 70% of the total number of epithelial cells in the rat prostate have died (Isaacs, 1984).

Response of the Normal Prostate to Androgen Ablation

Androgen has the dual ability to stimulate cell proliferation and inhibit cell death of normal prostatic glandular epithelial cells (Isaacs, 1984b; Kyprianou and Isaacs, 1988a). Androgen ablation induces a series of discrete biochemical events that lead to a cessation of cell proliferation and the death of these androgen dependent prostatic cells, ultimately resulting in involution of the gland. For example, within 12 hours of castration of the adult male rat, serum testosterone concentration falls to below 2% of the value present in an intact host. This rapid decline in serum androgen results in the ventral prostatic dihydrotestosterone concentration decreasing within the first 24 hours following castration to below a critical threshold value, and the result is cessation of proliferation and death of the androgen dependent ventral prostatic glandular epithelial cells (Kyprianou and Isaacs, 1988a).

Because transforming growth factor-β1 (TGF-β1) is a potent inhibitor of cell proliferation of both normal and malignant epithelial cells, the expression of TGF-β1 in the rat ventral prostate was studied after castration (Kyprianou and Isaacs, 1989). Steady state levels of TGF-β1 mRNA were determined by northern blot analysis and compared with mRNA levels for the C3 subunit of prostatein, the major androgen dependent secretory protein of ventral prostate. In the first day after castration, there is a dramatic increase in the levels of TGF-β1 mRNA in the ventral prostate (approximately 10-fold), and by 4 days after castration, TGF-β1 mRNA is maximally expressed (approximately 40-fold increase), by which time the androgen dependent C3 secretory protein mRNA transcripts diminish to undetectable levels. Androgen administration to rats 4 days after castration leads to a sharp decrease in TGF-β1 mRNA to a level comparable to its constitutive expression obtained in the intact control animals, indicating that expression of TGF-β1 in the rat ventral prostate is under negative androgenic regulation (Kyprianou and Isaacs, 1989). Scatchard analyses of the binding of TGF-β1 to membranes from rat ventral prostate reveal the presence of high affinity (kDa = 140 pM) saturable binding sites for ^{125}I-labelled TGF-β1, which are displaced in the presence of excess unlabelled TGF-β1 but are unaffected by epidermal growth factor, nerve growth factor, fibroblast growth factor or insulin, indicating the specificity of binding (Kyprianou and Isaacs, 1988b). Castration results in a significant increase in the total ^{125}I-labelled TGF-β1 binding per total prostate, with no apparent change in the affinity of membrane receptors for TGF-β1. These studies demonstrate that additional TGF-β1 receptors are synthesized during the first 4 days following castration, because the total number of receptors per gland increases two- to threefold even though the total number of cells per gland decreases by a third during this time period (Kyprianou and Isaacs, 1988b). The elevated TGF-β1 receptor and mRNA expression might be involved in the inhibition of cell proliferation and/or the induction of cell death observed following castration.

Attempts to demonstrate TGF-β1 inhibition of prostatic glandular cell proliferation during the regrowth of ventral prostate of castrated rats induced by exogenous androgen replacement have not been successful using either in vivo or in vitro exposure to exogenous TGF-β1 (Martikainen *et al*, 1990). This may be significant in that the in vitro growth of human neonatal prostatic epithelial cells has likewise not been shown to be inhibited by exposure to exogeneous TGF-β1 (Kaighn *et al*, 1989). As will be discussed below, there are studies, however, which suggest that changes in the TGF-β1 pathway may be involved in initiating prostatic glandular cell death following castration (Kyprianou and Isaacs, 1989a; Martikainen *et al*, 1990).

Interphase Death of Androgen Dependent Prostatic Cells following Androgen Ablation

The death of a cell can occur via several biochemically and morphologically distinct pathways (Kerr *et al*, 1972; Wyllie *et al*, 1980). One of these pathways has been termed "necrotic cell death". Necrotic cell death is elicited by any of a large variety of factors that lead to the permeabilization of the plasma membrane, with the resultant osmotic lysis of the cell and its internal membranes. In necrotic cell death, the cell has a passive role in initiating death. In contrast to this passively initiated necrotic cell death, there is a second pathway for cell death, termed programmed cell death, in which the cell actively participates in the initiation of its own death.

In programmed cell death, specific intracellular signals induce the cell to undergo an active energy dependent process of cell death that does not initially require a change in plasma membrane permeability (Wyllie *et al*, 1980). Once initiated, programmed cell death leads to a cascade of biochemical and morphological events that result in the irreversible fragmentation of the genomic DNA and then of the cell itself (Wyllie, 1980; Umansky *et al*, 1981; Cohen and Duke, 1984). In programmed cell death, fragmentation of DNA is an early event that irreversibly commits the cell to die and occurs before changes in plasma and internal membrane permeability. In many systems, this DNA fragmentation has been shown to result from activation of Ca^{2+}, Mg^{2+} dependent endonuclease present with the cell nucleus, which selectively hydrolyses DNA at sites located between nucleosomal units, thus resulting in a stereotypic nucleosomal ladder of DNA fragments (Wyllie, 1980; Umansky *et al*, 1981; Cohen and Duke, 1984; Wyllie *et al*, 1984). This nuclease activation is thought to be triggered by a sustained elevation in the intracellular free Ca^{2+} concentration initiated early in programmed cell death (Kaiser and Edelman, 1977; Nicotera *et al*, 1986; Poenie *et al*, 1987; Allbritton *et al*, 1988; McConkey *et al*, 1989a,b). DNA is also degraded during necrosis, but this is a late event in necrotic cells whose plasma and internal membranes have already lysed. In necrotic death, the DNA is degraded into a continuous spectrum of sizes as a result of the simultaneous action of both lysosomal proteases and nucleases released in cells already dead (Kyprianou and Isaacs, 1988a). The morphological pathway for programmed cell death is rather stereotypic and has been given the name "apoptosis" to distinguish this actively initiated process (ie early nuclear changes followed by eventual nuclear disintegration and fragmentation of the dying cell into a cluster of membrane bound apoptotic bodies) from the passively initiated process of necrotic cell death in which plasma, mitochondrial and lysosomal membrane changes precede changes within the cell nucleus (Kerr *et al*, 1972; Wyllie *et al*, 1980).

Biochemical and morphological studies have demonstrated that the involution of the normal prostate following androgen ablation is not the result of passively initiated necrotic cell death but is a process actively initiated by the cells themselves (Bruchovsky *et al*, 1975; Lee, 1982; Isaacs, 1984). This process involves a series of specific biochemical steps, ie enhanced expression of testosterone repressed prostatic message-2 (*TRPM-2*) (Montpetit *et al*, 1986; Rouleau *et al*, 1990) and a series of other genes (Saltzman *et al*, 1987; Buttyan *et al*, 1988); increased synthesis of new proteins including TRPM-2 (Lee and Sensibar, 1985; Buttyan *et al*, 1989; Grima *et al*, 1990); increase in intracellular free Ca^{2+} (Connor *et al*, 1988; Kyprianou *et al*, 1988; Martikainen and Isaacs, 1990); Ca^{2+}, Mg^{2+} dependent endonuclease induced fragmentation of DNA (Kyprianou and Isaacs, 1988a; Kyprianou *et al*, 1988; English *et al*, 1989) and development of apoptotic bodies (Kerr and Searle, 1973; Sanford *et al*, 1984; English *et al*, 1989), that result in the programmed death (apoptosis) of the androgen dependent glandular epithelial cells within the prostate following androgen ablation. This programmed death occurs in interphase and does not require these androgen dependent glandular prostatic epithelial cells to attempt to divide (Isaacs, 1984b).

Programmed Death of Human Prostatic Cancer Cells following Androgen Ablation

Additional studies have demonstrated that not only normal rat prostatic cells but also human androgen responsive prostatic cancer cells activate the pathway of programmed cell death following androgen ablation (Kyprianou *et al*, 1990). The PC-82 human prostatic cancer is highly androgen responsive when grown as a xenograft in nude mice (van Steenbrugge *et al*, 1984). If intact male nude mice are inoculated with human PC-82 prostatic cancer, continuously growing tumours are produced. If the host mice are castrated when the PC-82 tumour is approximately 0.5 cm^3 in size, the rate of cell proliferation decreases about 7-fold from 3.5% of the cells proliferating per day to 0.5%, and the rate of cell death increases approximately 11-fold from 0.5% of the cells dying per day to 4.7%. Because of these changes, the tumour involutes rapidly after castration, reaching approximately half its starting size within 3 weeks of castration. Biochemical analysis during this involution period has demonstrated that both TGF-β1 and TRPM-2 mRNA levels as well as DNA fragmentation into nucleosomal size pieces are detectably increased within the first day following castration (Kyprianou *et al*, 1990). The levels of all of these parameters increase to a maximum on the third day following castration. In addition, if exogenous androgen is given back to the castrated host, DNA fragmentation ceases, TGF-β1 mRNA and TRPM-2 mRNA levels drop, involution stops and tumour growth resumes.

Programmed Death of Proliferating Androgen Independent Prostatic Cancer Cells

Although androgen independent prostatic cancer cells do not activate the program of cell death following androgen ablation, these cells still retain the major portion of the programmed cell death pathway. This has been demonstrated using a series of Dunning R-3327 androgen independent prostatic cancers established as continuously growing in in vitro cell lines (Isaacs *et al*, 1986). For example, the Dunning AT-3 androgen independent, highly metastatic, anaplastic prostatic cancer cells have been treated in vitro with a variety of non-androgen ablative agents that induce "thymineless death" of the cells (eg cells treated with 5-fluorodeoxyuridine [5-Fdur] or tri-fluorothymidine [TFT]). Analysis has revealed that "thymineless death" results in an increase in the expression of the *TRPM-2* gene and an activation of the nuclear Ca^{+2} Mg^{+2} dependent endonuclease, with the resultant fragmentation of the genomic DNA of the AT-3 cells into a similar nucleosomal ladder, as seen in the death of androgen dependent prostate cells following castration (Kyprianou and Isaacs, 1989b). This cascade of events requires 6–18 hours before fragmentation of the DNA is complete. The AT-3 cells are not "dead", as defined by their ability to metabolize a mitochondrial vital dye, until 24 hours of treatment. This demonstrates that the fragmentation of the genomic DNA is an early, irreversible commitment step in programmed death of even androgen independent prostatic cancer cells. If the AT-3 cells are treated with osmotic shock induced by exposure to distilled water or agents that inhibit the plasma membrane ATPase activity, ie ouabain or iodoacetate, the cells rapidly lyse within less than 3 hours after treatment and do not metabolize the vital dye (ie they are dead) even though they do not fragment their DNA into nucleosomal size pieces nor do they elevate *TRPM-2* mRNA levels. These data demonstrate that agents that induce necrotic death of the AT-3 cells (ie osmotic effects) do not lead to the activation of the programmed death of these cells. Programmed death can be activated, however, even in androgen independent prostatic cancer cells, by specific agents, eg those able to induce a "thymineless" state (Kyprianou and Isaacs, 1989b).

Programmed Death of Interphase Androgen Independent Prostatic Cancer Cells

The problem with agents of this latter type, however, is that cell proliferation is required for the "thymineless" state to activate programmed death in these AT-3 cells. In this regard, it is interesting that in "thymineless" programmed death in the AT-3 cells, TGF-β1 mRNA is not enhanced. This may be significant in that in vitro untreated exponentially growing AT-3 cells produce and secrete substantial amounts of TGF-β1 (Matuo *et al*, 1990). At a concentration of 5 ng/ml, TGF-β1 has only a slight inhibitory effect on the growth of AT-3 cells in culture (ie <30% reduction in growth rate) (Matuo *et al*, 1990); TGF-β1, even at a concentration of 20 ng/ml, however, does not induce death of the AT-3. In contrast, both in vivo and in vitro studies have demonstrated that TGF-β1 can induce the programmed death of androgen dependent normal rat prostatic glandular cells even when physiological levels of androgen are present (Kyprianou and Isaacs, 1989a; Martikainen *et al*, 1990). This TGF-β1 induced programmed death does not require cell proliferation. These results suggest that the interphase death of androgen dependent normal and malignant prostate cells induced following androgen ablation may involve a TGF-β1 response and that androgen independent prostatic cancer cells have lost this coupled responsiveness.

One explanation for the inability of androgen ablation to induce programmed death in androgen independent prostatic cancer cells is that such ablation is not coupled to TGF-β1 changes and thus a sustained elevation in the intracellular free Ca^{2+} levels is not induced in these cells. This raises the issue of whether interphase androgen independent prostatic cancer cells can be induced to undergo programmed death if an elevation in the intracellular free Ca^{2+} is sufficiently sustained. To test this possibility, chronic exposure to a calcium specific ionophore was used to examine the temporal response of androgen independent, AT-3 rat prostatic cancer cells to a sustained elevation in intracellular free Ca^{2+}.

If AT-3 cells are treated in vitro with 10 μM calcium specific ionophore, ionomycin, cell death can be induced. Using microfluorescence image analysis (Tucker *et al*, 1989) of AT-3 cells loaded with the fluorescent dye, fura-2, to measure intracellular free Ca^{2+} level, such ionomycin treatment has been demonstrated to elevate the intracellular free Ca^{2+} levels from less than 50 nm to more than 400 nm within the first minute of treatment. After the first few minutes, the intracellular free Ca^{2+} returned to approximately 100–200 nm. Such sustained elevations in intracellular free Ca^{2+} result in cell proliferation stopping within 6 hours of treatment and the cells arresting in G_0 (ie the cells are in interphase). These interphase cells begin to die after about 48 to 72 hours. Biochemical analysis during this time course demonstrated that DNA fragmentation into nucleosomal oligomers begins as early as 6 hours after Ca^{2+} ionophore treatment (Martikainen *et al*, 1991).

The temporal pattern of DNA fragmentation is co-incident with these AT-3 cells losing their clonogenic ability. This demonstrates that once DNA fragmentation has occurred, the cell is irreversibly committed to death. DNA fragmentation is initiated at a time when plasma membrane permeability, mitochondrial function and cellular ATP content are all still maintained. Thus, the interphase death of AT-3 cells induced by 10 μM ionomycin treatment occurs via programmed, not necrotic, cell death (Martikainen *et al*, 1991).

Since the death of AT-3 cells induced by ionomycin treatment is via the programmed death pathway, it is noteworthy that no enhancement of *TRPM-2* gene expression occurs during this process (Martikainen *et al*, 1991). In all previous studies, in a large variety of cell types, expression of *TRPM-2* has been consistently enhanced when cells have been induced by a series of diverse means to undergo programmed death (Montpetit *et al*, 1986; Buttyan *et al*, 1989; Kyprianou and Isaacs, 1989b; Day *et al*, 1990; Kyprianou *et al*, 1990, 1991; Rouleau *et al*, 1990). Programmed cell death without enhancement of *TRPM-2* gene expression is even more significant in that when proliferating AT-3 cells undergo programmed death following exposure to chemotherapy agents that produce a "thymineless" state, enhanced *TRPM-2* mRNA expression is rapidly induced (Kyprianou and Isaacs, 1989b). These results suggest that enhanced *TRPM-2* expression either is an epiphenomenon not required for programmed cell death or is involved in the process that causes the initial elevation in intracellular free Ca^{2+}. The latter possibility, if correct, would explain why enhanced *TRPM-2* expression is not required in the programmed death of AT-3 cells induced by ionomycin, since the ionophore itself induces the required elevation in intracellular free Ca^{2+}, whereas it is required for programmed death induced by agents that produce a "thymineless" state, where presumably *TRPM-2* is involved in elevating intracellular free Ca^{2+}.

The possibility that enhanced *TRPM-2* expression is specifically involved in the elevation of intracellular free Ca^{2+} is further supported by the demonstration that the *TRPM-2* gene is identical to the previously identified sulphated glycoprotein-2 gene (*SGP-2*) (Bettuzzi *et al*, 1989). The encoded SGP-2 protein is secreted by Sertoli cells and binds to the acrosomal membrane of sperm (Sylvester *et al*, 1984). This might be significant, since the sperm undergoes an acrosomal reaction during penetration of the egg. This acrosomal reaction involves the breakdown of the acrosomal membrane, a process that is known to be initiated by an influx of extracellular Ca^{2+} (Thomas and Meizel, 1988). Recent immunocytochemical studies have demonstrated that TRPM-2 protein is localized to the apical cytoplasmic membranes of rat ventral prostatic glandular cells undergoing programmed cell death as early as 18–24 hours following castration. Western blot analysis has similarly confirmed that the TRPM-2 protein is associated with the cytoplasmic membranes. These results are consistent with the involvement of TRPM-2 protein in the influx of extracellular Ca^{2+} into prostatic glandular cells induced by androgen ablation, possibly by its interaction with plasma membrane slow calcium channels.

SUMMARY

To increase survival of men with metastatic prostatic cancer, a modality that can effectively eliminate androgen independent cancer cells is desperately needed. By combining such an effective modality with androgen ablation, all of the heterogeneous populations of tumour cells within a prostatic cancer patient can be affected, thus optimizing the chances of cure. Unfortunately, such effective therapy for the androgen independent prostatic cancer cell is not yet available. This therapy will probably require two types of agents, one having antiproliferative activity affecting the small number of dividing androgen independent cells, and the other able to increase the low rate of cell death among the majority of non-proliferating (ie interphase) androgen independent prostatic cancer cells present. Androgen dependent prostatic epithelial cells can be made to undergo programmed death by means of androgen ablation, even if the cells are not in the proliferative cell cycle. Androgen independent prostatic cancer cells retain the major portion of this programmed cell death pathway, only there is a defect in the pathway such that it is no longer activated by androgen ablation. If the intracellular free Ca^{2+} is sustained at an elevated level for a sufficient time, androgen independent cells can be induced to undergo programmed death. The long term goal is therefore to develop some type of non-androgen ablative method that can be used in vivo to induce a sustained elevation in Ca^{2+} in androgen independent prostatic cancer cells. To accomplish this task, a more complete understanding of the biochemical pathways involved in programmed cell death is urgently needed. At present, studies are focusing on the mechanism involved in the Ca^{2+} elevation in the normal and malignant androgen dependent cell induced following androgen ablation and the role of the TRPM-2 protein in this process.

References

Allbritton NL, Verret CR, Wolley RC and Eisen HN (1988) Calcium ion concentrations and DNA fragmentation in target cell destruction by murine cloned cytotoxic T lymphocytes. *Journal of Experimental Medicine* **167** 514

Bettuzzi S, Hiipakka RA, Gilna P and Liao S (1989) Identification of an androgen-repressed mRNA in rat ventral prostate as coding for sulphated glycoprotein 2 by cDNA cloning and sequence analysis. *Biochemical Journal* **257** 293–296

Bruchovsky N, Lesser B and Van Doorn E (1975) Hormonal effect on cell proliferation in rat prostate. *Vitamins Hormone Research* **33** 61–100

Buttyan R, Zaker Z, Lochshin R and Wolgemuth D (1988) Cascade induction of c-fos, c-myc, and heat shock 70K transcripts during regression of the rat ventral prostate gland. *Molecular Endocrinology* **2** 650–657

Buttyan R, Olsson CA, Pintar J *et al* (1989) Induction of the TRPM-2 gene in cells undergoing programmed death. *Molecular Cellular Biology* **9** 3473–3481

Carter HB and Coffey DS (1988) Prostate Cancer: the magnitude of the problem in the United States, In: Coffey DS, Resnick MI, Dorr FA and Karr JP (eds). *A Multidisciplinary Analysis of Controversies in the Management of Prostate Cancer*, pp 1–7, Plenum Press, New York and London

Catalona WJ and Scott WW (1979) Carcinoma of the prostate, In: Harrison JH, Gittes RF, Perlmutter AD, Stamey TA and Walsh PC (eds). *Campbell's Urology*, pp 1085–1124, WB Saunders & Co, Philadelphia

Cohen JJ and Duke RC (1984) Glucocorticoid activation of a calcium-dependent endonuclease in thymocyte nuclei leads to cell death. *Journal of Immunology* **132** 38–42

Connor J, Sawdzuk IS, Benson MC *et al* (1988) Calcium channel antagonists delay regression of androgen-dependent tissues and suppress gene activity associated with cell death. *Prostate* **13** 119–130

Day JR, Laping NJ, McNeill TH, Schreiber SS, Pasinetti G and Caleb EF (1990) Castration enhances expression of glial fibrillary acidic protein and sulfated glycoprotein-2 in the intact and lesion-altered hippocampus of the adult male rat. *Molecular Endocrinology* **4** 1995–2002

Ellis WJ and Isaacs JT (1985) Effectiveness of complete vs partial androgen withdrawal therapy for the treatment of prostatic cancer as studied in the Dunning R-3327 system of rat prostatic carcinomas. *Cancer Research* **45** 6041

English HF, Kyprianou N and Isaacs JT (1989) Relationship between DNA fragmentation and apoptosis in the programmed cell death in the rat prostate following castration. *Prostate* **15** 233–251

Grima J, Zwain I, Lockshin RA, Bardin CW and Cheng CY (1990) Diverse secretory patterns of clusterin by epididymis and prostate/seminal vesicles undergoing cell regression after orchiectomy. *Endocrinology* **126** 2989–2997

Helpap B, Steins R and Bruhl P (1974) Autoradiographic *in vitro* investigations on prostatic tissue with C-14 and H-3 thymidine double labeling method. *Beitrage Fur Pathologischen Anatomie Und Allgemeinen Pathologie* **151** 65–72

Isaacs JT (1981) Cellular factors in the development of resistance to hormonal therapy, In: Bruchovsky N, Goldie, J (eds). *Drug and Hormone Resistance in Neoplasia* **1** 139–156, CRC Press, Boca Raton

Isaacs JT (1984a) The timing of androgen ablation therapy and/or chemotherapy in the treatment of prostatic cancer. *Prostate* **5** 1–18

Isaacs JT (1984b) Antagonistic effect of androgen on prostatic cell death. *Prostate* **5** 545–558

Isaacs JT (1989) Relationship between tumor size and curability of prostate cancer by combined chemohormonal therapy. *Cancer Research* **49** 6290–6294

Isaacs JT and Coffey DS (1981) Adaptation vs selection as the mechanism responsible for the relapse of prostatic cancer to androgen ablation as studied in the Dunning R-3327 H adenocarcinoma. *Cancer Research* **41** 5070–5075

Isaacs JT, Isaacs WB, Feitz FJ, Scheres J (1986) Establishment and characterization of seven Dunning rat prostatic cancer cell lines and their use in developing methods for predicting metastatic ability of prostatic cancer. *Prostate* **9** 261–281

Kaighn ME, Reddel RR, Lechner JF *et al* (1989) Transformation of human neonatal prostate epithelial cells by strontium phosphate transfection with a plasmid containing SV40. *Cancer Research* **49** 3050–3056

Kaiser N and Edelman IS (1977) Calcium dependence of glucocorticoid-induced lymphocytolysis. *Proceedings of the National Academy of Sciences of the USA* **74** 638–642

Kerr JFR and Searle J (1973) Deletion of cells by apoptosis during castration-induced involution of the rat prostate. *Virchows Archives B* **13** 87

Kerr JFR, Wyllie AH and Currie AR (1972) Apoptosis: a basic biological phenomenon with wide ranging implications in tissue kinetics. *British Journal of Cancer* **26** 239–257

Kung TT, Mingo GG, Siegel MI and Watnick AS (1988) Effect of andrenalectomy, flutamide and leuprolide on the growth of the Dunning R-3327 prostatic carcinomas. *Prostate* **12** 357–364

Kyprianou N and Isaacs JT (1988a) Activation of programmed cell death in the rat ventral prostate after castration. *Endocrinology* **122** 552–562

Kyprianou N and Isaacs JT (1988b) Identification of a cellular receptor for transforming growth factor-β in rat ventral prostate and its negative regulation by androgens. *Endocrinology* **123** 2124–2131

Kyprianou N and Isaacs JT (1989a) Expression of transforming growth factor-β in the rat ventral prostate during castration-induced programmed cell death. *Molecular Endocrinology* **3** 1515–1522

Kyprianou N and Isaacs JT (1989b) Thymine-less death in androgen-independent prostatic cancer cells. *Biochemical and Biophysical Research Communications* **165** 73–81

Kyprianou N, English HF and Isaacs JT (1988) Activation of a Ca^{2+}-Mg^{2+}-dependent endonuclease as an early event in castration-induced prostatic cell death. *Prostate* **13** 103–118

Kyprianou N, English HF and Isaacs JT (1990) Programmed cell death during regression of PC-82 human prostate cancer following androgen ablation. *Cancer Research* **50** 3748–3753

Kyprianou N, Alexander RB and Isaacs JT (1991a) Activation of programmed cell death by recombinant human tumor necrosis factor plus topoisomerase II targeted drugs in L-929 tumor cells. *Journal of the National Cancer Institute* **83** 346–349

Kyprianou N, English HF, Davidson NE and Isaacs JT (1991b) Programmed cell death during regression of the MCF-7 human breast cancer following estrogen ablation. *Cancer Research* **51** 162–166

Lee C (1982) Physiology of castration-induced regression of the rat prostate, In: Murphy GP,

Sandberg AA and Karr JP (eds). *The Prostate Cell: Structure and Function, Part A, Morphology, Secretory, and Biochemical Aspects: Progress in Clinical and Biological Research* 74A, pp 145–159, Liss, New York

Lee C and Sensibar JA (1985) Protein of the rat prostate: synthesis of new proteins in the ventral lobe during castration-induced regression. *Journal of Urology* **138** 903–908

Lepor H, Ross A and Walsh PC (1982) The influence of hormonal therapy on survival of men with advanced prostatic cancer. *Journal of Urology* **128** 335–340

McConkey DJ, Hartzell P, Nicotera P and Orrenius S (1989a) Calcium-activated DNA fragmentation kills immature thymocytes. *FASEB Journal* **3** 1843–1849

McConkey DJ, Nicotera P, Hartzell P, Bellomo G, Wyllie AH and Orrenius S (1989b) Glucocorticoids activate a suicide process in thymocytes through an elevation of cytosolic Ca^{2+} concentration. *Archives of Biochemistry and Biophysics* **269** 365–370

Martikainen P and Isaacs JT (1990) Role of calcium in the programmed death of rat prostatic glandular cells. *Prostate* **17** 175–188

Martikainen P, Kyprianou N and Isaacs JT (1990) Effect of transforming growth factor-β1 on proliferation and death of rat prostatic cells. *Endocrinology* **127** 2963–2968

Martikainen P, Kyprianou N, Tucker RW, and Isaacs JI (1991) Programmed death of non-proliferating androgen-independent prostatic cancer cells. *Cancer Research* **51** 4693–4701

Matuo Y, Nish N, Takasuka H *et al* (1990) Production and significance of TGF-β in AT-3 metastatic cell line established from the Dunning rat prostatic adenocarcinoma. *Biochemical and Biophysical Research Communications* **166** 840–847

Meyers JS, Sufrin G, Martin SA (1982) Proliferation activity of benign human prostate, prostatic adenocarcinoma and seminal vesicle evaluated by thymidine labeling. *Journal of Urology* **128** 1353–1356

Montpetit ML, Lawless KR and Tenniswood M (1986) Androgen repressed messages in the rat ventral prostate. *Prostate* **8** 25–36

Nemoto R, Hattori K, Uchida K *et al* (1990) S-phase fraction of human prostate adenocarcinoma studied with in vivo bromodeoxyuridine labeling. *Cancer* **66** 509–514

Nicotera P, Hartzell P, Davis G and Orrenius S (1986) The formation of plasma membrane blebs in hepatocytes exposed to agents that increase cytosolic Ca^{2+} is mediated by the activation of a non-lysosomal proteolytic system. *Science* **209** 139

Poenie M, Tsien RY and Schmitt-Verhulsm A-M (1987) Sequential activation and lethal hit measured by $[Ca^{2+}]$, in individual cytolytic T cells and targets. *EMBO Journal* **6** 2233

Prout GR, Leiman B, Daly JJ, MacLoughlin RA, Griffin PP and Young HH (1976) Endocrine changes after diethylstilbestrol therapy. *Urology* **7** 148–155

Raghavan D (1988) Non-hormone chemotherapy for prostate cancer: principles of treatment and application to the testing of new drugs. *Seminars in Oncology* **15** 371–389

Redding TW and Schally AV (1985) Investigation of the combination of the agonist D-Trp-6 LHRH and the antiandrogen flutamide on the treatment of Dunning R-3328 H prostatic cancer model. *Prostate* **6** 219–232

Rouleau M, Leger J and Tenniswood M (1990) Ductal heterogeneity of cytokeratins, gene expression, and cell death in the rat ventral prostate. *Molecular Endocrinology* **4** 2003–2013

Saltzman AG, Hiipakka RA, Chang C and Liao S (1987) Androgen repression of the production of 29 kilodalton protein and its mRNA in the rat ventral prostate. *Journal of Biological Chemistry* **262** 432–437

Sanford ML, Searle JW and Kerr JFR (1984) Successive waves of apoptosis in the rat prostate after repeated withdrawal of testosterone stimulation. *Pathology* **16** 406–410

Schulze H, Isaacs JT and Coffey DS (1987a) A critical review of the concept of total androgen ablation in the treatment of prostatic cancer, In: Murphy GP, Khory S, Kuss R, Chatelain C and Denis L (eds). *Prostate Cancer Part A: Research, Endocrine Treatment, and Histopathology: Progress in Clinical and Biological Research* 243A, pp 1–19, Liss, New York

Schulze H, Isaacs JT, Senge T (1987b) Inability of complete androgen blockade to increase survival of patients with advanced prostate cancer as compared to standard hormonal therapy. *Journal of Urology* **137** 909–911

Scott WW, Menon M and Walsh PC (1980) Hormonal therapy of prostatic cancer. *Cancer* **45** 1929–1936

Shackney SE, McCormack GW and Cuchural GJ (1978) Growth rate patterns of solid tumors and their relationship to responsiveness to therapy. *Annals of Internal Medicine* **89** 107–115

Silverberg E and Lubera JA (1988) Cancer Statistics. *CA: Cancer Journal for Clinicians* **38** 14–19

Sinha AA, Blackhard CE and Seal US (1977) A critical analysis of tumor morphology and hormone treatment in the untreated and estrogen treated responsive and refractory human prostatic carcinoma. *Cancer* **40** 2836–2850

Smolev JK, Heston WDW, Scott WS and Coffey DS (1977) An appropriate animal model for prostatic cancer. *Cancer Treatment Reports* **61** 273–287

Sylvester SR, Skinner MK and Griswold MD (1984) A sulfated glycoprotein synthesized by Sertoli cells and by epididymal cells is a component of the sperm membrane. *Biology of Reproduction* **31** 1087–1101

Thomas P and Meizel S (1988) An influx of extracellular calcium is required for initiation of the human sperm acrosomal reaction induced by human follicular fluid. *Gamete Research* **20** 397–411

Tucker RW, Meade-Cobun K and Loats H (1989) Measurement of free intracellular calcium (Cai) in fibroblasts: digital image analysis of Fura 2 fluorescence, In: Fiskun G (eds). *Cell Calcium Metabolism*, pp 239–248, Plenum Press, New York and London

Umansky SR, Korol BA and Nelipovich PA (1981) In vivo DNA degradation in thymocytes of γ-irradiated or hydrocortisone-treated rats. *Biochimica Biophysica Acta* **655** 9–17

van Steenbrugge GJ, Groen M, Romijn JC and Schroeder F (1984) Biological effects of hormonal treatment regimens on a transplantable human prostate tumor line (PC-82). *Journal of Urology* **131** 812–817

Walsh PC and Jewett HJ (1980) Radical surgery for prostate cancer. *Cancer* **45** 1906–1910

Wyllie AH (1980) Glucocorticoid induces in thymocytes a nuclear-like activity associated with the chromatin condensation of apoptosis. *Nature* **284** 555–556

Wyllie AH, Kerr JFR and Currie AR (1980) Cell death: the significance of apoptosis. *International Reviews of Cytology* **68** 251–306

Wyllie AH, Morris RG, Smith AL and Dunlop D (1984) Chromatin cleavage in apoptosis: association with condensed chromatin morphology and dependence on macromolecular synthesis. *Journal of Pathology* **142** 67–77

The authors are responsible for the accuracy of the references.

Biographical Notes

Evelyn R Barrack, PhD, obtained a BSc in Biomedical Sciences at McGill University in Montreal and a PhD in Pharmacology at the Johns Hopkins University School of Medicine in Baltimore. She remained at Hopkins for postdoctoral training, then joined the faculty in the Department of Urology. She is Associate Professor of Urology in the Johns Hopkins University School of Medicine and Associate Director of Research in the James Buchanan Brady Urological Institute of the Johns Hopkins Hospital.

Terri H Beaty, PhD, received her undergraduate degree from the University of Texas at Austin and her doctorate in Human Genetics from the University of Michigan. She is currently an Associate Professor in the Department of Epidemiology at the Johns Hopkins University School of Hygiene and Public Health with research interests in genetic epidemiology and statistical genetics.

Bob S Carter is a graduate of Brigham Young University. He is currently a candidate for the MD and PhD degrees at the Johns Hopkins University School of Medicine and School of Hygiene and Public Health. His doctoral thesis concerns the genetic epidemiology and molecular genetics of prostate cancer.

Barton Childs, MD, is Emeritus Professor of Paediatrics at the Johns Hopkins University School of Medicine.

Leland W K Chung obtained his PhD at the University of Oregon Medical School and was trained at Johns Hopkins University, School of Medicine, and the James Buchanan Brady Urological Institute, Johns Hopkins Hospital, under Professor Donald S Coffey. He is Professor of Urology, Biochemistry and Molecular Biology and Director of the Urology Research Laboratory, University of Texas MD Anderson Cancer Center. His major research interests include the mechanisms of mesenchymal-epithelial interaction in genitourinary cancers and androgen regulation of gene expression by normal and neoplastic tissues.

Donald S Coffey, PhD, received his doctoral degree in biochemistry from the Johns Hopkins University School of Medicine. He is currently a Professor of Oncology, Urology, and Pharmacology and Molecular Sciences at the Johns Hopkins University School of Medicine. He is Director of the Research Laboratories of the Department of Urology at the Johns Hopkins Hospital and Deputy Director of the Johns Hopkins Oncology Center.

Gerald R Cunha, PhD, is Professor of Anatomy at the University of California, San Francisco. He trained in biology at the University of Santa Clara and received his PhD in anatomy at the University of Chicago in 1970. His early work at Stanford University dealt with mesenchymal-epithelial interactions in the developing male and female genital tracts. This basic theme was extended to an analysis of cell-cell interactions in hormonal response in developing and adult reproductive tracts while at the University of Colorado, Denver. In 1982 he joined the faculty at the University of California, where his group has established the idea that many effects of androgens on epithelial cells are elicited via mesenchymal androgen receptors and that adult epithelial differentiation and function can be altered by inductive mesenchymes. These findings have led to studies demonstrating that inductive mesenchymes can induce differentiation of prostatic carcinoma cells, an event associated with loss of tumorigenesis.

Lawrence Davis was a medical student in the Johns Hopkins University School of Medicine. After receiving his MD in June, 1991, he began his residency in internal medicine and hopes eventually to continue in clinical research.

Shin Egawa graduated in Medicine from Iwate Medical College, Japan, in 1981. He received his training in urology at Kitasato University School of Medicine, Japan. He is a research associate in the Scott Department of Urology, Baylor College of Medicine, Houston, Texas.

Hugh F English received his undergraduate degree from Georgia University, his PhD from the University of Virginia and a completed postdoctoral fellowship in the Department of Anatomy, Harvard School of Medicine. He is now a Research Associate in the Division of Endocrinology and Urology, Pennsylvania State University, College of Medicine, Hershey Medical Center.

Martin E Gleave, MD, completed his medical training at the University of British Columbia (UBC) in Vancouver, Canada, in 1984. Following an internship in Toronto, he returned to Vancouver to complete four years of surgical training at UBC and obtained his fellowship in urology (FRCSC) in 1989. Currently, he is at the University of Texas MD Anderson Cancer Center on a three year combined clinical/research fellowship. His current research interests include the role of growth factors in prostate cancer growth and metastasis, as well as the pharmacokinetics of prostate specific antigen.

Norio Hayshi received his MD in 1982 and his PhD in 1987 under the direction of Professor Juichi Kawamura, Department of Urology, Mie University, Mie, Japan. In 1988 he joined Dr Gerald Cunha's laboratory at the University of California, San Francisco, as a visiting fellow, and his work there focused on the role of stromal-epithelial interactions in the differentiation and growth of normal neoplastic epithelium. In 1990 he returned to the Department of Urology at Mie University as a member of the clinical staff.

Warren DeWayne Heston, PhD, is Director of Urologic Oncology Research, Memorial Sloan-Kettering Cancer Center, Attending Biochemist, Department of Surgery, Urology Service Memorial Hospital and Associate Laboratory Member of the Section of Molecular Pharmacology and Therapeutics, Sloan-Kettering Institute. He received his PhD from the University of Colorado in Pharmacology and Behavioural Pharmacogenetics. He established his research interest in Cancer Research using prostate based model systems during his postdoctoral training with Dr Donald S Coffey at the Johns Hopkins School of Medicine, Baltimore, Maryland. Dr Heston was Director of Urologic Research at Washington University in St Louis, Missouri, before joining the staff at Memorial Sloan-Kettering.

Soon-Joon Hong, MD, received his medical degree from the Yonsei University College of Medicine in Seoul, Korea. He is currently an Assistant Professor and Urologist at Yonsei University. Between 1988 and 1990 he was awarded a fellowship and trained at the Urology Research Laboratory, University of Texas MD Anderson Cancer Center. His major research interest is cell-cell interaction in bladder carcinogenesis and the development of a urine protein marker for early detection of bladder cancer.

Jer-Tsong Hsieh received his PhD from the University of Wisconsin-Madison in 1989. He is currently a postdoctoral fellow in the Department of Urology at the University of Texas MD Anderson Cancer Center. His primary research interest is the potential involvement of androgen repressed genes in the development of normal and neoplastic prostate gland.

Tomohiko Ichikawa received his MD from the School of Medicine, Chiba University, Chiba, Japan. During his residency programme in the Department of Urology, Chiba University Hospital, he also received his PhD from Chiba University. He completed postdoctoral studies with Dr John T Isaacs in the Johns Hopkins Oncology Center and is presently continuing his residency programme in the Department of Urology, Chiba University Hospital, Chiba, Japan.

Yayoi Ichikawa worked as a cytogenetic technician for eight years at the National Institute of Radiological Science, Chiba, Japan, before joining the Johns Hopkins Oncology Center for two years as a cytogenetic technician in Dr John T Isaacs' laboratory. She is presently continuing her cytogenetic studies in Japan.

John T Isaacs received his undergraduate degree from Johns Hopkins University and his PhD from Emory University. After completing his postdoctoral studies with Dr Donald S Coffey at the James Buchanan Brady Urological Institute at Hopkins, he joined the faculty of Johns Hopkins School of Medicine in 1980. He now has a dual appointment as an Associate Professor in the Johns Hopkins Oncology Center and the Department of Urology in the Johns Hopkins School of Medicine.

William B Isaacs received his PhD from the Department of Pharmacology and Experimental Therapeutics of the Johns Hopkins University School of Medicine in 1984, under the guidance of Dr Donald S Coffey. From then until 1988 he was a postdoctoral fellow with Dr Alice Fulton of the Department of Biochemistry at the University of Iowa. He is currently an Assistant Professor at the James Buchanan Brady Urological Institute at Johns Hopkins. His primary interest is the molecular biology of tumours of the genitourinary tract.

Dov Kadmon received his MD degree from the Hebrew University-Haddasah Medical School in Jerusalem, Israel. He subsequently trained in general surgery and urology at Barnes Hospital, Washington University School of Medicine in St. Louis, Missouri. After completing his urology training in 1980, he was awarded an AUA scholarship and spent two years studying animal models of prostate cancer. In 1982 he accepted a position on the faculty of Washington University Division of Urology, St. Louis, Missouri. He moved to Baylor College of Medicine, Houston, Texas, in 1986 where he is Associate Professor of Urology, Scott Department of Urology. His research interests include Positron Emission Tomography imaging of prostate cancer and other urological tumours, and the biology of early stage prostate cancer.

Thomas Krebs graduated MD in 1984 from the University of Berne, Switzerland. He received his training in pathology and urology in the Departments of Pathology and Urology at the same university. He is completing a research fellowship in the Scott Department of Urology at Baylor College of Medicine, Houston, Texas.

Natasha Kyprianou is a Greek Cypriot who received her undergraduate degree at Queen Mary College, London, and her PhD from the University of Wales College of Medicine, Tenovus Institute for Cancer Research, Cardiff. She completed postdoctoral fellowships at the Johns Hopkins Oncology Center and the Imperial Cancer Research Fund and is at present an Assistant Professor with the Department of Urology, University of Maryland School of Medicine.

Paula Martikainen received her MD from the University of Turku School of Medicine, Finland. She completed a Fogarty International Fellowship at Hopkins and is at present completing her residency programme in the Department of Pathology, University of Turku School of Medicine.

Wallace L McKeehan is a Senior Scientist and Deputy Director of the W Alton Jones Cell Science Center, Inc, in Lake Placid, New York. He trained in organic chemistry at the University of Florida and received his PhD in Biochemistry from the University of Texas (Austin). His PhD research and postdoctoral research at the Basel Institute for Immunology, Basel, Switzerland, were on the mechanism of translation level protein synthesis. He was a Research Associate in the Department of Molecular, Cellular and Developmental Biology at the University of Colorado (Boulder), where his research was on nutrient and growth factor control of cell growth in culture. His current research (since 1979) is on the mechanism of regulation of growth and function of the vascular system, liver and prostate, using isolated cells in culture.

Vincent W Merz received his MD from the University of Lausanne, Switzerland. He received his training in urology at the Department of Urology, University of Berne, Switzerland, and completed a research fellowship at the Scott Department of Urology, Baylor College of Medicine, Houston, Texas.

Sang Hee Park received BA and BS Pharmacy degrees from the University of Colorado, Boulder. She pursued her research interest in neuropharmacology at the University of Colorado and King's College, London. She is involved in studies concerning the molecular and cellular aspects of progression in prostate cancer.

Donna M Peehl was an undergraduate at Stanford University and received a PhD from the University of Colorado. There, from Richard Ham, she learned the principles of developing defined media for mammalian cells, which she later applied to the culture of human prostate cells. Postdoctoral fellowships at the University of California in Irvine and San Francisco with Eric Stanbridge and J Michael Bishop furthered her interests and expertise in the areas of somatic cell genetics and molecular biology. The goal of her current research at Stanford University is the identification of cellular and molecular markers of malignant potential in prostate cells.

Kenneth J Pienta, MD, is a graduate of the Johns Hopkins University School of Medicine. Currently, he is a Senior Clinical Fellow at the Johns Hopkins Oncology Center. His research interests are centred around dynamic cell structure and DNA organization and how cell organization is altered in cancer cells.

Marcus V Sadi, MD, received his MD and urology residency training at the Escola Paulista de Medicina in Sao Paulo, Brazil. He spent a year as a Research Fellow with Evelyn R Barrack in the Department of Urology, the Johns Hopkins University School of Medicine and the James Buchanan Brady Urological Institute of the Johns Hopkins Hospital. He is an Associate Professor of Urology at Paulista Medical School in Sao Paulo, Brazil.

Peter T Scardino graduated from the Duke University School of Medicine in 1971, completed surgical training at Massachusetts General Hospital and served as a Clinical Associate, Surgery Branch of the National Cancer Institute, Bethesda, Maryland. He was a urology resident at the UCLA School of Medicine where he became an instructor of urology. In 1979 he joined the faculty of the Baylor College of Medicine, and in 1989 he became the Russell and Mary Hugh Scott Chairman of the Scott Department of Urology. His major areas of research are urological oncology with emphasis in prostate cancer, ultrasonography, nerve-sparing techniques of radical cancer surgery and techniques of continent urinary diversion.

Jack A Schalken was trained as a biochemist at the University of Nijmegen and received his PhD in 1987. In his research he focuses on the molecular aspects of urological tumour progression. He was awarded a fellowship from the Royal Dutch Academy of Arts and Sciences (KNAW) in 1988. He currently works as Director of the Urology Research Laboratory, University Hospital Nijmegen, The Netherlands.

Fritz H Schröder, MD, has been Professor of Urology at Erasmus University, Rotterdam, The Netherlands, since 1977. He trained at the Saar University in Hamburg, Germany, and the University of California in Los Angeles and San Diego, where he was a Research Fellow in biology. After his return to Germany he was continuously involved in developing in vitro and in vivo (nude mouse) models of human prostate cancer. Four of six available permanent lines in nude mice were developed in his laboratory and by his associates. Endocrine dependence, its mechanisms, the impact on growth of endocrine factors and related clinical studies are his main scientific interests. He was Chairman and Secretary of the EORTC Genitourinary Group and has stimulated and contributed to a number of important clinical studies in the field of prostate cancer.

V Richard Sheridan is a postdoctoral associate in the Department of Pharmacology at the Fox Chase Cancer Center. He received his BA in biology at the University of Pennsylvania and a PhD from the University of Virginia. Dr Sheridan's doctoral work involved the analysis of temperature sensitive mutants in mitosis. He is currently studying the mechanism of action of estramustine on normal and estramustine resistant human prostatic carcinoma cell lines.

Gary D Steinberg, MD, received his undergraduate degree from Johns Hopkins University and his medical degree from the University of Chicago. He is currently a senior resident in urology at the James Buchanan Brady Urological Institute, Johns Hopkins Hospital, with research interests in prostate and bladder cancer.

Michael T Story received his BS from Loras College, his MA from Drake University and his PhD in microbiology from the University of Kansas. He was a Research Associate in the Cancer Research Laboratories in the Department of Gynecology and Obstetrics at the Medical College of Wisconsin. He joined the faculty in the Departments of Urology and Biochemistry at the Medical College of Wisconsin in 1980, where he is currently Associate Professor and Director of the Urology Research Laboratory.

Kenneth D Tew is Chairman of Pharmacology at the Fox Chase Cancer Center in Philadelphia. He received a BSc in microbial genetics from the University of Wales in 1973 and a PhD in the biochemical pharmacology of alkylating agents from the University of London (Chester Beatty Research Institute) in 1977. Following a postdoctoral appointment in the Department of Biochemistry at Georgetown University in Washington, DC, he joined the faculty in the Departments of Medicine and Pharmacology at the same institution until his move to Fox Chase in 1985. Dr Tew's research efforts have focused on understanding the mechanisms of action of the alkylating agent classes of anticancer drugs, with special emphasis on the biological determinants of tumour cell resistance to these agents.

Timothy C Thompson received the PhD degree in pharmacology from the University of Colorado at Boulder. He was a postdoctoral fellow at the Imperial Cancer Research Fund in London where he developed his interests in molecular carcinogenesis. He is an Assistant Professor in the Scott Department of Urology and the Department of Cell Biology at Baylor College of Medicine, Houston, Texas, where he continues to work in the area of molecular carcinogenesis with a special interest in prostate cancer.

Terry L Timme received his PhD in microbiology from Colorado State University in 1983. As a postdoctoral fellow in the Department of Cell Biology at Baylor College of Medicine, he developed gene transfer techniques for cells from patients with DNA damage-processing defects. He is affiliated with the Scott Department of Urology and has a primary appointment in the Urology Research Laboratory at the V.A. Medical Center, Houston, Texas. His research interests include genetic factors in initiation and progression of prostate cancer.

Patrick C Walsh, MD, is a graduate of Case Western Reserve University. Since 1974 he has been the Professor and Director of the James Buchanan Brady Urological Institute of the Johns Hopkins Medical Institutions. He is best known for his work on the surgical management of prostatic cancer.

George Wilding, MD, is Assistant Professor of Human Oncology at the University of Wisconsin Clinical Cancer Center and Chief of the Oncology Section of the Middleton Veterans Administration Hospital. He received an MS in pharmacology at Pennsylvania State University in 1976 and an MD from the University of Massachusetts in 1980. After internship and residency in internal medicine at the University of Massachusetts Medical Center, he trained in medical oncology in the Medicine Branch of the National Cancer Institute, where he remained in the Breast Cancer Section under Marc Lippman, MD, until 1988. He then moved to the University of Wisconsin. Clinically, he is the Principal Genitourinary Tract Medical Oncologist for the UWCCC. His laboratory focuses on the growth control of human prostate cancer and prostate carcinogenesis.

Y C Wong, PhD, is Reader in Anatomy and Sub-Dean of the Faculty of Medicine at the University of Hong Kong. He was born in Malaysia and graduated BSc from the Nanyang University in Singapore. He went to Canada in 1966 and obtained a PhD in anatomy in 1971 from the University of Western Ontario, London, Ontario. He joined the University of Hong Kong as Lecturer in Anatomy in 1971, was promoted to Senior Lecturer in 1977 and Reader in 1984. His research interests have been on reproductive biology with special emphasis on the role of stroma in functional differentiation of the prostatic epithelial cells.

Haiyen E Zhau received her MS from Boston University and her PhD from McGill University, Montreal, Canada. She is an Assistant Professor in the Department of Urology, University of Texas MD Anderson Cancer Center. Her research interests include the investigation of the mechanisms underlying cellular interaction, roles of oncogenes and tumour suppressor genes in genitourinary cancer growth and progression and the development of relevant biological markers for an early diagnosis and prognosis of human bladder and prostate cancers.

LIST OF PREVIOUS ISSUES

VOLUME 1   1982

No. 1: Inheritance of Susceptibility to Cancer in Man
Guest Editor: W F Bodmer

No. 2: Maturation and Differentiation in Leukaemias
Guest Editor: M F Greaves

No. 3: Experimental Approaches to Drug Targeting
Guest Editors: A J S Davies and M J Crumpton

No. 4: Cancers Induced by Therapy
Guest Editor: I Penn

VOLUME 2   1983

No. 1: Embryonic & Germ Cell Tumours in Man and Animals
Guest Editor: R L Gardner

No. 2: Retinoids and Cancer
Guest Editor: M B Sporn

No. 3: Precancer
Guest Editor: J J DeCosse

No. 4: Tumour Promotion and Human Cancer
Guest Editors: T J Slaga and R Montesano

VOLUME 3   1984

No. 1: Viruses in Human and Animal Cancers
Guest Editors: J Wyke and R Weiss

No. 2: Gene Regulation in the Expression of Malignancy
Guest Editor: L Sachs

No. 3: Consistent Chromosomal Aberrations and Oncogenes in Human Tumours
Guest Editor: J D Rowley

No. 4: Clinical Management of Solid Tumours in Childhood
Guest Editor: T J McElwain

VOLUME 4   1985

No. 1: Tumour Antigens in Experimental and Human Systems
Guest Editor: L W Law